HYPOTHERMIA AND COLD STRESS

HYPOTHERMIA AND COLD STRESS

EVAN L. LLOYD

Department of Anaesthetics,
Princess Margaret Rose Orthopaedic Hospital
Edinburgh

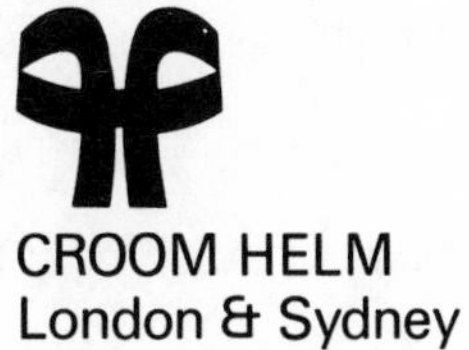

CROOM HELM
London & Sydney

Croom Helm Ltd, Provident House, Burrell Row,
Beckenham, Kent BR3 1AT

Croom Helm Australia Pty Ltd, Suite 4, 6th Floor,
64–76 Kippax Street, Surry Hills, NSW 2010, Australia

British Library Cataloguing in Publication Data

Lloyd, Evan L.
Hypothermia and cold stress.
1. Hypothermia
I. Title
616.9'88 RC88.5
ISBN 0-7099-1665-5

Phototypeset by Words & Pictures Ltd. Thornton Heath, Surrey
Printed and bound in Great Britain
by Billing & Sons Limited, Worcester.

CONTENTS

LIST OF FIGURES

LIST OF TABLES

PREFACE

Environmental cold is a problem faced by people in many parts of the world, and hypothermia and frostbite have become terms which are widely known even among the lay public. However, what is much less well known even among the medical profession is that cold stress can have profound effects on the body even before hypothermia develops. Some of these effects are transient and merely inconvenient but others may contribute to chronic disability leading to death, or may cause death acutely. Unfortunately the severity of the cold may be relatively mild and in these cases cold is never considered as a causative factor in the illness or death.

Even when hypothermia has developed, the correct management of the case depends not only on the type of hypothermia, i.e. the way it developed, but also on any other factors which may be present because of the circumstances in which the hypothermia occurred. These factors may not only complicate the management of the hypothermia but may also require specific treatment. As if these problems are not enough, the management team at each stage of treatment has to decide which methods of rewarming are the best for the particular case, also taking into account what is practical under the circumstances.

This book will attempt to deal with the practical problems and possibilities, for prevention as well as treatment, and only cover the underlying physiological changes to the extent necessary to help the understanding of any particular problem.

PART 1: MEASUREMENT, MECHANISMS AND MYTHS

INTRODUCTION

Despite the fact that people living in cold, hostile environments have probably been aware since the beginning of time that cold kills, accidental hypothermia is possibly one of the most underrated killers in modern medicine. This sad state is partly due to under-reporting or incorrect diagnosis and partly due to a terrifying lack of awareness among the lay public and the medical profession of the many ways that cold stress and hypothermia can contribute to death, illness or injury. This lack of awareness is true over a wide range of environmental situations.

Temperature affects all living tissues and not only are man's efficiency and well-being profoundly affected by the thermal stresses of the environment in which he lives and works but, if the thermal stresses become too extreme, the normal physiological responses may be overwhelmed. If the stressor is heat, heatstroke and other problems may arise, while cold stress may lead to hypothermia.

The subject of temperature regulation has been extensively and well reviewed and similarly the clinical features of hypothermia and the physiological changes of the functions of the different systems and organs of the body during cold stress and hypothermia have also been well reviewed (Burton and Edholm, 1955; Danzl, 1983; Grayson and Kuehn, 1979; Holdcroft, 1981; Hornback, 1984; Horvath, 1981; Keatinge, 1969; Kew, 1976; Lagerspetz, 1982; Maclean and Emslie-Smith, 1977; Paton, 1983a and b). The individual aspects of physiological changes will only be detailed where they are relevant to some particular aspect of the clinical management of a patient or where such information is necessary for the understanding of particular findings or the particular aspect is controversial or recent information has become available.

One area of physiological/pathological change is that which accompanies cold stress. While the acute effects are usually identified in the physiological changes accompanying thermoregulation the possible effects of prolonged exposure to cold stress which are not severe enough to cause hypothermia are either ignored or overlooked. Cold may affect superficial tissues as in frostbite but it may also affect the skin and superficial tissues in other ways. In addition the important systems of the body, e.g. cardiovascular system, respiratory system and nervous system both peripheral and central, may also be affected in subtle ways which may not be readily recognisable as being due to cold. This aspect will be covered in Part 2.

The effects of cold medically recognised in antiquity were limited to the observation of an increased risk of constipation in people whose houses faced east or north and it does not appear that cold injuries as such were recognised. There is certainly no mention of cold in the Hippocratic Collection which probably included the library of the medical school at Cos, where Hippocrates (460–377 BC) taught, as well as his own writings (Encyclopaedia Brittanica, 1973a). This is strange since his contemporary, the historian Herodotus (484–420 BC) could differentiate between drowning and hypothermia at sea. When a Persian fleet under Darius's general Mardonius was wrecked by a strong northerly gale and 20,000 men died, Herodotus says that some men 'were seized and devoured by sea monsters while others were dashed violently against the rocks; some who did not know how to swim were engulfed and some died of the cold'. Later when the Greek fleet defeated Xerxes's Persian fleet at Salamis Herodotus said: 'Of the Greeks there died only a few; for, as they were able to swim, all those that were not slain outright by the enemy escaped from the sinking vessels and swam across to Salamis. But on the side of the Barbarians more perished by drowning than in any other way, since they did not know how to swim' (Rawlinson, 1910).

In 1796 James Currie in Britain was an observer at a shipwreck and he noticed that sailors hanging onto a lifeboat became confused and drifted away (Keatinge, 1969). He followed this observation with some human research and proved that hypothermia could precede drowning (Currie, 1798). Despite this evidence, by the turn of the century it was well established in the official mind that deaths at sea were almost invariably due to drowning, with thirst and attacks by sharks being other causes of death respectable enough to be put on a death certificate (Keatinge, 1969). Therefore when the *Titanic* sank in 1912, the disaster inquiry confined itself to trying to fix the blame for the accident, and in the return from the Superintendent of the Port of Southampton 19 pages of names are recorded in careful handwriting, with drowning as the cause of death in every case (Mersey, 1912). However, the facts of the accident could lead to a different diagnosis of death. The night was fine and calm with no swell running in the sea. There were 3,560 lifebelts available and yet all 1,489 passengers who entered the water were dead when SS *Carpathia* reached them one hour and 50 minutes later. Since they were in the water very close to a number of icebergs, it is reasonable to presume that the water was very cold and that hypothermia was in fact the cause of death. This fact was recognised by a non-medical survivor (Beesley, 1912), but ignored by the medical and administrative authorities. Further suggestive evidence of the importance of hypothermia in causing death at sea came in the report of the sinking of the *Gneisnau* in the area of the Falkland Islands in December 1914 but again the report appeared in a non-medical publication (Scott-Daniell, 1965).

The hazards of cold water immersion were recognised by German workers before and during the Second World War (Grosse-Brockhoff, 1950) though it is unfortunate that this appreciation was at least partly responsible for the infamous experiments at Dachau (Alexander, 1945). An inquiry by a committee under Admiral Talbot into naval life-saving during the just-ended Second World War found that two-thirds of the total naval casualties died after escaping from their sinking ships, the majority from immersion hypothermia (Admiralty Papers, 1946). Even in the sheltered waters of Scapa Flow, hypothermia was a major cause of deaths among those who escaped from the sinking *Royal Oak* (McKee, 1966). These deaths occurred in the water and after reaching land. A thorough investigation following the sinking of SS *Lakonia* in the relatively warm waters off Madiera confirmed the importance of hypothermia as a cause of death at sea with 111 out of the 120 deaths being due to this cause (Keatinge, 1965). Nevertheless habits are hard to break and ten years later when SS *Lovat* sank off the south coast of England, the BBC news, from the warmth and comfort of London, reported that all the crew had drowned except for four survivors, apparently ignoring the evidence of a helicopter crewman who, through an accident, landed in one of the life-rafts. This crewman reported that two of the *Lovat*'s crew had died in the raft while he was present. Since they were uninjured, out of water and thinly clad, death was obviously from hypothermia and not drowning. Also the deaths of two boys who died in the English Channel were diagnosed as due to drowning though their temperatures were never measured (Golden, 1973b), and this pattern continues to be repeated (Karhunen and Cazanitis, 1983).

Inland waters — lochs, rivers, canals, disused quarries — are other sites of many deaths from hypothermia which are again usually wrongly attributed. In the early months of every year there are reports in the papers of people misled by warm air temperatures diving into inland waters, or being thrown in because of boating mishaps, and dying because of hypothermia or the more immediate effects of immersion in very cold water. It is salutary to think that a police doctor reported on hypothermia in drunken sailors falling into the harbour and canals of Hamburg as long ago as 1875 (Reinke, 1875). The lack of awareness of the possibility of hypothermia as a cause of death is well illustrated in an incident described by Thomas Firbank (1940). In this episode the author and his farm bailiff, Caradoc, go for a swim across a small north Wales lake. It is August but the waters of the lake are still cold. Caradoc dies during the swim and the cause is given as heart failure because his lungs were dry. In an attempt to rationalise the cause, a childhood warning against swimming is taken as indicating a weak heart which had been unable to sustain the effort of the swim. This seems unlikely since Caradoc had been brought up on a hill farm and had been successfully managing Firbank's farm which rose to 3,000 feet altitude with gradients of 1 in 2. There was no evidence of cardiac weakness during his work and a reconsideration of the description suggests that hypothermia could have been the cause of death.

Baron de Larrey gave an authoritative account of mass casualties due to cold exposure in Napoleon's army on the retreat from Moscow (Werner, 1885) and similar observations were made by Killian (1966) about casualties among Hitler's armies on the Russian front. However even on land there may be problems of diagnosis. For example, if a climber falls and is injured and is dead by the time a rescue team reaches him that person is inevitably entered in the register as a fatality due to trauma even though he may have been alive immediately after the fall. However under certain circumstances and at particular times of the year, there is a high degree of probability that the deaths would be due to hypothermia, but usually no attempt is made to assess the injury and decide if death would have occurred with equal rapidity in a warm environment.

Problems in Investigating Hypothermia

It is incredibly difficult to achieve meaningful results in experiments with accidental hypothermia. The results from animal experiments cannot be directly related to the human situation because the morphology and thermoregulatory physiology of the animals may differ greatly from that of man. Also most animal experiments are carried out under general anaesthesia which introduces another complication which may be compounded by possibly variable pharmacological effects on different animals and the fact that different animal experiments may utilise different anaesthetic techniques. Finally animal experiments are usually carried out with endotracheal intubation which, by by-passing the naso-pharynx, alters the hydrodynamics of respiration and transfers the major site of respiratory heat and moisture loss from the nose to the trachea and main bronchi, which in turn may alter the effect on the rest of the body.

Studies on man do not ease the problem. Results obtained by observations made during hypothermia induced for medical or surgical reasons are suspect for the same reasons as results from animal experiments, viz. anaesthesia, endotracheal intubation and the variety of drugs used to assist the anaesthetist, e.g. muscle relaxants and phenothiazines. In conscious subjects ethical considerations prevent core temperatures below 34 °C being achieved with volunteers and at this temperature the subject will shiver and there will therefore be no problem in rewarming. In addition at 34 °C the full physiological response to hypothermia is not present and the shivering itself prevents some of the vasoconstriction associated with cold exposure. Another criticism against using even human experiments as a guide to field work is that the method of inducing hypothermia — immersion in cold water — may produce changes which differ markedly from those which may occur in the field. The obvious difference is with hypothermia occurring in the hills where exhaustion is usually an important factor. However, the experimental immersion may differ even from accidental immersion in that, in the accidental situation, fear is probably present and possibly injury with resulting alteration of vasomotor control. In fact the only experiments on man which have been taken to meaningful temperatures have been those performed by the Nazis at Dachau (Alexander, 1945). Though the temperatures reached were comparable to those seen in cases of accidental hypothermia, there could be dangers in accepting the results uncritically since the experimental subjects were malnourished, emaciated and with very little hope to provide the incentive to live, which contrasts with the well-fed, mildly plump people who are the main customers of the rescue services. It is now being suggested that the Dachau experiments in fact contributed little to the general knowledge of hypothermia (Paton, 1983a) and it is possible that they have delayed progress.

There is also unfortunately a continuing discrepancy in the knowledge of the effects of cold between lay people, who have had outdoor experience of cold climates, and the medical profession. This gap in knowledge is obvious when one considers that Herodotus, a historian, by listening to people could differentiate between drowning and hypothermia whereas one of his contemporaries, the academic physician Hippocrates, made no mention of hypothermia. More recently the writings of Jack London (1876–1916) gave many physiological and psychological reactions to cold stress and hypothermia in such stories as 'To Build a Fire', 'The Law of Life' and 'An Odyssey of the North' at a time when the bulk of the medical profession was blissfully ignorant of the existence of hypothermia. Even the few doctors who travel into the hostile environments are usually practical men concerned with immediate care, and they generally have neither the time nor the inclination to do research or publish results. If clinical observations are made, the nonentity of the observer, at least in medical eyes, or the lack of scientific 'measurement' may mean that the information is ignored or dismissed as anecdotal or hearsay. On the other hand the academics, of sufficient standing to command medical attention to their publications and pronouncements, are located in large centres of population and live and work in well-heated buildings and this insulates them from personal experience of the hostile environments. Even when there was a marked increase in deaths associated with a winter smog in London in 1952, it was assumed that the effects were due to atmospheric pollution. Of the three major publications dealing with that episode, only the paper written from a general practice and a later *Lancet* editorial mentioned the associated cold (Pemberton, 1984). The insulating effect of upper-class urban living was one of the factors which saved the lives of many MacDonalds in the Glencoe massacre. When the Marquis of Stair in Edinburgh ordered the massacre in the depths of winter, he was under the impression that highlanders could not survive for long in harsh weather. In fact the coincidental snow storm probably saved lives since the MacDonalds, cold acclimatised and familiar with the terrain, were able to escape detection and travel whereas the Government troops were delayed and hampered. Though many of the very young or very old and the wounded probably died of hypothermia, only 38 were killed by the troops. Some of the credit for this must also go to the Campbell troops, including their chief Glenlyon, who were sickened by the slaughter and the treachery to the highland traditions of hospitality (Linklater, 1982). Future progress in the treatment of accidental hypothermia in the field may come when researchers decide to investigate the reasons for the clinical cases and responses noted by the rescuers and physicians in the field (Leathart, 1971) rather than dismissing them as anecdotal if the responses are not understood by the academics.

There is a scientific desire for controlled studies (Chinard, 1979), but it would be very difficult to achieve in accidental hypothermia. One only has to consider the many variables such as the predisposing factors, the type of onset, the age and build of the victim, the unpredictability of cases, and the time interval and management of the case between discovery and reaching hospital, to appreciate the difficulties in obtaining proper comparisons.

One final difficulty associated with the study of hypothermia is that any piece of research may be interpreted in different ways. For example when Talbot *et al.* (1941) reported the death of a patient with profound circulatory collapse during rewarming from induced hypothermia, they suggested that 'the mechanisms of vasomotor collapse are different in rewarming from hypothermia as compared with those in surgical or medical shock' and concluded that 'in retrospect it is thought that sudden vasodilatation was responsible for the cardiovascular breakdown'. This retrospective thought became incorporated in the literature as the cause of death during rewarming from acute hypothermia (Behnke and Bauer, 1970; Keatinge, 1969; Maclean and Emslie-Smith, 1977) even though the case had been one of prolonged hypothermia, rewarming was spontaneous with no surface heat and the description was more like that of cardiac failure with pulmonary oedema ('Cyanosis with gasping and shallow respiration and congestion of the lungs on post-mortem' (Talbot *et al.*, 1941)). Even the Dachau experiments have had opposite interpretations put on the results. Whereas the conclusion by most authorities is that they show that rapid rewarming in a hot bath is the best treatment for immersion hypothermia (Burton and Edholm, 1955; Keatinge, 1969), one author has stated that the results show that slow rewarming is superior to rapid rewarming (Zingg, 1966).

1 MEASUREMENT OF BODY TEMPERATURE

Instruments

There are a number of devices which can record temperature.

The commonest instrument is a *mercury-in-glass thermometer* but in hypothermia it is essential to have a low-reading one. The normal clinical thermometer does not record lower than 35 °C and therefore cannot be used to diagnose hypothermia. The special low-reading thermometer records down to 27 °C but there are occasions when even this is not low enough. The mercury-in-glass thermometers have other disadvantages:

(1) They are fragile, and may therefore be broken in use or found to be broken when needed.
(2) They are rigid, and this limits the sites from which temperatures can be taken and if the rectal site is being used the patient has to be repeatedly disturbed to take the reading.
(3) They cannot be used to measure skin temperature.
(4) To record an accurate temperature the mercury has to be shaken down and it was found that a low-reading thermometer needed to be shaken down 30 times before it was able to record a low temperature (Mills, 1979; Thomas and Green, 1973). If this is not done a low core temperature may be missed.

The most useful instrument is an *electronic thermometer*. The great advantage of this device is that the temperature range to be covered is almost limitless, ranging from temperatures approaching absolute zero to several thousand degrees above zero. Most people choose a narrower range to suit their particular needs. However, it is worth remembering that the wider the range covered by any individual instrument, the less the accuracy within that range. This system has another advantage that the actual probes, which use either *thermistors* or *thermocouples*, can be made in a variety of shapes and the one instrument can therefore be used to record environmental temperature, skin temperature and core temperature from any site including the blood leaving the heart. This device can also be utilised in a radio-telemetric system (Higgens *et al.*, 1978).

There are other specialised techniques for measuring core temperature (Wedley, 1979) such as the *radio-pill* (Wolff, 1961) which transmits the core temperature from the intestinal tract after being *swallowed* (Hayward *et al.*, 1984a), and other radio-telemetric devices have been *implanted* and used to follow core temperature changes of dogs during simulated deep diving (Verlander *et al.*, 1978). Another method uses *colour changes in chemicals* with an array of dots changing colour at different temperatures and the final changed dot giving the reading (McAllister, 1975). Unfortunately this system is only available covering the normal clinical range, i.e. above 35 °C, and each device can only be used once. A more promising system is that which uses a servo-controlled heating pad on the surface of the body. This gradually balances the temperature of the skin surface until a stable balance is reached with the deep body temperature. The two systems which have been developed so far are one which is applied to the skin surface of the trunk (Fox and Solman, 1970; Fox *et al.*, 1973c) and one which is used for tympanic temperature measurement (Keatinge and Sloan, 1975). While these systems are non-invasive their disadvantages are expense, bulk, possible fragility and the fact that there is an appreciable time lag before the reading can be taken.

There are other methods which can be used to assess temperature on the surface of the body. *Thermography*, which records radiant heat (Leese *et al.*, 1978; Park and Reece, 1976), can be read using either a television camera system in black and white or colour, or *liquid crystals* (Yoder, 1979) which are painted directly on to the skin and differences in colour give differences in temperature. This is inaccurate in absolute temperature but can show relative differences in temperature and has been used in physiological studies, e.g. the sites of high heat loss at rest (Hayward *et al.*, 1973), during swimming (Wade and Veghte, 1977) or running (Clark *et al.*, 1974a, b; Veghte *et al.*, 1979), and has been used in frostbite to provide clinical evaluation of the depth of damage (Hamlet, 1976) and to study the physiological alterations after immediate recovery (Nair *et al.*, 1977). Even in the controlled thermal environment of the operating theatre, liquid crystals, even on the forehead, gave no indication of the true changes in core temperature (Lacoumenta and Hall, 1984) and they are therefore not even useful as a screen for malignant hyperpyrexia.

Heat flow discs can detect the flow of heat through the skin covered by the disc and the *Schlieren* device can be used to observe patterns of heat flow around a solid object.

The *hands* are instruments which are often ignored but can give a useful and easy check on the temperature status of the patient, e.g. in the home. If the doctor slides his hand between the patient's trunk and the clothing or bed, he will get a quick check and can often exclude hypothermia (Danzl, 1983; Houlsby, 1979). This could be of use for example in an elderly patient who has suddenly become confused, which may be due to hypothermia, a cerebrovascular accident or may even be the only sign of an unsuspected infection. If, however, the patient felt warm in this region hypothermia can be excluded as the cause of the confusion and similarly in the field a hand in the axilla might exclude hypothermia as a cause of unconsciousness. If the patient felt cold to the hand in these regions a thermometer would be needed.

Uses of Temperature Measurement

The usual reason for measuring temperature is to identify changes in body temperature, e.g. fever, hyperthermia or hypothermia. However, the measurement of skin temperature has been used to assess changes in environment, e.g. the efficacy of the modifications carried out on helicopters for arctic use (Higgenbottom *et al.*, 1977) and measurement of the temperature of the skin of the great toe has been advocated as a guide to the degree of peripheral vasodilation and perfusion, particularly after cardiac surgery (Brock, 1975; Matthews *et al.*, 1974a, b). Heat flow discs can be used to adjust an environment to give thermoneutral conditions for a patient, e.g. after extensive burns (Bittel *et al.*, 1977) and the Schlieren device has been used to observe the patterns of heat flow around a human body (Clark and Toy, 1975a, b) and this can provide information about heat loss as affected by posture or clothing, and it has several other research applications.

Sites of Core Temperature Measurement

Since the definition of hypothermia specifies a core temperature of below 35 °C, measurement of core temperature is obviously essential and this is usually made at easily accessible sites.

The *oesophagus* is the preferred site since it provides an indirect measure of the temperature of the blood leaving the heart (Cooper and Kenyon, 1957; Stupfel and Severinghaus, 1956). It is essential that the temperature probe is placed in the lower oesophagus since the oesophagus near the tracheal bifurcation is uniformly 1 °C cooler, either due to the direct cooling effect of inspired gases below the endotracheal tube (Whitby and Dunkin, 1969; 1970) or to evaporation in the trachea at that site (Stupfel and Severinghaus, 1956). However, during normal respiration without the presence of an endotracheal tube, the oesophageal temperature was found to be identical to the cardiac temperature as measured by a thermistor in the pulmonary artery (Hayward *et al.*, 1984a) and the correlation was found to be particularly good during the first vital 30 minutes after a person was removed from the cold and treatment started. Unfortunately practical difficulties encountered with temperature measurement in the oesophagus often mean that other sites have to be used.

The *rectal* temperature is often used as a core temperature but even in the same subject a rectal probe may record different temperatures at different sites (Burton and Edholm, 1955). An additional danger in the use of rectal temperature is that, while it is adequate for initial assessment when the person is found (Hayward *et al.*, 1984a), it may neither record a true core temperature nor bear a constant relationship to the core during rewarming. In one study (Hayward *et al.*, 1984a) with the subject's rewarming in a hot bath the pulmonary artery temperature reached normothermia before the after-drop in the rectal temperature had been completed.

For practical purposes the *mouth* temperature is often used in the field and it has been criticised for not giving a true reading of core temperature in hypothermia (Collins and Exton-Smith, 1979). It has been claimed that local heat on the head and neck invalidate oral temperature measurements as a true core reading (McCaffrey *et al.*, 1975a; Marcus, 1973a, b) but this view has been challenged (Collis *et al.*, 1977). Nevertheless for normal clinical conditions, unless someone has taken hot food or drink within the previous 30 minutes, a mouth temperature of 37 °C must indicate that the person is normothermic. As the person is exposed to cold stress and the core temperature drops, the mouth temperature may drop faster, but the true core temperature will never be lower than the mouth temperature and therefore the mouth temperature can be used as an initial screening measurement. It is probably also true that the lower the mouth temperature the more severe the effects of the cold stress and the greater the danger for the person (Lloyd, 1979c).

Measurement of the temperature of *freshly voided urine* has been advocated as an accurate measurement of core temperature and is especially advised for use with the elderly (Brooke *et al.*, 1973; Collins, 1983b; Collins and Exton-Smith, 1979; Fox *et al.*, 1975). This measurement is useful as a screening test but suffers from the practical disadvantages that it cannot be repeated at short intervals and cannot be done if the patient is incontinent or unconscious.

The *nasopharynx* is a site often used in anaesthesia though it is less reliable than the oesophageal temperature in estimating cerebral temperature (Whitby and Dunkin, 1971) since the probe is subject to inadequate exclusion from the outside air, a leakage of gas from the endotracheal tube and accidental displacement.

The *tympanic membrane* is another site often suggested as giving a true core temperature reading. There is, however, normally a steep gradient of temperature along the auditory canal during exposure to cold air (Cooper *et al.*, 1964a; Greenleaf and Castle, 1972) and many investigators have found the accuracy to be questionable and affected by the ambient temperature and local blood flow (Bradbury *et al.*, 1964; Greenleaf and Castle, 1972; Hayward *et al.*, 1984a; Keatinge and Sloan, 1975; McCaffrey *et al.*, 1975a, b; McCook *et al.*, 1961; Marcus, 1973a, b; Nadel and Horvath, 1970; Randall *et al.*, 1963; Sloan and Keatinge, 1975), though one reported a good correlation with the oesophageal temperature (Webb, 1973a). This last was in cardiopulmonary bypass during which the ambient temperature is fairly high. The probe can be uncomfortable (Hayward *et al.*, 1984a) and there is the danger of perforating the ear drum or causing bleeding if the probe is pushed in too hard, and anything less is liable to be measuring the temperature of the wall of the auditory canal or even the air in the canal. The system using a servo-controlled heating pad on the outside of the ear (Keatinge and Sloan, 1975) is probably the only reliable method of accurately measuring core temperature by this route, and measurements of auditory canal temperature by this method gave good correlation with oesophageal temperature (Holdcroft and Hall, 1978).

It has been noted that differences exist between temperatures measured at the various sites (Kerslake, 1972) and that the time and amplitude of the response to thermal stimuli may vary between these sites (Hayward *et al.*, 1984a; Piironen, 1970). Now the temperature of the blood leaving the heart is probably the closest approximation of a true core temperature (Bligh, 1973) but, since this site is impractical for routine use, though used occasionally in research (Hayward *et al.*, 1984a), the accuracy of the measurement at any other site must be compared with the temperature of the blood leaving the heart, and in fact many attempts have been made to compare the values obtained from the different sites (Collins and Exton-Smith, 1979; Cooper and Kenyon, 1957; Cranston, 1966; Edwards *et al.*, 1978; Holdcroft and Hall, 1978). In clinical practice a high degree of accuracy is not necessary and there may be as great a difference in accuracy between different measuring devices as there is between the different core sites and, provided the attendant is aware of how the various sites differ in accuracy and response, a site should be used which is most practical in the particular situation, taking into account the environment and the device available.

In these circumstances it might be better to use the concept of TOTAL BODY HEAT which is determined by the core temperature being taken along with mean skin temperature and a formula is used to calculate total body heat. Because of the great variation in skin temperature on different sites of the body and at different times of the day (Aschoff *et al.*, 1974) the calculation of mean skin temperature is determined by measurements at a number of different sites with the results being weighted. The numbers of sites measured have varied from 15 down to 3 (Holdcroft, 1981) and the various combinations have been considered (Colin *et al.*, 1971; Ramanathan, 1964; Shanks, 1975c; Teichner, 1954) and the difficulties discussed (Aschoff *et al.*, 1974). Though the formula for 15 points is undoubtedly the most accurate, the 3 and 4 point formulae are sufficient for practical purposes. The 3 point (Burton and Edholm, 1955) uses the formula T mean skin = (0.14 × T forearm) + (0.36 × T calf) + (0.5 × T abdomen), with the mean body temperature = (0.7 × T core) + (0.3 × T mean skin), and a nomogram has been developed using this 3 point system (House and Vale, 1972). The 4 point formula (Holdcroft and Hall, 1978; Ramanathan, 1964) is T mean skin = 0.3 (nipple + upper outer arm) + 0.2 (anterior mid thigh + lateral mid calf). The mean body temperature = (0.66 × T core) + (0.34 × T mean skin) and from this the body heat content (Joules) = mean body temperature (°C) × 0.83 (specific heat of tissues) × weight (kg) × 4.18. This is of most use in following change rather than obtaining absolute values. The use of this concept means that though a person in a sauna and a person in a cold room may have the same core temperature, calculation of the total body heat shows that the person in the cold room has less total body heat. It can also show that though the core temperature of a person may drop on induction of anaesthesia there is no immediate loss of total body heat since the skin temperatures rise at the same moment and the changes are merely a redistribution of body heat (Holdcroft, 1981).

2 METHODS AND ROUTES OF HEAT LOSS

Because the body temperature of man is higher than the environment, human beings are constantly losing heat and the routes of heat loss are the normal physical ones which apply to any object animate or inanimate, viz. convection, radiation, conduction and evaporation, and each can be affected by a number of factors.

Convective heat loss is increased by wind, and wind speed is more important for heat loss than temperature or humidity (Iampietro *et al.*, 1958, 1960; Maclean and Emslie-Smith, 1977) and this has resulted in the use of the term 'wind chill' index (Siple and Passel, 1945). The various rates of heat loss can be allocated to zones indicating the danger of cold-induced damage and the precautions that should be taken (Adam, 1981; Maclean and Emslie-Smith, 1977). It has been claimed that convective heat loss increases with the square of wind velocity up to 60 mph after which there is very little increase (Hornback, 1984) but certainly the greatest increase is as the wind speed increases from 0 to 20 mph. The maximum danger is likely to be at moderate temperatures because people do not think there is any danger, e.g. −1 °C with no wind is 'cool' but a 10 mph wind will more than double the rate of heat loss. Convective heat loss is increased by movement, through the 'pendulum' movement of the limbs and through a bellows effect in the clothing (Clark *et al.*, 1974b). Body posture will also alter convective heat loss by varying the convective currents round the body (Clark and Toy, 1975a, b).

Radiation is often poorly understood. Radiation heat loss has been measured as being 55 to 65 per cent of the total heat loss (Danzl, 1983; Maclean and Emslie-Smith, 1977) but this is usually measured in a nude subject in a moderately cold room. However, radiation only occurs from the surface of an object and therefore the lower the temperature difference between the surface of a person and nearby solid objects, the less heat will be lost by radiation. The purpose of wearing clothing is to insulate the body and therefore the outside temperature drops, reducing the radiant heat loss. Similarly in the cold, vasoconstriction can result in the outer one inch of body tissue having a thermal conductivity equivalent to that of cork (Maclean and Emslie-Smith, 1977) and therefore radiant heat loss is minimised. Two good examples of radiant heat transfer are when a church stands empty and unheated from Monday to Saturday in winter and though the heating may be started early on the Sunday morning the fabric of the building has not had time to warm. Therefore when the congregation arrive they may feel the air to be warm but then after an interval they will start to feel cool as they lose radiant heat to the building. The same phenomenon is seen in reverse in the tropics where, though the night air is cool, the radiant heat from the walls makes sleeping difficult. The body can also gain radiant heat from the sun, 460 kcal/hour at sea level with a clear sky or 700 kcal/hour in the Antarctic and at 19,000 feet in the mountains. The quantities can be reduced by climatic factors such as clouds and increased by reflection from snow, sand or sea, and clothing modifies the effects.

Conductive heat loss is normally a fairly small part of the total because it only occurs with substances in direct contact with the body. Since air, which is the substance in contact with most of the body surface trapped under the clothing, has a very low thermal capacity it does not remove much heat by conduction. Water, however, has a very high heat transfer coefficient (Horvath, 1984) and in fact conducts heat 10 to 25 times better than air (Hirvonen, 1982) and therefore someone immersed in water has no insulation at the skin/water interface (Horvath, 1981). As a result, conductive heat loss is very important for someone immersed in water, but there is a similar problem for someone in a high pressure atmosphere, e.g. diving, where the thermal conductivity of the compressed gases is equivalent to that of water. On land conductive heat loss is increased by wet clothing because water accelerates the transfer of heat between the body and the surface of the clothing. Another time conductive loss is often forgotten is when a casualty is well covered with blankets but continues to lie with nothing between him and the ground.

Evaporative heat loss occurs through insensible moisture loss (or sweating), through evaporation from clothing which has become wet from outside, e.g. from rain, or from inside by sweating, and, in these circumstances, wind will increase the rate of evaporation and therefore the rate of heat loss which may reach catastrophic levels. Evaporative heat loss also occurs through breathing and some animals, e.g. dogs, use panting as a major route for heat loss. Panting is a rapid blowing of air over the moist mucosa of the tongue and oropharynx not to be confused with tachypnoea.

In man *respiratory* heat is lost through warming and humidifying the inspired air, with humidification normally being the greater (Burton and Edholm, 1955). However, at −40 °C the heat loss from warming the inspired air is almost equal to the heat lost by humidifying the inspired air (Webb, 1955). Even in man the volume of fluid lost through respiration may amount to about 33 per cent of the normal total evaporative loss (Burton and Edholm, 1955) and the proportion is the same even for neonates (Soulski *et al.*, 1983). Air, which is relatively dry even during rain, is humidified to 100 per cent saturation by the lungs, accounting for the major proportion of respiratory heat loss (Burton and Edholm, 1955). An average of 32 mg of water per litre of ventilation is lost by breathing whether at rest (Webb, 1955) or during exercise (Brebbia *et al.*, 1957) and vapour loss is proportional to the respiratory minute volume. During vigorous exercise the person has to breathe fast and deep and this obviously increases the total quantity of heat lost through the respiratory tract. The higher the altitude or the colder the temperature, the drier the air and therefore the greater the respiratory moisture loss (Heath and Williams, 1981). If a person is exercising or working in cold temperatures at altitude the volume of body water lost through breathing may be large enough not only to cause dehydration of the upper respiratory tract secretions (McFadden, 1983) but also whole body dehydration (Heath and Williams, 1981). Caldwell *et al.* (1969) estimated that it required more than 0.5 kcal of heat to vaporise 1 g of mucosal water from the respiratory tract and it has been estimated that in resting subjects 10 to 15 per cent of the total heat loss would be from the respiratory tract (Caldwell *et al.*, 1969; Webster, 1952) and Brebbia *et al.* (1957) calculated that respiratory heat loss alone was about 9 per cent of the total energy expenditure. However, the quantities of heat lost during respiration are not usually excessive and can easily be replaced by increased metabolic heat production. There are times when the respiratory heat loss may become very important such as when metabolic heat production is impaired, e.g. under anaesthesia or in hypothermia, and, as discussed later, when the atmospheric air is very dry especially if cold as well. When there is an abnormal constitution of the respired gases, e.g. in deep diving where the diver is in a heliox atmosphere, the oxygen/helium mixture has such a tremendous heat transfer capacity at pressure that there are complex changes in the proportions of heat lost through the different routes — convection, conduction, radiation and evaporation — and respiratory heat loss alone may precipitate hypothermia. There is also a suggestion that helium resets the central thermostat (Hayes, 1977). Despite extensive physiological knowledge, the potential use of the respiratory tract in the prevention and treatment of hypothermia was largely ignored until it was suggested (Lloyd, 1971) following a disaster in the Cairngorm Mountains in Scotland in which seven children lost their lives.

Urine is another route by which heat is lost from the body though it is not usually noticed (Burton and Edholm, 1955). However, if there is a diuresis as occurs on exposure to cold the increased volume will increase the heat loss especially since even in the cold the urine is voided at core temperature (Collins and Exton-Smith, 1979). The effect of the urinary heat is noticed if someone urinates in the water, when the person experiences a warm feeling in the area of the groin, hips and legs (Lehrmann, 1982; Low, 1982). By collecting the urine from an uninjured normothermic person in bags it is possible in an emergency to use the heat to try to prevent hypothermia developing in an injured survivor (Gavshon and Rice, 1984).

In the outdoors it is reasonably easy to identify cold stress environments. Cold temperatures and wind are easily recognised and quantified. Wetness, however, is more difficult. Rain can increase cold stress by wetting the clothing of individuals but there may be other elements. A humid environment increases the thermal conductivity of air (Lahti, 1982) and produces an increase in heat production even though it has no apparent effect on heat exchange or subjective sensations (Iampietro *et al.*, 1958). In addition a high level of moisture content in the ambient air will penetrate the clothing and therefore reduce the insulative value of the clothing.

In the domestic environment, it is sometimes assumed that cold stress is absent. However, cold stress may occur in a number of ways. Obviously absolute temperature is one factor and draughts will provide the wind-chill factor. The fact that bedrooms and bathrooms often remain totally unheated, with a window open even at night in winter, may result in repeated exposures to severe cold stress especially if only one room in the house is heated. This would be exaggerated if that one room was overheated.

Dampness is another poorly understood problem. As in the outdoors, if there is a high moisture content of the air, the moisture will percolate the clothing and reduce the insulating properties of the clothing. The term 'relative humidity' can cause confusion since it only refers to the moisture content of the air as a percentage of the moisture content which is carried when the air is fully saturated. However, warm air can carry more water in vapour form than can cold air and therefore air which has a comfortable relative humidity of 50 per cent when warm may have a relative humidity of 100 per cent or more when cold. Unfortunately if the water vapour content reaches a relative humidity of more than 100 per cent, the excess water vapour condenses as liquid. In a house, water vapour is constantly being released into the air from cooking, boiling a kettle, hot water from washing dishes or clothes, baths or showers and from gas burners used for cooking or for heating, especially if non-flued. Despite all these possibilities one of the biggest sources of water vapour is the human body from breathing and perspiration, and the more bodies the more water vapour.

One of the worst scenarios is if a lot of people are concentrated in one room which is overheated. There will be a lot of water vapour being poured into the air but because the room is hot the air feels dry though the windows may have condensation. Then when the person leaves the warm room and goes into a cold room or out of doors, the water vapour in the clothes will condense and additional body heat will be needed to evaporate the moisture and dry the clothes. It is unfortunate that the lower social classes are likely to be the group with the greatest financial difficulty. They are therefore likely only to heat, or overheat, one room and the houses are likely to have small rooms, with less air volume for the moisture vapour to disperse in, and the humidity will therefore rise faster and higher. The housing occupied by the lower social classes is unfortunately also likely to be poorer quality with poor wall, roof and window insulation, and therefore any unheated rooms will be colder in winter with greater condensation.

Bedrooms may be one of the most hazardous rooms for cold stress, and it was found that the night bedroom temperature in London was 8 to 9 °C and even when people lived and slept in the same room it was only 9 to 13 °C (Eddy *et al.*, 1970). Many bedrooms are totally unheated and therefore a person is exposed to the greatest degree of cold at a time when he is dressing and undressing and the insulation from clothing is reduced. Even when he gets into bed he may have cold stress because the bedding is cold, and if the bedding is damp as well, the cold stress is increased because damp bedding will increase conductive heat loss and body heat is needed to evaporate the moisture from the bedding and this requires a lot of heat. If the bedroom is cold, it will almost inevitably be damp from condensation. During the day warm moist air comes from the kitchen and bathroom, and at night from breathing and from insensible water vapour loss from the body. The moisture condenses most obviously on walls and windows but, if the bedroom is totally unheated, it will also condense on the bedding.

The bathroom is another danger room from cold. It is a room which is seldom heated and, after a bath, the person is totally naked, vasodilated and wet. There is therefore a tremendous heat loss potential — total surface area exposed for convection, conduction and radiation, no vasoconstriction and therefore a maximal heat gradient and rate of loss, plus evaporation. After the heat loss the clothing may prevent the body rewarming in the warm part of the house and this is a greater risk for babies.

There are a number of things which can be done to reduce the hazards of the bedroom (Stephens, 1982). Four-poster beds, bedsocks and nightcaps or a cellular blanket over the head will increase warmth, but, if the bedding is damp, there is still the risk of hypothermia. The dampness can be reduced by pre-warming the bed by using warming pans, hot water bottles or electric blankets, though to be effective these must be used several hours before the person goes to bed. The ideal way to prevent condensation is to improve the insulation of the walls and windows and provide central heating throughout the house. A simpler measure is to have the bedroom door shut during the day, to prevent the warm moist air from getting into the room, and to have the bedroom window open during the day to dry out all the moisture released at night (Stephens, 1982).

It is also possible to improve matters by the use of different materials for bedding (Stephens, 1982). Natural fibres such as cotton and wool absorb water vapour from the air, whereas nylon, acrylic and polyester are non-hygroscopic and lightweight. A polythene sheet above the mattress will prevent the body moisture reaching the mattress but this is sometimes uncomfortable to sleep on. Comfort can be improved by having a cellular nylon/acrylic underblanket above the polythene. The conventional interior sprung mattress is an important item in which water vapour condenses and the lower layers have a higher moisture content because they are colder and because moisture will drain by gravity. However, if a plastic foam mattress is used, it is hydrophobic and any condensation drains through it and out at the bottom. There is a great resistance to foam mattresses in the UK where they account for only 10 per cent of the market. One reason for this is that the foam used in the UK is low grade and non-fire resistant. On the continent of Europe, where high-grade fire-resistant foam is used, plastic foam mattresses account for 85 per cent of the market (Stephens, 1982).

Therefore the way to reduce the damp problem of a bedroom to the minimum (Stephens, 1982) is to keep the bedroom door shut and the window open during the day, and to sleep on a high-grade fire-resistant plastic foam mattress in a nylon/polyester sleeping bag. This type of mattress and sleeping bag have the additional advantage that they can be easily washed. Unfortunately it is the lower socio-economic classes who are probably in the poorest quality housing, who cannot afford the cost of central heating and improved insulation, who may only be able to afford to heat one room, who are likely to keep the bedroom windows shut to conserve heat while leaving the bedroom door open to allow heat to reach the bedroom from the rest of the house and who are likely to be most resistant to change as far as traditional bedding is concerned.

3 REGULATION OF BODY TEMPERATURE

Introduction

As soon as man is exposed to cold physiological changes for regulating body temperature are brought into play and complex equations have been developed (Rivolier *et al.*, 1984) to fit round human heat balance. However, for practical purposes it is probably more useful to realise that the human body loses heat through the normal physical routes discussed earlier and that man in a cold environment normally maintains his body temperature by balancing the rate of heat loss with heat production with the control being through a central thermostatic mechanism in the brain (Burton and Edholm, 1955; Maclean and Emslie-Smith, 1977).

Central Thermostat

The primary control of body temperature is through a central thermostat situated in the hypothalamus and this regulates the body temperature within a narrow range. This thermostat is not a simple on/off device but is in fact more akin to a 'black box' with a complex system of neurones linking the sensory input and the effector output. There are many cross linkages and a number of neurochemical transmitters. This is a growing field of investigation and it is not certain whether all the transmitters have been identified and their interrelationships, control mechanisms and sites of action are also still being clarified (Cooper *et al.*, 1977; Cox *et al.*, 1980; Lomax, 1985; Lomax and Schonbaum, 1979, 1983; Milton, 1982). Despite this complexity and all the theories about the control of body temperature, in practical terms the system works like a thermostat (Danzl, 1983; Satinoff, 1979).

The thermostat is activated by impulses from central receptors, which respond to changes in the temperature of the blood and are situated along the distribution of the internal carotid artery, the reticular area of the midbrain and the pre-optic and posterior hypothalamus. Information is also supplied by peripheral receptors situated mainly in the skin, but some in deeper tissues such as the stomach. There is also clinical evidence which suggests that there may be temperature-sensitive receptors in the interior of the peripheral veins (Lloyd, 1979e). In addition to the central thermostat there are spinal thermostatic reflexes though these alone are insufficient to control body temperature (Downey *et al.*, 1967).

The thermostat regulates the temperature of the body by adjusting heat production and heat loss, but the setting of the thermostat itself may be altered. There is a normal diurnal variation in core temperature and the range can vary between individuals. In young adults the diurnal range can be as small as 0.7 °C or as large as 2.1 °C and the average is 1.49 °C for males and 1.2 °C for females (Maclean and Emslie-Smith, 1977). The lowest temperature is usually at 5 a.m. and the highest at 8 p.m. The normal circadian rhythm can be upset, e.g. by prolonged undersea voyage (Colquohoun *et al.*, 1978), by arctic exploration during prolonged daylight (Simpson, 1981) or by the long arctic winter, i.e. situations in which the normal night/day cycle is disturbed, or even by travel across a number of time zones (Colquohoun, 1984) and desynchronisation of the normal circadian rhythms has been suggested as a cause of hypothermia in the elderly (Moore-Ede, 1983). In women ovulation causes a temporary alteration of the thermostatic set-point and the set-point is also lowered during sleep (Maclean and Emslie-Smith, 1977). The lowered temperature commonly found in myxoedema may be due to a direct effect on the thermostat or to an inability to increase heat production in response to a cold stress. Mental depression also affects diurnal rhythm (Crawford, 1979) and there are cases where recurrent admissions to hospital with mental problems have been associated with a cerebrally mediated lowering of core temperature (Maclean and Emslie-Smith, 1977; Thomas and Green, 1973) but the problem still is unresolved as to the exact mechanism.

Heat Production

Basal Metabolic Heat

This is the minimum heat produced by the vital basal functions of the body, but the absolute body temperature can alter the level of basal heat production (Burton and Edholm, 1955). Eating food increases basal heat through the energy required for digestion and absorption, and in hypothermia associated with malnutrition the absence of food intake is an important factor. Emotion also increases heat production under basal conditions.

Shivering

When the person is exposed to cold, heat production rises by increased muscle metabolism and tone leading eventually to shivering (Schneider and Brooke, 1979) but any increase in heat production is always accompanied by a rise in oxygen consumption and shivering may double or treble oxygen consumption and carbon dioxide output (Lim, 1960). Shivering is progressive, starting in the neck muscles and moving to the abdominal and pectoral muscles and finally reaching the extremities (Horvath, 1981). The onset of shivering is controlled by central and peripheral stimuli working independently (Lim, 1960) but may also be triggered by extraneous stimuli such as touch or a loud noise. Shivering metabolism is proportional to decreased core temperature when the mean skin temperature is constant (Buguet *et al.*, 1967; Cabanac and Massonet, 1977) and proportional to the lowered mean skin temperature when the core temperature is constant (Hong and Nadel, 1979). The intensity of shivering is affected by the rate of change which has important clinical implications (see pp. 39–41).

Non-shivering Thermogenesis (NST)

Heat may also be produced without shivering — so-called NST. This has traditionally been associated with brown fat (brown because of the high concentration of iron-containing cytochrome which only becomes evident after fat depletion). It used to be thought that brown fat only occurred in rodents, small mammals and neonates, but the subject is more complicated than that and has been reviewed (Alexander, 1979; Maclean and Emslie-Smith, 1977).

NST is a complex problem which seems to encourage workers to take sides. However, the fact that one good study in Antarctica found no evidence of noradrenaline-induced brown fat activity in man (Budd *et al.*, 1984) does not prove conclusively that there is no mechanism in man for an increased heat production that does not include shivering (NST). Shivering thresholds tend to be at higher body temperatures in leaner individuals (Hong and Nadel, 1979) and there is in fact a suggestion that obesity and NST may be interlinked (Jung and James, 1980). Whereas fat people are less at risk from hypothermia in a cold environment because of the insulating effect of the subcutaneous adipose tissue (Jequier *et al.*, 1974) — a possible factor in the ability of the female to withstand cold better than the male — this may not be the whole story. Obese and post-obese people have a much lower NST response than lean people, as measured in the metabolic response to cold stress and to an injection of noradrenaline. All lean individuals respond by a large increase in metabolic rate whereas obese people have a lower response and show a fall in deep body temperature especially on food deprivation. However, a complicating factor in this is that the intake of food itself has an effect on the metabolic rate. The metabolic rate increases after a meal (Rothwell and Stock, 1979) and overfeeding results in an increase in the resting metabolic rate (Garrow, 1983), while conversely, fasting results in a decrease in the resting metabolic rate (Garrow, 1983) and in prolonged cold, a restricted calory intake results in a lowering of the core temperature (Iampietro and Bass, 1962). This problem is still unresolved.

Activity

Deliberate activity will also increase heat production, which may rise 10 to 15 fold during hard physical exercise, and this rate of heat production may be maintained for several hours (Maughan, 1984). However, under conditions of great cold stress, additional heat may be needed from shivering to maintain normothermia (Horvath, 1981). Though shivering can coexist with exercise, and the increase in metabolism due to exposure to cold is normally additive to the metabolism of exercise (Goode and McDonald, 1982), increasing exercise intensities have the effect of increasingly suppressing the shivering response (Hong and Nadel, 1979) but shivering continues in submaximal exercise and therefore for any level of exercise the oxygen consumption is higher in a cold environment than in a warm one (Horvath, 1981).

There are, however, limitations in heat-production capabilities. If hypoxia is present as occurs at high altitude, there is a limit in the maximum oxygen uptake and there will therefore be a decrease in the total possible heat production and shivering may be inhibited (Alexander, 1979). In conditions of very severe cold, there will obviously be a great need for heat production which may utilise most of the maximal possible oxygen uptake. If the person then has to undertake very vigorous exercise, the maximal oxygen uptake may be insufficient to provide for the high demand of both the exercise and the severe cold stress and therefore a person can develop unexpected and unsuspected hypothermia despite vigorous muscular exercise (Hirvonen, 1982). Finally, if the person is exhausted or suffering from malnutrition he cannot increase heat production because of the lack of substrate (fuel) for metabolism (Wang, 1978).

Activity and shivering are not economical in thermoregulation because they are accompanied by an increased blood supply to the muscles and this increases heat loss. In fact only 48 per cent of the extra heat generated is retained in the body (Jansky, 1979).

Regulation of Heat Loss

When a subject is exposed to cold stress the body responds by vasoconstriction of the peripheral vessels mainly via the sympathetic nervous system. However, even after surgical division and subsequent degeneration of the sympathetic nerve supply to the fingers, moderate local cooling will greatly reduce the blood supply (Lewis and Landis, 1929) through a direct vasoconstrictor action on the blood vessels (Smith, 1952) though there may be some effect through cold sensors, which it has been suggested may lie in the superficial veins in the limbs (Lloyd, 1979e). This vasoconstriction reduces heat loss by direct limitation of blood flow to the periphery, thus increasing the depth of shell insulation and reducing the temperature differential between the skin and the environment. It also allows a counter-current exchange of heat between the arteries and veins in the distal half of the limbs. Below a temperature of 10 to 12 °C the peripheral vasoconstriction fails and 'hunting' occurs, i.e. alternating vasodilatation and vasoconstriction. There may actually be very little increase in the volume of blood circulating in the skin during the vasodilatation (Hayward, 1983), thus preserving the insulating effect of the vasoconstriction.

However, the rate of heat loss from the head cannot be reduced because there is minimal vasoconstrictor activity, if any (Froese and Burton, 1957), and in fact facial temperatures stabilise well above freezing (Steegman, 1979). Though this makes the head relatively resistant to frostbite as compared with the limbs, the rate of heat loss through the head increases in a linear manner between +32 °C and −20 °C, and at rest in −4 °C the heat loss from the head may equal half the total heat production (Froese and Burton, 1957). Other examples illustrating the importance of the head as a route for heat loss are given in the discussion of the diving reflex. In cold weather a hat or woolly bonnet is of great benefit in reducing heat loss and improving comfort. Finally, one woman, who had been smuggling frozen chickens, collapsed unconscious and the diagnosis of hypothermia was made, probably caused by her method of smuggling, which was to carry the frozen chickens on her head under the hat (*Scotsman*, 1977).

In animals horripilation — raising of the hairs — is a very effective means for controlling heat loss by varying the insulating depth of the hair coat, and in man, piloerection or goose-pimples is a vestigial remnant of this mechanism.

The body may be exposed to heat by being in a hot environment or, in a cold environment, by vigorous exercise with too much protective clothing. When the body temperature rises heat must be lost and the body reacts with vasodilatation which raises the superficial temperature of the body and, the greater the temperature differential between the skin and the air temperature, the greater the heat loss through radiation, conduction and convection. The vasodilatation also increases the transfer of heat from the core to the shell, and the amount of fluid available to the sweat glands. Sweating is an important route for heat loss, with evaporation of one litre of sweat requiring 580 kcal (Maughan, 1984). In vigorous exercise, such as the marathon, there is a correlation between the sweat rate and the running speed (Guezennec and Pesquies, 1985), but maximum sweat production can only be maintained for a limited period before being reduced (Leithead, 1965). Sweating may be impaired by dehydration, by drugs such as atropine, hyoscine and the antihistamines, by some skin diseases such as eczema, and some people have an absence of sweat glands (Hertzman, 1957).

One of the methods of regulating body temperature is behavioural. For example, in the cold a man will curl up into the fetal position and not only does this reduce the total body surface exposed to the cold environment by 30 to 40 per cent (Pugh, 1968) but the areas of high heat loss from the body surface (Hayward *et al.*, 1973) are protected. The area of increased heat loss recorded from the lateral thorax by Hayward *et al.* (1973) has not been substantiated (Reed *et al.*, 1984) and the probable explanation is that when the person was standing normally the arm was against the lateral thorax and there was a total increase in temperature due to the body crease/skin fold contact effect. Then when the subject lifted his arm for thermography the camera recorded this effect (Reed *et al.*, 1984). By contrast, if the person is overheating the core/shell temperature gradient decreases, the skin becomes redder, the amount of activity decreases and the posture is changed from flexion to extension, and this happens even in immature babies (Harpin *et al.*, 1983). Therefore when sunbathing on a hot beach the person naturally adopts a spreadeagled position and, though it is often assumed that this is to allow maximum tanning of the skin, it also allows the body the greatest potential for heat loss by convection, conduction, radiation and also evaporation of sweat.

Man has an extraordinary ability to adapt to all stressful environments (Le Blanc, 1966) and prolonged exposure to cold stress results in an alteration of responses — adaptation, acclimatisation, conditioning, habituation, tolerance (Bodey, 1978; Cooper, 1976; Horvath, 1981; Houdas *et al.*, 1985). These are not well understood and there is some argument as to their existence. However, despite the extensive and complex physiology involved in thermoregulation (Maclean and Emslie-Smith, 1977), the factors which have had the greatest influence in allowing man to live in and explore very hostile areas of the world are in fact the way man can limit his time of exposure to cold, and man's technological ability to manipulate his thermal environment by the use of clothing, heating and shelter (Maclean and Emslie-Smith, 1977). The proof of the success of the technology is that the skin temperature of man in the Arctic is the same as that of man in the Tropics.

4 FACTORS ALTERING NORMAL TEMPERATURE REGULATION

General

There are a number of ways that the normal control of body temperature can be disrupted. Mental stress even of as mild a degree as mental arithmetic increases the heat loss, as also do nausea, vomiting, fainting, trauma and haemorrhage. Exhaustion, as well as reducing the heat-generating capacity, is also associated with a maximal rate of heat loss (Witherspoon *et al.*, 1971). (This is independent of any reduction of heat-generating capacity.) Sleep, alcohol and anaesthesia also affect temperature regulation.

As will be discussed later, at the extremes of age there is an increased risk of hypothermia and there are also racial variations in the response to cold. The Aborigines in Australia can sleep comfortably on nights when a European is shivering with the cold because the core temperature of the Aborigine drops further than that of the European before causing discomfort, and the Aborigine then utilises the heat of the sun to rewarm. The Aborigines, the Bantu and the Kalahari bushmen also have morphological differences as compared with Caucasians who have more subcutaneous fat (Wyndham *et al.*, 1964). However, the 'primitive' groups are not noted for having an abundance of food, and this food shortage may not only cause lowering of the core temperature directly through lack of energy but may also act through the decreased fat layer. Another group, the natives of Tierra del Fuego, astonished visitors such as Charles Darwin by their ability to appear comfortable, though half naked, in a snowstorm, and their physiological adaptation is to maintain a constant high metabolic rate.

Many medical disorders predispose to hypothermia (Braun, 1982; Maclean and Emslie-Smith, 1977) and as medical awareness of the possibility of hypothermia has increased, so has the range of drugs, either alone or in combination, which have been shown to increase the risk of an individual developing hypothermia (Holdcroft, 1981; Maclean and Emslie-Smith, 1977). Some of these drugs are prescribed for some of the medical disorders which themselves predispose to hypothermia.

In the practical situation the hypothermia risk will inevitably be multifactorial. For example in a lifeboat following the sinking of a ship during war or peace, heat loss will be increased by mental stress but there will be additional varying combinations of nausea, vomiting, fainting, trauma, haemorrhage and exhaustion all contributing to an increased heat loss. An additional complication is that the best anti-seasick remedy — hyoscine (Laitinen *et al.*, 1981) — also decreases the metabolic rate (Keatinge and Evans, 1960). The possible contribution of alcohol and the availability of protection from the elements increase the difficulties of understanding any particular situation. The emergency operating theatre is another place of complex interactions as the effects of fear, haemorrhage, trauma, etc. compound the difficult thermal picture produced by the various drugs and techniques used during the anaesthetic.

Food Deprivation and Oxygen Lack

It is known that a restriction of calories results in a lowering of the core temperature on exposure to cold (Iampietro and Bass, 1962) and below an effective critical temperature extra food is necessary to allow continuing growth and at the same time to meet the needs of increased heat production (Close and Mount, 1978). As will be discussed later, energy is produced not only through the metabolism of glycogen but also through lypolysis and gluconeogenesis, and, as the exercise becomes more prolonged, the glycogen source becomes much less important (Guezennec and Pesquies, 1985). Fatigue and exhaustion are the result of complex changes (Guezennec and Pesquies, 1985) but, though the depletion of the glycogen stores by fasting results in the person being more sensitive to fatigue, exercise can still be carried out after hepatic and muscle glycogen depletion (Guezennec and Pesquies, 1985). The lipid stores of the body are depleted by prolonged starvation but the rate of depletion is faster if the starvation is accompanied by cold exposure and exercise (Guezennec and Pesquies, 1985). The metabolic demand of cold exposure is similar to that of prolonged exercise, though less marked (Guezennec and Pesquies, 1985), and the combination of cold exposure and fasting produces a severe metabolic strain on the organism (Guezennec and Pesquies, 1985). It is therefore not really surprising that malnutrition and hypothermia are often seen together (Howitt, 1971; Sadikali and Owor, 1974).

Sleep

When a person falls asleep the cerebral thermostat is reset to a new low level (Hey, 1972; Maclean and Emslie-Smith, 1977) and sleep also causes a reduction of the basal metabolic rate (Adams, 1970; BMJ, 1973; Shapiro *et al.*, 1984). However, sleep can be divided into two main types (Wilkinson, 1965) differentiated by the EEG patterns. In one type there is a burst of fast cortical activity which looks similar to that of an alert awake pattern and is accompanied by rapid eye movements (REM) and this type is called paradoxical or REM sleep. In the other predominant type there is a slow wave pattern and this type is called slow wave or non-rapid-eye-movement (NREM) sleep (Adams, 1970). The heat production during sleep is 9 per cent lower than the heat produced when the person is awake and at rest, even taking into account movements during sleep and periods of awakening at night (Shapiro *et al.*, 1984). During NREM sleep oxygen consumption (Oswald, 1975) and metabolic rate are at their lowest (Shapiro *et al.*, 1984) and if NREM sleep is divided into four types or grades (Shapiro *et al.*, 1984) the heat production during NREM4 sleep is 14 per cent lower than awake resting (Shapiro *et al.*, 1984). During the night there is a gradual reduction in heat production which rises again before wakening, i.e. similar to the temperature cycle (Shapiro *et al.*, 1984), though whether the heat production follows the changing settings of the central thermostat or is the prime cause of the temperature changes is not known. The onset of sleep is also associated with a slight degree of alveolar hypoventilation and carbon dioxide retention (Phillipson, 1978).

When a person falls asleep there is an immediate rise in skin temperature which occurs in both thermoneutral and cold environments (Buguet *et al.*, 1979a) though this may be merely a redistribution of the total body heat (Lunn, 1969). During REM sleep, the skin temperature rises in both thermoneutral and cold environments if the rectal temperature is high, whereas REM sleep causes a drop in skin temperature if the rectal temperature is low (Buguet *et al.*, 1979a). When the person wakes during the night or shows marked body movements the skin temperature drops, especially in the cold (Buguet *et al.*, 1979a). When this observation is taken with the one that in the cold a person wakes more often and moves about more often than at thermoneutral (Buguet *et al.*, 1979a) it is likely that the body is aware of cold discomfort and in wakening and body movement the body is trying to restore the total body heat content. It has been stated (Pugh, 1968) that there is no danger from falling asleep in the extreme cold since each bout of shivering will wake the person (Pugh, 1968) and certainly this has been the experience of scientists carrying out research in the Antarctic and in 1902 a man slept in the open for 36 hours in Antarctica during a blizzard and survived though he had been covered by snow (Brent, 1974). There is the caveat about the situation if the person is exhausted (Pugh, 1968). Not only may the exhausted person not be wakened by a bout of shivering but the exhausted person may not in fact shiver.

There are therefore several risk factors occurring when a person falls asleep in a cold environment:

(1) The initial redistribution of body heat will increase the heat loss from the body surface.
(2) The lowered set point of body temperature will allow the total body heat content to fall before the cold causes discomfort.
(3) The lowered metabolic rate, especially in NREM sleep, will increase the danger of the rate of heat loss from the body being greater than the metabolic heat production.
(4) During REM sleep the skin temperature rises if the core temperature is normal, and this will again increase heat loss. The fact that this does not occur during REM sleep if the core temperature is low is of some safety value but by this time the person is already in danger.

The folk-lore among climbers in a cold environment, where members of a group will do everything in their power to prevent anyone falling asleep, may therefore have a sound physiological basis. It is probably true that staying awake may make the difference between survival and death (Clarke, 1976), especially at high altitude where the alveolar hypoventilation at the onset of sleep may also be fatal. The other phenomenon, of a person falling asleep in a warm room and inexplicably feeling cold on waking, is also understandable.

Alcohol

It is common practice in northern countries for a host to greet his guest on a cold night with a full glass of alcoholic beverage (Vanggaard, 1978). In a cold person the intake of alcohol results in a feeling of warmth spreading through the body which has been attributed to an increase in the circulation in the skin (Vanggaard, 1978). The redness of facial skin after alcohol intake is an indication of an increase in skin blood flow but it may not cause any increase in heat loss (Vanggaard, 1978). There are two other situations in which a similar increase in skin blood flow occurs without increased heat loss. These are following nicotinic acid (Vanggaard, 1978) and in the 'hunting' vasodilatation phenomenon (Hayward, 1983) (see p. 28). After a drink the alcohol is distributed round the body in relation to the blood flow in the various body compartments. Exercise can therefore alter the arterial alcohol levels by increasing the distribution into the muscles (Vanggaard, 1978).

World wide it is now recognised that alcohol is a very important cause of death in water (BMJ, 1979) and on land (Weyman *et al.*, 1974), and, in one study, alcohol was a contributing factor in 91 per cent of cases of urban hypothermia (Fitzgerald and Jessop, 1982). However, the role of alcohol in hypothermia is complex. It was traditionally taught that alcohol intake increased heat loss from the body because of the vasodilatation it induced (Victor and Adams, 1958) and in support of this view is the fact that many cases of accidental hypothermia have been found to have an elevated blood alcohol level (Maclean and Emslie-Smith, 1977). Nevertheless many studies have failed to demonstrate that alcohol ingestion increased heat loss in:

(1) resting men during cold air exposure (Anderson *et al.*, 1963; Livingstone *et al.*, 1980);
(2) resting men during cold water immersion (Fox *et al.*, 1979; Keatinge and Evans, 1960; Martin *et al.*, 1977; Vanggaard, 1978);
(3) exercising men during cold water immersion (Fox *et al.*, 1979).

It has been suggested (Fox *et al.*, 1979) that the failure of the cold water studies to demonstrate enhanced heat loss may be due to the very intense stress of cold water. Cold air coupled with the internal heat production of exercise would create a thermal situation that is much less stressful and therefore any tendency for peripheral vasodilatation would not have to overcome extreme vasoconstriction. Alcohol ingestion prior to exercise and a cold air stress has been shown to enhance heat loss (Graham, 1981; Graham and Dalton, 1980; Haight and Keatinge, 1973; Juhlin-Dannfelt *et al.*, 1977). This is associated with a decrease in blood glucose (Graham, 1981;

Graham and Dalton, 1980; Haight and Keatinge, 1973; Juhlin-Dannfelt *et al.*, 1977) and whether this is due to alcohol inhibiting gluconeogenesis (Juhlin-Dannfelt *et al.*, 1977; Krebs *et al.*, 1969) or interfering with insulin secretion (Singh and Patel, 1978; Singh *et al.*, 1980) is not important in practical terms. Post-alcoholic hypoglycaemia may occur even without exercise and result in hypothermia (Duckworth and Cooper, 1964) and the lowering of blood glucose, which itself impairs thermoregulation (BMJ, 1979), is also liable to lead to early exhaustion, e.g. in hill walking, as another factor promoting hypothermia which will itself then aggravate the impaired gluconeogenesis (Krarup and Larsen, 1972). Alcohol may also act by resetting the central thermostat to a lower level (Lomax, 1983). Another danger of alcohol consumption is that the awareness of cold stress is impaired with subjects all registering a greater degree of thermal comfort than controls exposed to the same cold stress or with similar temperature readings (Graham, 1981; Graham and Baulk, 1980; Keatinge and Evans, 1960; Vanggaard, 1978) and exercise itself impairs the little awareness of cold stress that survives the alcohol (Graham, 1981). Possibly through this increased tolerance to cold, alcohol decreases shivering thermogenesis even during immersion (Lomax, 1983; Pozos and Wittmers, 1983; Vanggaard, 1978), leading to an increased heat loss during immersion, a greater drop in core temperature during the post-immersion recovery period and a decrease in the total body heat regained (Graham and Baulk, 1980). Even after cessation of cold exposure taking alcohol provides prompt subjective relief and shivering stops very rapidly (Vanggaard, 1978). Therefore alcohol even in quantities which result in blood levels below those of legal intoxication (Graham, 1981) are dangerous before activity in a cold environment because:

(1) Alcohol causes an increased level of bravado (BMJ, 1979) while impairing the ability to assess risks.
(2) Impaired shivering during the cold stress may result in an increased rate of cooling.
(3) The lowering of blood glucose levels will increase the risk of exhaustion leading to hypothermia and a further impairment of gluconeogenesis, and if hypoglycaemia occurs (Haight and Keatinge, 1973) this will cause vasodilation and increased heat loss.
(4) The increased tolerance to cold will leave the person unaware of

the severity of the cold stress and may lead to unnecessary risks being taken during exposure and after recovery from immersion.
(5) Heat production is impaired after removal from the cold stress and this increases the dangers of continued cooling after rescue.
(6) Since alcohol is a sedative, another danger may lie in its tendency to make people fall asleep with the increased dangers of failure to maintain body heat.
(7) A final danger is that alcohol causes a diuresis (Hamlet, 1983) and therefore increases the risk of dehydration which increases the risk of hypothermia and frostbite.

The only possible value of alcohol might be just before abandoning ship where the increased tolerance to cold might be of value in reducing panic and, if this resulted in the person staying still instead of swimming, heat loss would be minimised and there might be an improved chance of survival. Modest quantities of alcohol taken at night during high altitude appears to be a safe and valuable hypnotic in a situation where problems with sleep are very common (Clarke, C., personal communication, 1984).

Fitness

There is disagreement about the effects of fitness in thermal regulation and its role in the prevention of hypothermia.

Cold causes a sympathetic response and catecholamine release (Goode and McDonald, 1982; Hartung *et al.*, 1984) which induces a release of free fatty acids (FFA) into the circulation (Hanson and Johnson, 1965) and some FFA is utilised by shivering muscles, with a proportion going to the liver where it is converted into low-density lipoprotein (LDLP) which is an important source of energy in thermogenesis (Alexander, 1979). Contrary to popular belief the main source of energy in endurance activity, e.g. marathon running, is not glucose/glycogen but is in fact FFA and LDLP, especially after two hours of activity (Guezennec and Pesquies, 1985), and increasing fitness results in an increased ability to utilise FFA and LDLP for energy (Alexander, 1979; Hartung *et al.*, 1984; Moriya, 1984). Therefore since the main endurance muscles are the large limb muscles, which are the same as used in shivering, increased fitness should result in an increased ability to generate heat over prolonged periods. In the normal ranges of cold stress as experienced by hill walkers, the fit person will be able to continue much further and may be able to reach safety before he becomes exhausted (Brotherhood, 1975; Edwards, 1975), whereas the unfit person may become exhausted in the open and he will then not only be unable to produce heat but the rate of heat loss will be maximal (Witherspoon *et al.*, 1971). Fatigue/exhaustion is a complex phenomenon related not just to a diminution in the fuel supply but also to electrolytic changes and mechanisms in the central nervous system (Guezennec and Pesquies, 1985).

Physical fitness improves the thermal response to exercise in temperate climates but has no effect on exercise in the cold, and the thermoregulatory mechanisms are unchanged (Schwartz *et al.*, 1977). However, though increasing fitness causes a lessening of the insulating layer of fat, it also results in a diminution of shivering on exposure to cold (Budd, 1965) and it has been suggested that, though the cooling rate does not change, the increased fitness allows an increased metabolic rate to be sustained without shivering. Improving fitness results in an increase in the maximum oxygen uptake and therefore fit people can work better and are more comfortable in the cold than unfit people (Horvath, 1981). The maximum work capacity in cold water is reduced more in thin people than in fat people and it is suggested that the increased heat loss from the thin person produces a drop in body temperature and this results in a decreased work capacity (Horvath, 1981). However, it could also be that, while the thin person does lose more heat than the fat one, the decrease in work capacity is because a higher proportion of the total oxygen uptake is having to be diverted into heat production with less being available for work. In this second possibility increased fitness would obviously allow more oxygen to be available for work and therefore increase the work capacity.

On immersion fit people increase their metabolic rate to values 50 per cent greater (Jacobs *et al.*, 1984; Johnson *et al.*, 1977) than those predicted by the use of equations developed by Hayward *et al.* (1975a) and the time taken to cool 1 °C was directly related to the level of endurance fitness (Jacobs *et al.*, 1984). Golden and Hervey (1972) found that on immersion, the very fit males produced a very high metabolic rate accompanied by a running type of movement but cooled faster than the unfit, fat females who stayed still in the water and cooled least, though this finding was probably entirely due to the decrease in heat loss because of the fat in the women and an increase in heat loss due to the movement of the limbs in the men.

Certainly one fit man managed to maintain a high rate of heat production by shivering and as a result there was no cooling of core temperature despite exposure to 12 °C water for two hours (Golden and Hervey, 1981). Despite this it is often the fit person who succumbs first in cold water (Lehrmann, 1982), though this may be related to total body mass as much as fat (Lehrmann, 1982).

Improved fitness also results in an improved ability to sleep in the cold and an increase in the person's peripheral temperature in the cold (Horvath, 1981).

Symptomless Cooling

The normal responses to cold can also be modified. For example in one experiment a man, who was used to being exposed to 0 °C air, was seated in water at 29 °C and cooled to hypothermic temperatures without shivering and without being aware of feeling cold (Hayward and Keatinge, 1979). It was suggested that some people, especially those regularly exposed to cold, were susceptible to progressive symptomless hypothermia. The reason for concern is that divers are regularly exposed to cold, and progressive, symptomless hypothermia might be the cause of confusion, bad judgement and resulting death which is known to occur in diving (Hayward and Keatinge, 1979; Keatinge *et al.*, 1980). However, other experiments showed that, though subjects who were used to cold exposure (acclimatised) cooled faster when sitting in cold water than did subjects who were unused to cold, if the subjects were active in cold water, e.g. swimming, those who were unused to cold cooled faster than the cold acclimatised (Hampton *et al.*, 1979).

The state of peripheral vasomotor tone depends on an interaction of peripheral and central temperatures (Reaves and Hayward, 1979). However, it is also true that the central thermostat responds to the rate of firing of the temperature-sensitive neurones and the rate of firing of receptor neurones is at least partially dependent on the rate of change of the stimulus. Therefore if the peripheral and central temperatures change slowly, the body may cool to much lower temperatures than if the temperatures change rapidly. During experimental cooling, it is possible, by slightly raising the skin temperature at the onset of shivering, to abolish shivering and the sensation of cold without stopping continued cooling (Harnett *et al.*, 1980; Kaufman, 1983; Keatinge *et al.*, 1980). This effect can be produced even though the increased water and skin temperature is in fact cold enough to cause continued cooling and the effect is therefore due to perceived warmth.

This phenomenon has a number of clinical implications:

(1) It is known that divers can become hypothermic despite having warm water supplied to the skin (Keatinge *et al.*, 1980) and it has been suggested that the reason divers can develop symptomless hypothermia is because of the high level of respiratory heat loss in this situation, but studies have shown that this is not the main cause (Hayes *et al.*, 1981). Thermoregulation for the deep diver is different from the normal situation (Vanggaard, 1985). For divers, the environment, especially in heliox, while not being unduly cold, has the capacity to transfer a great deal of heat but the protective clothing prevents profound cold shock and in fact the skin temperature remains relatively high (Hayes *et al.*, 1981). The core temperature therefore has to drop further before shivering is provoked. It is also possible that the perception of peripheral temperature may be modified by changes in core-skin temperature gradients (Hayes, 1979). In heliox atmospheres the normal routes of heat loss continue but the quantities lost through each route are greatly altered from those under normal conditions (Hayes, 1979). It has also been suggested that the provision of warmed humidified air for divers may cause symptomless hypothermia by suppressing shivering (Pozos and Wittmers, 1983).

(2) The suggestion has been made that the reason elderly people can become hypothermic without discomfort or warning is that the normal mechanisms for preserving and restoring body temperature are ineffective. While the normal mechanisms are undoubtedly impaired, it is also true that the elderly hypothermics have probably been exposed to cold environments for some considerable time and the rate of cooling is very slow. The tendency for some of the elderly to put on small inefficient heaters at irregular intervals may compound the problem by causing perceived warmth sufficient to overcome peripheral vasoconstriction while not providing sufficient heat to rewarm the person.

(3) A similar phenomenon can occur if someone repeatedly moves in and out of a refrigerated room. The warmer air outside, which may still be below freezing, gives a sensation of perceived warmth and this prevents the activation of the heat conservation

mechanisms, and leaves any heat debt uncorrected. Return to the cold room causes further cooling (Kaufman, 1983), and the person can therefore slide into hypothermia. Failure to rewarm completely between dives may be one possible cause of hypothermia and sudden death in divers (Hayes, 1985).

(4) During rewarming the maintenance of vasoconstriction is dependent on a cold skin (Hayward *et al.*, 1984a) and the perception of warmth by the skin results in a reduction of the heat conservation mechanism (Kaufman, 1983). This is the situation if people are warmed by an outdoor fire or warmed blankets. In both there is perceived warmth but not much actual heat. In body-to-body warming the actual skin temperature of the rescuer is low but is enough to provide perceived warmth (Kaufman, 1983). It is interesting that the total removal of peripheral cold stress results in the same increase in hand blood flow as does cervical sympathectomy (Grayson and Kuehn, 1979).

5 DEFINITIONS AND CLASSIFICATION

HYPOTHERMIA could be defined as 'the clinical state of subnormal body temperature' (Benazon, 1974). However 'normal temperature' and 'body temperature' are not precise terms since *normal* temperature in man has a diurnal variation of 1 to 2 °C. In addition skin temperature, even in protected locations such as the axilla, is almost always different from the temperature at deeper body locations. This led Bergman in 1845 (Aschoff and Wever, 1958) to propose that the body could be divided into a homiothermic core and a poikilothermic shell, a concept later elaborated and refined (Aschoff and Wever, 1958). The body core consists of the deeper tissues of the body, and within the core are to be found all the vital organs, e.g. heart and brain, and, since human cells appear to function most efficiently at the normal body temperature, the body tries to keep the temperature of the vital organs as stable as possible and succeeds over a surprising range of environmental thermal stresses. The shell is composed of the superficial tissues and the size and temperature of the shell may vary considerably according to the external environment, the degree of protection and the activity of the individual, but, in extremis, the tissues in the shell are thermally expendable. There is, however, a great deal of argument as to the respective proportions of core and shell. It has been suggested that the shell is limited to 1.6 mm depth from the skin surface, i.e. about 10 per cent of the body mass, with the rest being core (Danzl, 1983). On the other hand it has been calculated that in a man resting at 21 °C environmental temperature, more than 50 per cent of the body tissue will be at a temperature lower than that of the core (Burton and Edholm, 1955). In the hypothermia environment the ambient temperature will be much lower than 21 °C and therefore the proportion of tissue at a temperature lower than the core is likely to be much greater than 50 per cent, especially if the person is not shivering. Shivering and activity require circulation to the muscles and this therefore raises the temperature of a proportion of the muscle bulk to that of the core and increases the effective size of the core. Despite the complexities and disagreements, the basic concept is of practical value for understanding thermal physiology.

A more precise definition of significant hypothermia therefore is 'that condition of a temperature regulating animal when the core temperature is more than one standard deviation below the mean core temperature of the species in resting conditions in a thermoneutral environment' (Bligh and Johnson, 1973). However, for practical purposes in man, it has now been agreed that a person is considered to be in a state of hypothermia if the core temperature is below 35 °C (Holdcroft, 1981; Maclean and Emslie-Smith, 1977; RCP, 1966). The lower the core temperature the greater the danger for the person but the definition of hypothermia, using only the measurement of the core temperature, may mislead people into a false sense of security. When the core temperature is above 35 °C but below 37 °C the person cannot be diagnosed as suffering from hypothermia but is obviously being affected by the cold, i.e. is suffering some degree of COLD STRESS. The term 'cold stress' can also be applied to any degree of environmental cold which causes the physiological thermoregulatory mechanisms to be activated. The significance of cold stress lies not in any absolute measurements but on the effects produced on the body.

A related concept is that of THERMAL COMFORT, which could be defined as being the environmental situation in which there is neither heat nor cold stress. The problem is that what is comfortable for one individual is uncomfortable for another, and this is affected by many factors, e.g. size, age, activity and degree of adiposity. This variation causes many problems for doctors, architects and engineers (Bedford, 1946; Edholm and Lobstein, 1981; Fanger, 1970).

The effect of cold exposure can therefore be divided into grades of severity:

(1) Mild cold stress — core temperature normal with normal total body heat.
(2) Moderate cold stress — core temperature normal but with reduced total body heat.
(3) Severe cold stress — core temperature < normal to 35 °C.
(4) Mild hypothermia — core temperature < 35 to 32 °C.
(5) Moderate hypothermia — core temperature < 32 to 28 °C.
(6) Severe hypothermia — core temperature < 28 °C.

This division is based on the observations that at a core temperature below 32 °C disturbances of cardiac conduction become more common and below 28 °C the risk of ventricular fibrillation rises more rapidly.

Hypothermia, even as defined above, is not a diagnosis in itself but merely a symptom and even the addition of a gradation of degrees of severity is not sufficient since a person with a core temperature of 29.5 °C who is shivering vigorously (Golden, 1979) is in a far less parlous state than someone not shivering even though his core temperature is 32 °C. There are in fact different types of hypothermia. The body temperature is sometimes lowered deliberately as part of a therapeutic regime (INDUCED HYPOTHERMIA) but hypothermia may also occur without deliberate intention (ACCIDENTAL HYPOTHERMIA) and there are many subtypes of accidental hypothermia (Foray and Salon, 1985; Golden, 1983; Lloyd, 1979a). It is useful to differentiate between PRIMARY ACCIDENTAL HYPOTHERMIA, in which the body possesses normal thermoregulation but the exposure to cold is overwhelming, and SECONDARY ACCIDENTAL HYPOTHERMIA in which mild to moderate cold exposure leads to hypothermia because of abnormal thermogenesis (Golden, 1983). This division will be of great value in the assessment of the cause of any particular incident so that where possible appropriate measures may be taken to prevent a recurrence. The causes of secondary hypothermia can be subdivided in a number of different ways (Fitzgerald and Jessop, 1982; Golden, 1983), but whichever divisions are used, there will be an overlap in any individual case, and it is probably safer to consider that a number of diseases and drugs may precipitate hypothermia (Braun, 1982; Holdcroft, 1981; Maclean and Emslie-Smith, 1977). Injury may also precipitate hypothermia (Sefrin, 1982) and hypothermia is a common problem in patients who are critically ill from any cause (Chernow *et al.*, 1983). Another classification is by the rate of cooling, though a simple division into rapid and slow on the basis of an arbitrary figure, e.g. six hours (Golden, 1973a), does not match the physiological changes. There is another possible classification (Lloyd, 1979a):

(1) Very rapid or 'Immersion' hypothermia, where the cold stress is so great that the body's resistance is overwhelmed and the core temperature is forced down despite the heat production of the body being at or near the maximum possible. Hypothermia therefore occurs before the body becomes exhausted. The commonest cause of this type is falling into cold water but deep diving (below 150 metres) with the use of oxyhelium gas mixtures may also cause immersion hypothermia because of the tremendous respiratory heat loss which occurs under these conditions and the heat transfer capacity of the compressed gas.

(2) Intermediate or 'Exhaustion' hypothermia, where the critical

factor is depletion of the body's food (fuel) stores and the core temperature falls because the supply of heat has failed. The cold exposure is such that the body's heat production has been able to maintain the body temperature as long as sufficient energy sources were available in the body. This is the type most commonly found in mountaineers or hill walkers (Andrew and Parker, 1978; McInnes, 1979).

(3) Slow or 'Subclinical chronic' hypothermia, where there has been a prolonged exposure to cold of a mild degree and, while the cold has not overwhelmed the heat production of the body, the thermogenesis has not been sufficient to completely counteract the cold. The core temperature has remained normal (35 °C or above) possibly for days, weeks or even months but it may eventually drift into the hypothermic range, or frank hypothermia may be precipitated by some other factor such as a fall. This is the most usual type found in the elderly or in association with malnutrition.

(4) 'Chronic' hypothermia, where the core temperature remains below normal for long periods, sometimes even in summer. There are a number of possible causes, all with some physiological abnormality (Maclean and Emslie-Smith, 1977).

(5) 'Intermittent' hypothermia, where episodes of hypothermia recur at intervals. The problems seems to be that though the temperature-controlling mechanisms seem to function normally the central thermostat has an abnormally low set-point. This abnormality lasts for from a few minutes to several hours or days before the thermostat setting returns to normal (Maclean and Emslie-Smith, 1977).

Of these (4) and (5) fall into the category of secondary hypothermia (Golden, 1983). Types (1), (2) and (3) are the groups most likely to be encountered by the emergency services and it is important to differentiate between them because the physiological changes are different and therefore not only may the clinical management vary but interpretation of experimental work must consider the method of inducing hypothermia. In 'immersion' hypothermia the heat-generating capacity of the body remains unimpaired and therefore the person will have very little difficulty in rewarming once he has been removed from the environment in which the severe rate of heat loss is occurring. In 'exhaustion' hypothermia, on the other hand, the capacity of the body to generate heat is reduced through exhaustion, and even a relatively mild degree of cold exposure may be sufficient to cause continued cooling. Thermal protection must therefore consider every avenue of heat loss however small the absolute quantities, and even small quantities of additional heat supplied, if safe, may make the difference between life and death. The important factor in the 'subclinical chronic' hypothermia is the fact that during cooling there is a complex movement of the fluids in the body (Hamlet, 1983; Harnett *et al.*, 1983a; Maclean and Emslie-Smith, 1977) (see below).

The different types can only be distinguished by the case history. For example a climber in a snowstorm disabled by a broken leg will probably cool as rapidly as if immersed, because the shock of the injury will increase the rate of heat loss (Sefrin, 1982), and the secondary factor of the fracture will prevent the person generating heat to his full capacity and may therefore prevent exhaustion. Similary a diver may suffer 'immersion' hypothermia even in a dry pressure chamber. On the other hand, a swimmer lost overboard in relatively warm water is a candidate for 'exhaustion' hypothermia (Beckman and Reeves, 1966). A middle-aged man or a child with severe malnutrition is likely to develop 'subclinical chronic' hypothermia (Sadikali and Owor, 1974; Maclean and Emslie-Smith, 1977) whereas a fit 70-year-old out walking in the hills probably has 'exhaustion' hypothermia.

Fluid Shifts

When man is exposed to cold there is a constriction of the peripheral blood vessels and, because the peripheral veins normally contain a considerable volume of blood, the vasoconstriction results in a shunting of this blood into the deep capacitance vessels (Hayward, 1983). This results in an increased circulating volume in relation to the available vascular bed, and an increased arterial pressure, and, to remove the relative excess of volume, the body responds with a diuresis (Burton and Edholm, 1955; Collis *et al.*, 1977; Danzl, 1983; Hamlet, 1983; Hayward, 1983; Hervey, 1973; Keatinge, 1969). This cold-induced diuresis results from a failure of tubular reabsorption of sodium (Rogers, 1971) and/or water (Coniam, 1979; Danzl, 1983; Hamlet, 1983) and occurs in spite of diminished glomerular filtration and renal blood flow (Tansey, 1973). It may act through the inhibition of Anti-diuretic Hormone (ADH) (Danzl, 1983), though the changes in renal function tend to be masked by circulatory changes (Kanter, 1962; Moyer *et al.*, 1956). Nevertheless the net result of the diuresis is that there is a contraction of the extracellular fluid volume though it remains isotonic (Rogers, 1971). The most obvious aspect of the fluid loss is a severe weight loss experienced by people exposed to cold over prolonged periods (Rogers, 1971).

There are other complicating factors. Moisture is also lost through respiration (Burton and Edholm, 1955; Collis *et al.*, 1977; Hamlet, 1983; Keatinge, 1969; Maclean and Emslie-Smith, 1977) and the volume lost is increased by exercise or work (Hamlet, 1983) and by breathing cold dry air (Hamlet, 1983) as occurs in the polar regions and at high altitude. Vigorous exercise in the cold can also produce a marked fluid loss through sweating (Budd, 1984; Hamlet, 1983) and, because the air is dry, evaporation is rapid and the person may not notice the amount of sweating, even though it may amount to 1 to 2 litres/day (Hamlet, 1983), and the total fluid loss working in the cold may amount to 0.74 to 3.4 per cent of the total body mass in one day (Budd, 1984). Exercise also causes an increase in the intravascular fluid volume despite a decrease in fluid intake and this effect still occurs even in the presence of total body dehydration (Tappan *et al.*, 1984), and any increase in intravascular volume is liable to increase the diuresis. It is therefore not surprising that dehydration is a common problem in mountain patients (MacInnes, 1979; Mills, 1983a). As a final problem, cold itself has a tendency to depress the sensation of thirst (Hamlet, 1983), and there may also be problems with the availability of water in the mountains. In winter or in high mountains the only source of water may be by the laborious means of melting snow. The depression of thirst could be a factor in the low fluid intake found in the elderly (Hamlet, 1983).

Alcohol is a dangerous fluid in the cold because, in addition to its other effects, it causes a diuresis (Hamlet, 1983) even without cold stress. Immersion also seems to have a diuretic effect (Greenleaf *et al.*, 1981) and people in water are aware of this because of the need to urinate (Lehrmann, 1982; Low, 1982). Whether this is due to haemodilution (Greenleaf *et al.*, 1981) or is a result of the hydrostatic squeeze, prolonged immersion results in a person becoming dehydrated (Low, 1982).

As patients and animals are cooled to low temperatures the blood volume decreases to 60 per cent of normal volume after six to eight hours at a body temperature of 15 °C (Popovic and Popovic, 1974). This decrease in blood volume is accompanied by an associated concentration of the blood (Burton and Edholm, 1955; Hervey, 1973; Keatinge, 1969; Popovic and Popovic, 1974) resulting in haematocrits approaching 60 per cent (Hervey, 1973; Roberts *et al.*, 1985) and the blood viscosity increases 2 per cent for each 1 °C decrease in temperature (Hedley-Whyte *et al.*, 1976). The haemoconcentration may be due to shifts of fluid (Barbour *et al.*, 1943) as a result of increased cellular activity in the cold producing osmotically active metabolic end products that require the movement of water into the cells, but the mechanism of the haemoconcentration has not yet been clarified (Popovic and Popovic, 1974). It may be partly related to the fact that, on normal exposure to cold, plasma is sequestered in the periphery (Hamlet, 1983; Roberts *et al.*, 1985) with a decrease in local haematocrit (Schmid-Schonbein and Neumann, 1985), while the cells are retained in the active vascular bed. The severity of these fluid shifts is directly related to the duration of cold exposure and therefore to the rate of onset of hypothermia (Burton and Edholm, 1955; Keatinge, 1969; Tansey, 1973).

During rewarming the circulating blood volume increases and this increase in volume may be up to 130 per cent of the value prior to cooling (Popovic and Popovic, 1974). This increase in volume is probably due to a reversal of the fluid shifts which occurred during cooling (BMJ, 1978b; Burton and Edholm, 1955; Linton and Ledingham, 1966) and therefore the potential volume of fluid available to return to the circulation during rewarming will depend on the duration of cooling. The clinical implication of this is that in cases of prolonged hypothermia if the rewarming is too rapid the volume of fluid returning to the circulation may cause an overload and result in cerebral and/or pulmonary oedema (Bloch, 1965; Lloyd, 1973).

6 HYPOTHERMIA

Symptoms and Signs

One of the earliest signs of hypothermia is a change in personality and a person may become unco-operative and may develop inco-ordination (Danzl, 1983). A variety of signs and symptoms have been described (Harnett *et al.*, 1983a; Pugh, 1964, 1966) (Table 6.1) in an attempt to give a clinical guide to the level of hypothermia, but these can only be a very general guide since individuals show a great range of responses, e.g. loss of consciousness may occur as high as 33 °C (Holdcroft, 1981) or as low as 27 °C (Cooper *et al.*, 1964b). A person may even be conscious though confused down to a temperature of 26 °C (Paton, 1983b), and in one case consciousness was still present at a rectal temperature of 24.3 °C (Lloyd, 1972) though this patient was confused. It is, however, probably true that if a person is unconscious with a core temperature above 33 °C, then hypothermia is unlikely to be the cause (Paton, 1983b).

Similarly shivering is considered to cease at 30 °C (Pozos and Wittmers, 1983) but a 14-year-old boy was shivering with a core temperature below 29 °C (Golden, 1979). In another case a misdiagnosis was made because since the victim was shivering his temperture was not taken at first but was then found to be 30 °C (Karhunen and Cazanitis, 1983), and shivering has even been recorded at a core temperature of 24 °C (Alexander, 1945). At the other extreme some experimental subjects can cool without shivering, many mountain rescue cases never shiver (Jones in Marcus, 1979a) and one immersion victim did not start shivering till the core temperature reached 37 °C (Theilade, 1977).

Despite the fact that hypothermia protects the brain from the effects of anoxia (Carlsson *et al.*, 1976), in clinical practice survival in hypothermia is almost totally dependent on having sufficient cardiac function and output to maintain a high enough blood pressure to give adequate perfusion of the heart and brain and therefore cardiac function has more relevance to ultimate survival than brain temperature.

Table 6.1: Signs and Symptoms at Different Levels of Hypothermia

°C		
37.6	'Normal' rectal temperature	
37	'Normal' oral temperature	
36	Increased metabolic rate in attempt to balance heat loss	
35	Shivering maximum at this temperature. Hyperreflexia, dysarthria, delayed cerebration	
34	Patients usually responsive and with normal blood pressure, lower limit compatible with continued exercise	
33	Retrograde amnesia	Pupils dilated. Most shivering ceases.
32	Consciousness clouded	
31	Blood pressure difficult to obtain	
30 29 28	Progressive loss of consciousness Increased muscular rigidity Slow pulse and respiration Cardiac arrhythmia develops Ventricular fibrillation may develop if heart irritated	
27	Voluntary motion lost along with pupillary light reflex, deep tendon and skin reflexes Appear dead	
26	Victims seldom conscious	
25	Ventricular fibrillation may appear spontaneously	
24 23 22 21	Pulmonary oedema develops. 100% mortality in shipwreck victims in Second World War (Molnar, 1946)	
20	Heart standstill	
18	Lowest *accidental* hypothermic patient with recovery (Laufmann, 1951)	
17	ISO-ELECTRIC EEG	
9	Lowest artificially cooled hypothermic patient with recovery (Niazi and Lewis, 1958)	
4	Monkeys revived successfully (Niazi and Lewis, 1957)	
1 to −7	Rats and hamsters revived successfully (Smith, 1959)	

Source: Adapted from Harnett *et al.* (1983a)

Death and Revival

Profound accidental hypothermia may show a clinical picture very difficult to distinguish from death:

(1) Skin is ice-cold.
(2) Body core temperature is low.
(3) Muscles and joints are still and simulate rigor mortis.
(4) Respiration is difficult to register.
(5) The peripheral pulse is impossible to feel and the blood pressure is impossible to measure.
(6) Pupils are without reaction to light stimulus.
(7) Other reflexes are absent.
(8) Heart sounds are inaudible.
(9) ECG shows a slow rhythm with broad complexes, multifocal ventricular extrasystoles and atrial flutter, a pattern easily misinterpreted as electrical artefacts (Jessen and Hagelsten, 1978).

Even when there has been definitive evidence of total cessation of cardiorespiratory activity (Kugler-Podelleck *et al.*, 1965; Niazi and Lewis, 1958; Siebke *et al.*, 1975) the victim can survive. Nor is a flat EEG a certain indicator of death in hypothermia. It is now generally agreed that the only certain diagnosis of death in hypothermia is failure to recover on rewarming (Danzl, 1983; Frankland, 1975; Freeman and Pugh, 1969; Golden, 1973a; Hillman, 1971; Leathart, 1971; Lilja, 1983; Welton *et al.*, 1978; Zingg, 1966). This point has become so well recognised that an official circular (NHS, 1974) has stated that before brain death can be diagnosed the doctor must check that the core temperature is normal (Item, 1976b). Unfortunately brain death may itself be the cause of the hypothermia even in the Tropics (Johnson, 1983). One final problem in diagnosing death is the fact that even after death the body does not cool by Newtonian Laws (Kuehn *et al.*, 1980).

Diagnosis

In cases of hypothermia where life is still present the diagnosis of other conditions is difficult because the features of hypothermia mask the clinical features of other disorders (Ledingham and Mone, 1980; Maclean and Emslie-Smith, 1977). Gastrointestinal motility slows and may cease during cooling (Paton, 1983b) and as a result gastric dilatation and decreased or absent bowel sounds are common in hypothermia (Danzl, 1983). Figure 6.1 is the X-ray of the silent abdomen of an 86-year-old patient who was conscious but disorientated and had a totally irregular ECG with multifocal ventricular and

Figure 6.1: Plain X-ray of a Silent Abdomen in a Patient with a Core Temperature of 24.3 °C Showing Gaseous Distension, Mainly Gastric

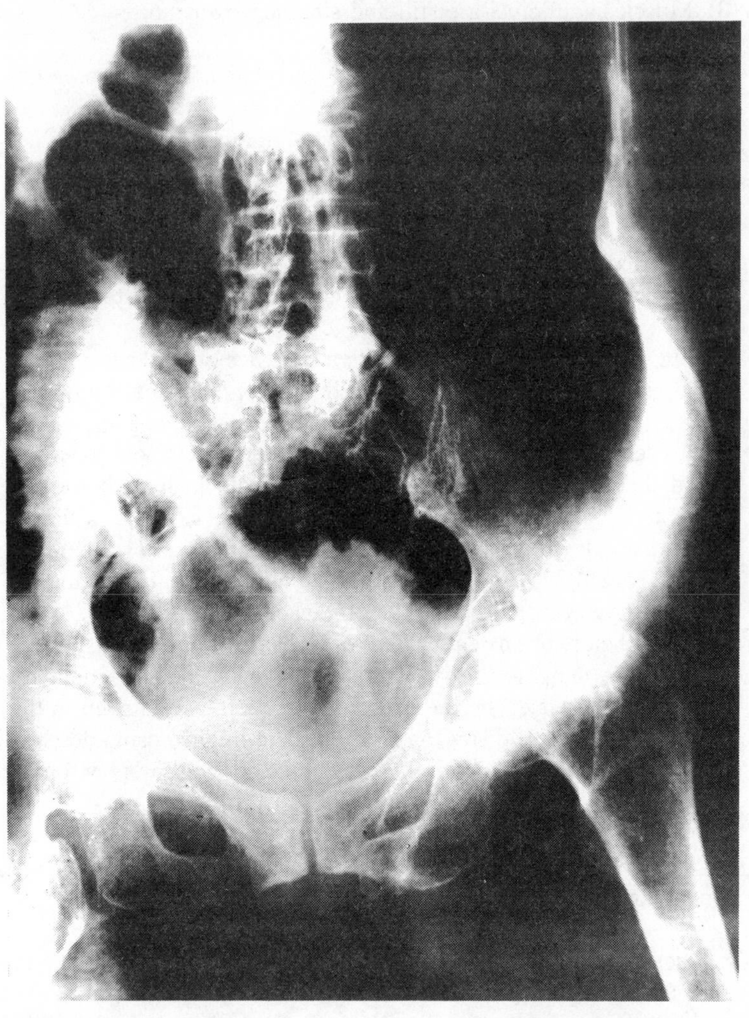

supraventricular extrasystoles, and a broken ankle (Lloyd, 1972). Initial diagnosis was of some cardiac or abdominal catastrophe in a senile patient. However, when her core temperature was raised from its initial 24.3 °C, conscious level returned to normal as also did the ECG, and the gaseous distension (mainly gastric) disappeared and bowel sounds returned, leaving only the fracture.

Figure 6.2: X-ray Chest on Admission Showing Pneumonic Changes at a Core Temperature of 32.5 °C

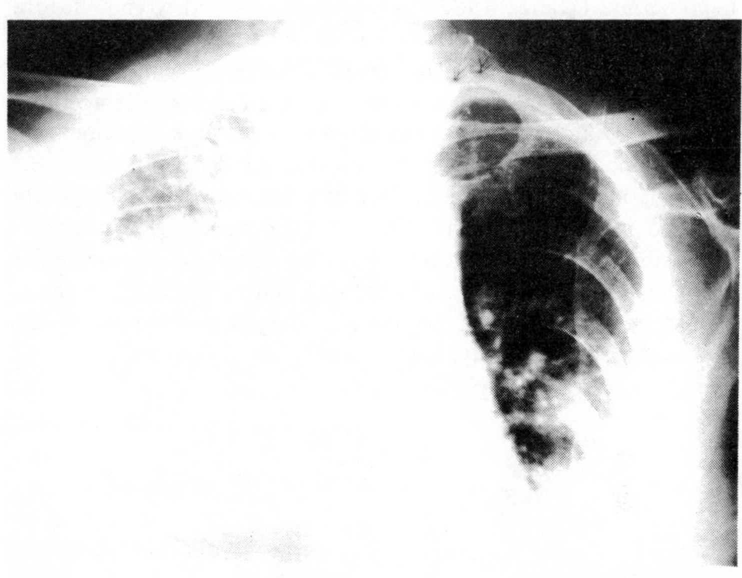

Figure 6.3: X-ray Chest of Same Patient as Figure 6.2 Showing Marked Improvement on Reaching Normothermia After 24 Hours' Airway Warming Treatment

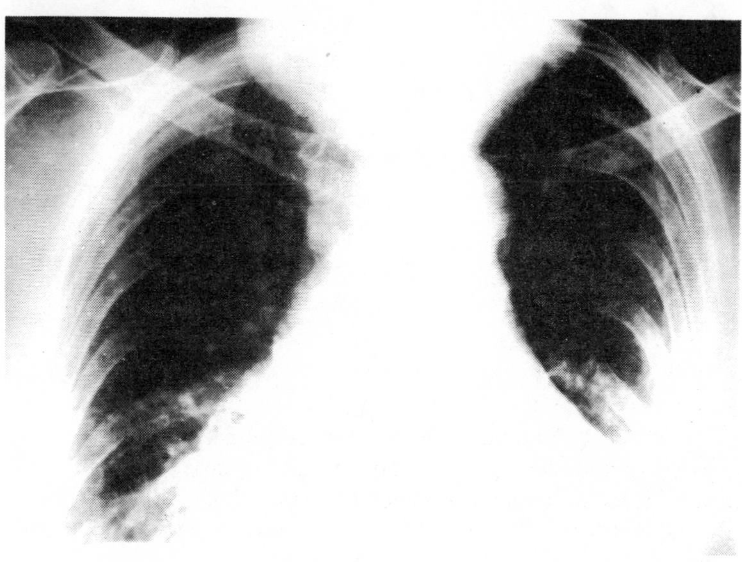

Slurred speech and ataxia may be diagnosed as being the result of a cerebrovascular accident (CVA) whereas the true cause may be hypothermia (Danzl, 1983). Another 75-year-old woman seen in hospital (Lloyd, 1972) was unconscious, cyanosed, with an unrecordable blood pressure and an X-ray as in Figure 6.2 with a suspected diagnosis of CVA and pneumonia. However, the core temperature was 32.5 °C and, on rewarming, the patient became conscious with normal blood pressure and a much improved X-ray (Figure 6.3).

In hypothermia the reflexes are affected and there is a general increase in rigidity which makes accurate neurological diagnosis impossible, and the alterations in cardiac conduction cause similar problems for cardiologists. It is therefore important that the patient should be normothermic before any diagnosis is made or any irrevocable method of treatment started.

7 THE CAUSE OF DEATH AFTER RESCUE

Introduction

Sixteen people fell into the water off Greenland. The rescue ship reached them quickly and all 16 were capable of climbing on to the rescue ship. Once on board they were given hot drinks and wrapped in warm covers, and they all died (case report, Hervey in Marcus, 1979a).

This is fairly typical of the problem faced by rescuers and causes a lot of frustration to the rescue teams who feel helpless and cannot understand the reason.

During the Dachau experiments the Nazis noticed that after the person had been removed from the cold water the core temperature continued to drop for a while before starting to rise again (Alexander, 1945; Burton and Edholm, 1955) and they called this phenomenon the 'after-drop'. Because many of the deaths which occur after a person has been removed from the cold stress situation happen shortly after rescue, and the time of post-immersion collapse happened to coincide with the time the rectal temperature is at its lowest (Golden, 1983), it has been assumed that death and the after-drop are connected and the traditional explanation is that death is due to ventricular fibrillation precipitated by the continued cooling of the heart (Alexander, 1945; Burton and Edholm, 1955; Collis *et al.*, 1977; Freeman and Pugh, 1969; Golden, 1974; Hirvonen, 1979; Keatinge, 1969; *Lancet*, 1972a; Lloyd, 1973; Maclean and Emslie-Smith, 1977; Mountain Rescue, 1968; Mountain Rescue and Cave Rescue, 1972). However, one ECG obtained during rewarming showed that the heart stopped in asystole (Mills, 1983a). Because of these assumptions, the danger of the after-drop has been so emphasised that it has now almost reached the state of a mythical ogre, so much so that any explanation of death occurring after rescue had to invoke the after-drop, e.g. slow rewarming is dangerous because it allows the person to shiver which will aggravate the after-drop and therefore cause death (Lloyd, 1964). There are some aspects which deserve to be looked at in more detail before the true significance can be assessed:

(1) The phenomenon of the after-drop.
(2) The mechanism for the precipitation of ventricular fibrillation.
(3) The contribution of the after-drop to the post-rescue deaths.
(4) Other possible causes.

(1) The 'After-drop'

When a variety of core temperatures were measured while cooling pigs (Golden, 1979; Golden in Marcus, 1979a) there was a variation in the after-drop at the different sites with a large drop at the rectal level but a negligible drop in the central venous blood. Indeed, the temperature of the central venous blood was rising at a time when the rectal temperature was still falling. This phenomenon was also noted in a human subject (Hayward *et al.*, 1984a). When the circulation was arrested during cooling the changes in core temperature which then occurred supported the view that the after-drop is only obvious in those sites where conductive heat transfer is primarily responsible for changes in temperature (Golden and Hervey, 1977, 1981), i.e. the temperature changes can be explained by the normal physics of heat transfer (Golden and Hervey, 1977, 1981; Kaufman, 1983; Savard *et al.*, 1984). The generally accepted belief that the after-drop is caused by cold blood returning to the core from the cooler peripheral circulation (Alexander, 1945; Burton and Edholm, 1955; Collis *et al.*, 1977; Lilja, 1983; Maclean and Emslie-Smith, 1977) can no longer be supported since there was no evidence of any cold bolus in the central venous circulation though an after-drop was being recorded in the rectum (Golden, 1979; Hayward *et al.*, 1984a) and experimentally, even during rewarming in a hot bath, the cardiac temperature had returned to normal while the rectal temperature was still completing the after-drop (Hayward *et al.*, 1984a). On theoretical grounds this absence of a cold bolus should not be surprising since in hypothermia the peripheral circulation is reduced to an absolute minimum with the blood being sequestered in the central capacitance vessels and there is therefore insufficient blood volume in the periphery to produce a bolus (Paton, 1983b). An additional piece of evidence is that in young volunteers being rewarmed by surface heat (radiant or hot bath) there was no increase in the limb and extremity blood flow during the after-drop (Cooper and Ferguson, 1983; Savard *et al.*, 1984). Research using mechanical and mathematical models confirmed the fact that most of the

Figure 7.1: Temperature Gradients in Sheep During Cooling and Spontaneous Rewarming

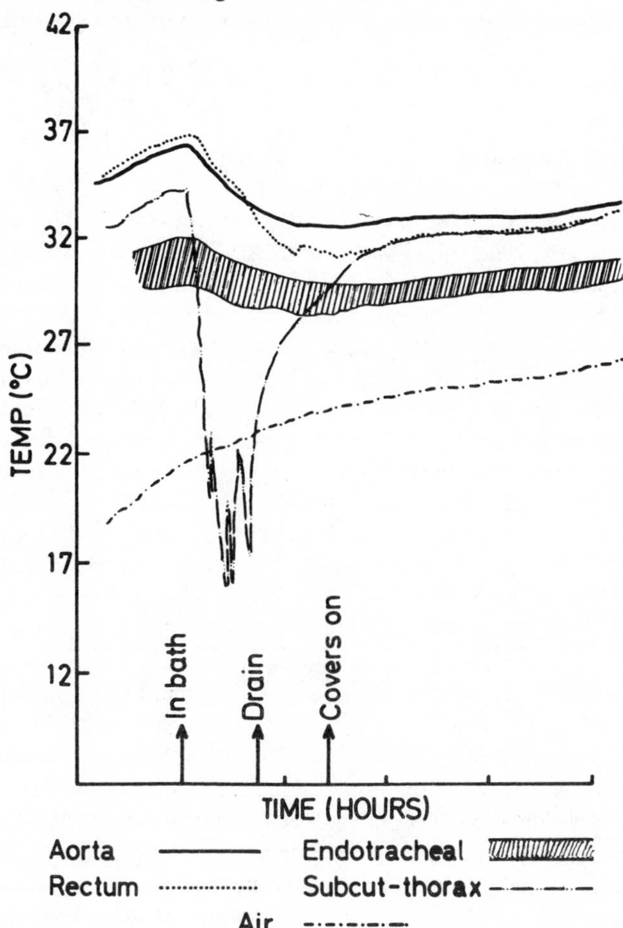

temperature curves seen during cooling and rewarming can be observed without the necessity for circulation (Golden and Hervey, 1981; Golden *et al.*, 1977; Hervey in Marcus, 1979a). These models have been criticised as being too simplistic (Harnett *et al.*, 1983a) and it is suggested that much more complex models are required to take into account the inter-tissue variation and the effect of circulation.

The absence of circulation means that not only do the temperature changes occur more slowly but in the pigs in which the circulation was stopped the central venous temperature drop stopped at once whereas

Figure 7.2: Temperature Gradients in Sheep During Cooling and Treatment with Airway Warming

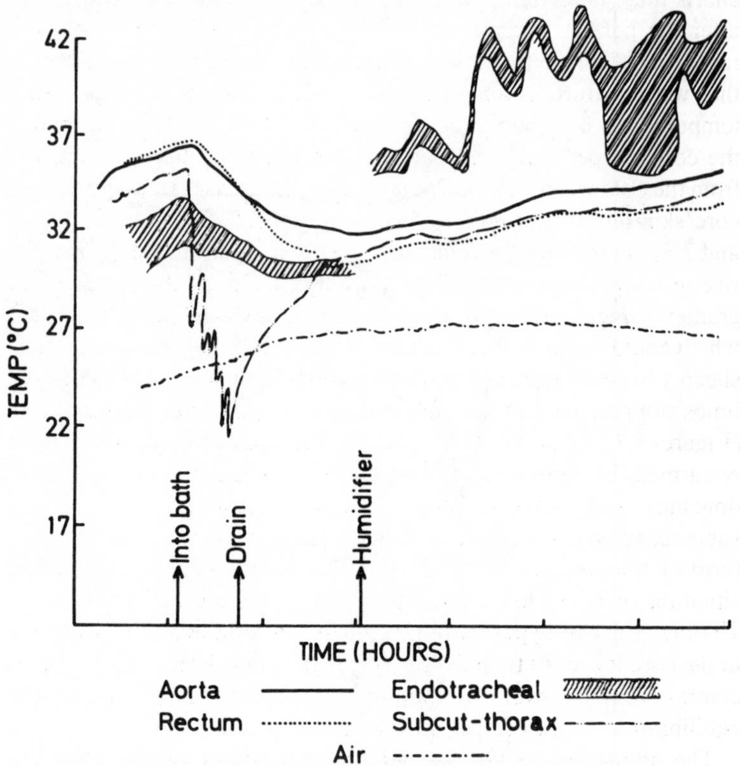

Note the intra-tracheal tracings show the temperature during inspiration at the lower part of the hatched zone with the temperature during expiration at the upper part. During use of the humidifier in airway warming the positions are reversed, the inspired temperature being higher than the expired.

with the live pigs there was a slight after-drop of the central venous temperature. Similar changes were noticed in sheep being cooled by immersion (Figures 7.1 and 7.2) where the aortic and rectal temperatures were cooling at the same rate until the cold water was drained after which the rectal temperature continued to drop whereas the drop in the aortic temperature slowed and levelled off higher and sooner than the rectal (Lloyd *et al.*, 1976a). In fact if the rate of heat production is high enough to balance the heat flow from the core to the shell, there is no after-drop (Golden and Hervey, 1981; Hayward *et al.*, 1984a; Savard *et al.*, 1984).

There is another aspect of the after-drop for which an intact circulation may be necessary. In the original Dachau temperature charts there is certainly a continued drop in rectal core temperature after the person is removed from the water but unfortunately the recording of skin temperatures ceased at the moment of removal from the water (Burton and Edholm, 1955). However, when skin temperatures continue to be recorded (Lloyd *et al.*, 1976a), though the core temperature continues to drop after the sheep is removed from the cold water, the skin temperature in fact rises until the normal core/skin temperature difference is re-established (Figures 7.1, 7.2 and 7.3). Thereafter the after-drop in core temperature stops and the rise in temperature starts. The re-establishment of the temperature gradients might just be the redistribution of the same total body heat which could occur without a circulation but during the cooling of the sheep whenever agitation of the water and douching of the exposed limbs stopped the skin and subcutaneous temperatures started to rise (Figures 7.1, 7.2 and 7.3). Similarly in the group of sheep which were rewarmed by immersion in hot water (Figure 7.3), whenever douching and agitation of the hot water stopped the skin and subcutaneous temperatures, which had been higher than the core (aortic) temperature, dropped till they reached the more normal situation of being lower than the core temperature (Lloyd *et al.*, 1976a). Since in hypothermia the main heat production is occurring in the core it is easy to understand why the after-drop at the aortic or central venous level is minimal and ceases even before the equilibration of the temperature gradients is complete.

The after-drop so far discussed is that which occurs when the person is left undisturbed. However, one of the worries associated with the use of any particular treatment is that it may aggravate the after-drop. One of the advantages claimed for the hot bath treatment is that it reduces the magnitude of the after-drop (Burton and Edholm, 1955; Keatinge, 1969; Light *et al.*, 1983). This claim originated from the Dauchau experiments (Alexander, 1945) though these only concerned immersion hypothermia. An alternative view is that while rapid rewarming does not affect the magnitude of the after-drop it reduces its duration (Cooper and Ross, 1960; Freeman and Pugh, 1969). However, a mathematical model predicts that both duration and magnitude should be reduced (Golden and Hervey, 1981). These conclusions are based on the assumption that the core temperature remains uniform at all sites and this is manifestly not the case (Golden, 1979). In an experiment on himself Hayward found that

Figure 7.3: Temperature Gradients in Sheep During Cooling and Rewarming in a Hot Bath

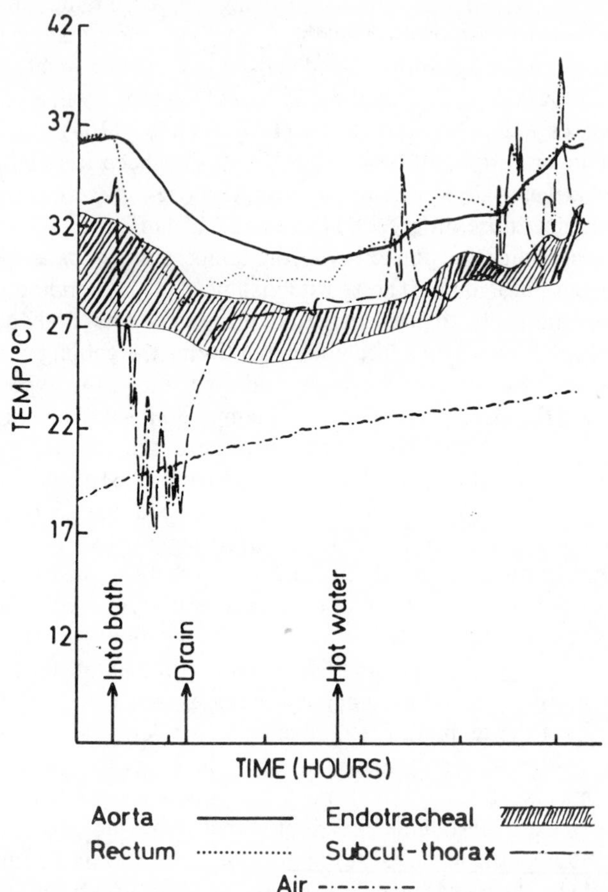

when he was rewarming spontaneously, the expected after-drop was recorded from the rectal probe whereas, as in Golden's work, the probe in the right pulmonary artery recorded a negligible after-drop. However, though rewarming in a hot bath reduced the magnitude and duration of the after-drop recorded from the rectal probe, the pulmonary artery probe recorded a definite though small after-drop (Hayward *et al.*, 1984a). This finding suggests that an intact circulation may add a contribution to any after-drop recorded in the central vascular system, the extent being determined by the level of heat supplied to the surface. The occurrence of this 'secondary after-drop' in the presence of an intact circulation is confirmed by Hong and Nadel (1979). Subjects were cooled while sitting at rest on a bicycle ergometer and when they were asked to pedal the exercise caused a redistribution of body heat and a drop in the core temperature as recorded in the oesophagus, the size of the drop being proportional to the intensity and magnitude of the exercise (Glaser and Holmes-Jones, 1951; Hong and Nadel, 1979). In one case, treatment was started half an hour after rescue using blankets plus hot-water bottles in the groin and axilla and there was a 1 °C drop in core temperature (Vaagenes and Holme, 1982) and since the body temperature gradients usually stabilise in 20 to 30 minutes, this drop was probably caused by the treatment and could therefore be a 'secondary after-drop'.

(2) The Mechanism for the Precipitation of Ventricular Fibrillation (VF)

Many theories have been advanced to explain the onset of VF but extensive studies have so far failed to define the precise mechanisms involved in the production of VF in hypothermia. In hypothermia induced for medical or surgical reasons, and in laboratory animals, drugs (Angelakos, 1959) or the choice of anaesthetic agent may either enhance or reduce the likelihood of VF (Wylie and Churchill-Davidson, 1966), but this factor is obviously not involved in cases of accidental hypothermia.

Alterations in the concentration of individual electrolytes have been noted (Beavers, 1959; Beavers and Covino, 1959; Beavers and Rogers, 1959; Buky, 1970; Elliott and Crismon, 1947; Fisher *et al.*, 1955; Platner and Hosko, 1953; Swan *et al.*, 1953; Taylor, 1956), and relative ionic imbalance (Cooper, 1961) has also been postulated as a cause of VF in hypothermia, but there is no general agreement as to the direction of the changes or their interpretation. Sudden changes of the hydrogen ion concentration in either direction, and sudden raising or lowering of the $PaCO_2$ have been know to precipitate VF (Cooper, 1961; Covino and Hegnauer, 1955; Good and McDonald, 1982; Keatinge, 1969; Malamos *et al.*, 1962; Osborn, 1953; Osborn *et al.*, 1961; Swan *et al.*, 1955).

Hypoxia of the myocardium has also been proposed as a precipitating cause (Bigelow *et al.*, 1950; Edwards *et al.*, 1954; Hegnauer *et al.*, 1951; Penrod, 1951) but, while initial experiments supported this hypothesis, later work suggested that in hypothermia the oxygen carried in the blood is sufficient for the reduced myocardial work (Fairley, 1961; Keatinge, 1969; Wylie and Churchill-Davidson, 1966). Sudden hypoxia as a consequence of the reduction in the level of inspired oxygen or increased demand (Keatinge, 1969) may, however, precipitate VF in the hypothermic heart.

The Role of Temperature

Information from the 1939–45 war and other reports suggested that the lethal lower limit for cardiac temperature was 23 to 25 °C (Keatinge, 1969; Molnar, 1946) but individual case reports have shown that the core temperature may be very low without VF occurring (Laufman, 1951; Lloyd, 1972; Niazi and Lewis, 1958). VF is not brought about by the direct effect of the cold on the cell membrane of the cardiac muscle (Hoff and Stansfield, 1949; Keatinge, 1969; Scherf *et al.*, 1953) and indeed the end result of hypothermia alone is often asystole (Keatinge, 1969; Niazi and Lewis, 1958; Paton, 1983b). A rapid infusion of cold blood is a known precipitating factor for the onset of VF (Wylie and Churchill-Davidson, 1966) and a high potassium content, an acid pH of the stored blood, or even citrate intoxication (Wylie and Churchill-Davidson, 1966) have been implicated. Since there is no evidence of there being sufficient blood in the periphery to produce a cold bolus to return to the heart, these three factors are unlikely to be the cause of VF during rewarming from accidental hypothermia. The effect of a fall in temperature on cardiac muscle, which possesses intrinsic potential for electrical activity (Brash, 1951), is to increase the refractory period and to slow conduction and thus hinder the development of fibrillation (Keatinge, 1969). Warming the muscle increases the risk of fibrillation (Keatinge, 1969).

Temperature Gradients

In dogs there is a normal temperature gradient across the myocardium, the epicardium being 0.5 to 1 °C lower than the intramyocardial temperature and therefore the normal T wave and the normal electrical ventricular gradient could depend on the temperature difference between the subendocardial ventricular layers which are surrounded by blood and the subepicardial solid portions of the myocardium (Lepeschkin, 1951). It was found that the larger the intramyocardial temperature gradient the higher the mean temperature at which VF occurred, and the onset of VF was not related to whether the right or left ventricular myocardium was the colder (Mouritzen and Andersen, 1965). At increasingly lower temperatures fibrillation tended to occur with progressively smaller gradients and below 20 °C fibrillation sometimes occurred with no measurable gradient. It was further noted that electrical fibrillation by a standardised technique was readily accomplished, even at very low temperatures if the intramyocardial temperature gradients were below 1 °C, but defibrillation was difficult or impossible with gradients over 2 °C (Mouritzen and Andersen, 1965). Intramyocardial temperature gradients occur routinely during the induction of hypothermia by the commonly used clinical or experimental methods (Bonnabeau *et al.*, 1963) and the hypothesis has been advanced (Lloyd and Mitchell, 1974) that VF supervenes when it becomes more efficient for intracardiac electrical conduction to occur through the muscle tissue rather than by the normal neuromuscular mechanism. In hypothermia, neuromuscular conduction is impaired and from the evidence it was suggested that selective cooling of the endocardium and subendocardial conducting system in relation to the myocardium increases the risk of VF and vice versa (Lloyd and Mitchell, 1974).

Clinical Evidence

The observation of the relation between the onset of VF and a rapid infusion of cold blood (Wylie and Churchill-Davidson, 1966) tends to support the hypothesis and further evidence may be found in case reports of treatment. Mediastinal irrigation with warm saline would warm the myocardium more than the subendocardial conducting tissue, and defibrillation was in one case not achieved until the mediastinal temperature reached 28 °C (Linton and Ledingham, 1966) and was difficult in another (Althaus *et al.*, 1982).

Other available methods of central rewarming would tend to return warmed blood to the heart and warm the endocardium more than the main mass of the cardiac muscle. In cases rewarmed by the heart/lung machine, cardiac rhythm has reverted spontaneously to sinus (Kugelberg *et al.*, 1967), or defibrillation has been readily achieved (Althaus *et al.*, 1982; Fell *et al.*, 1968; Kenyon, 1961). Similarly peritoneal dialysis has caused asystole to change to regular sinus rhythm at 27 °C (Jessen and Hagelsten, 1978), has allowed defibrillation and restoration of sinus rhythm at a rectal temperature of 21.1 °C (Lash *et al.*, 1967) and has been shown to improve the configuration of the ECG (Patton and Doolittle, 1972).

The stabilising effect of airway warming on myocardial rhythm

(Lloyd, 1973) must be through selective endocardial warming via the pulmonary venous blood (Lloyd *et al.*, 1976a; Shanks and Marsh, 1973), and it has resulted in the restoration of normal sinus rhythm at an oesophageal temperature below 27 °C (Lloyd, 1972). In rabbits cooled by heliox (rectal temperature 19.5 to 23.5 °C), a blast of hot (43 °C) humidified heliox (80 per cent helium, 20 per cent oxygen) occasionally produced VF (Beran and Sperling, 1979). However, this was a sudden surge from a ventilator through an endotracheal tube and suggests either that too rapid change even of endocardial temperature may be dangerous or that the VF was triggered by a nervous reflex provoked by the excess heat on a cold trachea. In dogs the addition of airway warming via an endotracheal tube to rewarming with water-circulating blankets caused occasional ventricular extrasystoles below 30 °C and these continued over several degrees, though there were no cases of VF (Roberts *et al.*, 1983). The fact that in a similar experiment with dogs cooled to a lower temperature, the heat remained in sinus rhythm throughout rewarming with airway warming or diathermy (White *et al.*, 1984) suggests that the extrasystoles may have been due to the combination of hot water rewarming plus airway warming.

The available evidence suggests therefore that during the development of or rewarming from hypothermia, any factor which alters the intracardiac gradient, so that the subendocardial and neuromuscular conducting system becomes significantly different from the main mass of cardiac muscle, increases the risk of VF. Sudden marked changes of ionic or blood gas status or temperature, by first affecting the subendocardial conducting system, may cause a temporary cessation of normal neuromuscular transmission and thus enhance transmission by the intramuscular route and increase the risk of VF. The hypothesis that for maximal cardiac benefit there should be a slight myocardial temperature gradient with the endocardium warmer, still appears valid.

One fact known from hypothermia induced for cardiac surgery (Wylie and Churchill-Davidson, 1966) is that mechanical irritation of the heart is liable to precipitate VF. The main argument used for not using external cardiac massage in accidental hypothermia is that the mechanical irritation may precipitate VF in a heart which was previously beating normally even though no pulses could be felt (Golden and Rivers, 1975; Mills, 1983a). The heart is not held rigidly in the mediastinum, and the mediastinum itself can move within the chest, and it is therefore likely that if a patient is being moved vigorously (Golden, 1973a; Lloyd, 1973), e.g. rolled while bed-making, handled roughly while being lifted on to a stretcher, or bounced during evacuation on foot or in a vehicle driving over rough ground, there may be sufficient movement of and trauma to the heart to provoke VF from mechanical irritation. This is a more likely explanation than that cold blood from the limbs cools the heart further and thus causes VF (Mountain Rescue, 1968).

(3) The Contribution of the After-drop to Post-rescue Deaths

It is true that the lower the cardiac temperature the greater the cardiac irritability and below the range 27 to 30 °C the risk of VF rises rapidly (Fell *et al.*, 1968; Sellick, 1963; Wylie and Churchill-Davidson, 1966). Therefore any after-drop of cardiac temperature will increase the irritability (Kaufman, 1983) and the risk of ventricular fibrillation but, as can be seen from the involved discussions above, there is very little evidence to support the idea that post-rescue deaths are due to ventricular fibrillation precipitated by the occurrence of the after-drop. Indeed, logic dictates that since cooling of the body and therefore the heart does not itself provoke ventricular fibrillation there is no reason why cooling of the heart through the same temperature range during the after-drop should alone provoke ventricular fibrillation. This is especially true when one considers that some of the post-rescue deaths occur at relatively high core temperatures whereas other patients survive from very low core temperatures. There is in fact no correlation between the depth of hypothermia and cardiac arrest (Lee and Ames, 1965). It could be suggested that a return of cold blood from the periphery might increase the irritability of the heart and therefore the risk of ventricular fibrillation by creating intra-myocardial temperature gradients with the endocardium cooler than the myocardium. However, there is no evidence that cold blood returns to the heart in a sufficient bolus (Golden, 1979; Hayward *et al.*, 1984a; Lloyd *et al.*, 1976a). Since disturbance of cardiac rhythm has been excluded as the major cause of post-rescue death it is necessary to consider if some other aspect of cardiac function is involved in the post-rescue cardiovascular collapse.

(4) Other Possible Causes

One suggestion to explain the collapse of people following rescue from the sea is a removal of the hydrostatic squeeze as the person is removed from the water (Golden, 1980). On transition from air to 'head-out immersion in thermoneutral (35 °C) water the pressure squeeze on the peripheral tissues of man increases the venous return and produces a rise in cardiac output of 35 per cent (Arborelius *et al.*, 1972; Begin *et al.*, 1976). On removal from the water this process is reversed and the sudden drop in venous return may be sufficient to cause a devastating drop in arterial pressure with unconsciousness and possible cardiac arrest (Golden, 1980) especially since baro-receptor responses are impaired in hypothermia (Kaul *et al.*, 1973). If the person is being lifted vertically, gravitational effects could further impair venous return, and the use of a lifting loop round the trunk, as used by helicopters, could cause further obstructive problems (Golden and Hervey, 1981). However, the strap may not be as dangerous as expected since it may prevent hypotension by a Valsalva manoeuvre type of action (Merrifield in Marcus, 1979a). It has also been suggested that part of the success of the hot bath treatment is due to the early restoration of the hydrostatic squeeze (Golden, 1980). Unfortunately since a body lying in water tends to lie horizontally near the surface of the water and the position is similar in a hot bath the magnitude of the hydrostatic squeeze is relatively small (Golden, 1980) and may be too small to be important. Though removal of the hydrostatic squeeze might provide an explanation for deaths occurring while victims are being hauled out of the water, it cannot explain the similar cases of collapse and death which can occur following rescue on land.

In sheep (Figure 7.4) during spontaneous rewarming from hypothermia the blood pressure dropped despite a rise in cardiac

Key to Figure 7.4

B	Base line readings before cooling by immersion. Each sheep was considered to have a reading of zero, and changes are recorded as changes from the base line
SH	Stable hypothermia after removal from cold water and after the after-drop has occurred
I	Intermediate temperature during rewarming
N	Normothermia
●—·—·—●	Changes during cooling
x ------------ x	Changes during rewarming in a hot bath
□·············□	Changes during spontaneous rewarming
●————●	changes during airway warming

Standard errors are indicated.

Figure 7.4: Cardiovascular Changes During Cooling and Rewarming Sheep — a comparison of three methods

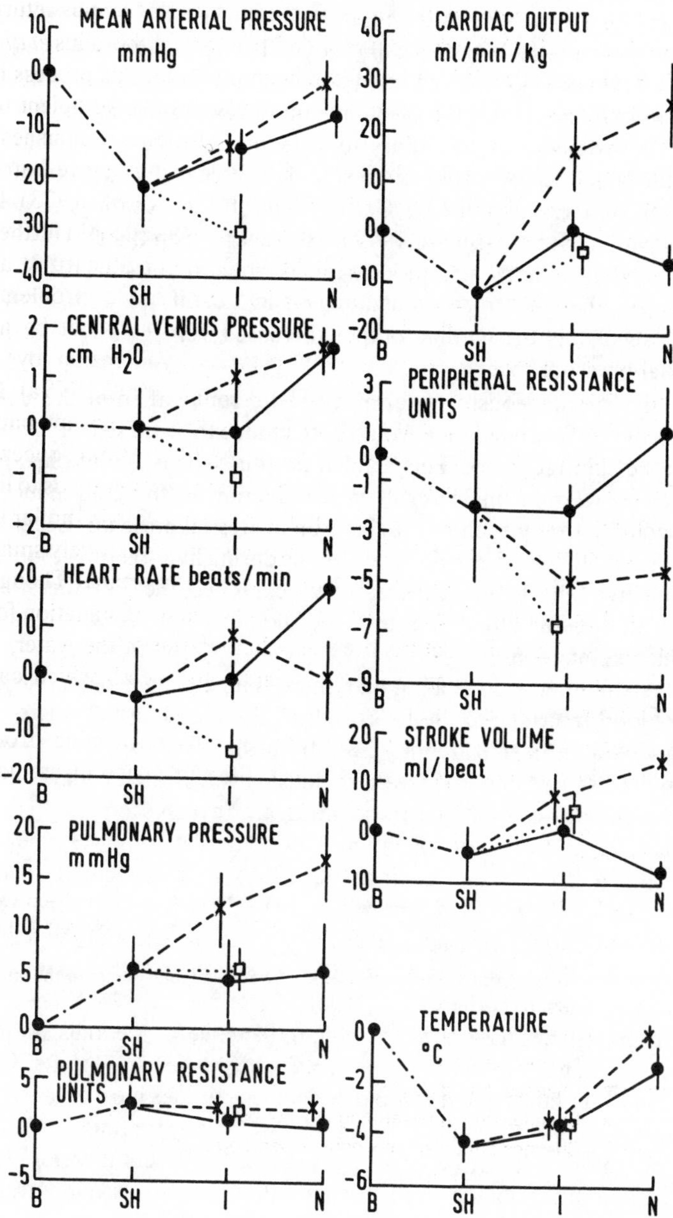

output (Lloyd *et al.*, 1976b). The cause was a drop in peripheral resistance which could not be compensated for by the small rise in cardiac output and the cold heart is unable to produce a sufficient compensatory increase in output (Paton, 1983a). Since the central venous pressure (CVP) also fell (Lloyd, 1986) the drop in arterial pressure was obviously due to hypovolaemia. This fits in with the current explanation for the phenomenon of rewarming collapse, i.e. that hypovolaemia is secondary to a decrease in the central blood volume which has occurred as a result of the cold-induced fluid shifts (Burton and Edholm, 1955; Collis *et al.*, 1977; Keatinge, 1969; Maclean and Emslie-Smith, 1977). However, when the sheep were immersed in a hot bath, though the peripheral resistance fell as expected, the CVP rose immediately and steadily (Lloyd, 1986). Because of this the cardiac output increased very greatly and the arterial pressure rose.

In the spontaneously rewarming group, removal from the cold water and surface insulation would both reduce the cold sensory input from the skin receptors. This sudden drop in sensory input plus the perceived warmth might result in a reduction in the cold-induced vasoconstrictor tone leading to the drop in arterial pressure. Because there is no blood in the peripheral vessels during hypothermia there is no fluid available to fill the increased vascular bed, the CVP therefore falls and then the blood pressure, and the other findings would also fit this explanation.

Even on immersion in a hot bath there is no evidence of a bolus of cold blood returning to the heart, but as discussed earlier, there is, during cooling, a shift in body fluid from the intravascular into the interstitial spaces and into the cells, causing generalised oedema and slight cellular oedema, and these shifts are reversed on rewarming (BMJ, 1978b; Burton and Edholm, 1955; Hamlet, 1983; Harnett *et al.*, 1983a; Linton and Ledingham, 1966; Maclean and Emslie-Smith, 1977; Popovic and Popovic, 1974). These fluid shifts must be considered during rewarming especially as the severity of the shifts which occur during cooling are directly related to the duration of cold exposure (Burton and Edholm, 1955; Keatinge, 1969). Since the superficial tissues have been exposed to the cold for the longest time during cooling they will have experienced the greatest fluid shifts. The surface heat of the hot bath would affect these tissues most and would therefore reverse the shifts very rapidly and this extra fluid could fill the increased vascular bed causing a rise in CVP, and therefore the cardiac output is able to rise sufficiently to produce a rise in arterial pressure despite the fall in peripheral resistance caused by the substitution of a warm stimulus for a cold one (Figure 7.4). The fact that in the hot bath the pulmonary arterial pressure remained higher than in the group warming spontaneously may indicate a slight degree of pulmonary fluid overload which could possibly be precipitated into pulmonary oedema by any cardiac inefficiency or extra fluid.

Hypothesis

Survival during rewarming from accidental hypothermia is dependent on a balance being achieved between the size of the vascular bed, controlled by the vasomotor tone, and the circulating blood volume which is partly dependent on the extent of the dehydration often found in hypothermia but is also affected by the extent and rate of reversal of the fluid shifts which have occurred during cooling. If the relaxation of the vasoconstrictor tone predominates death will occur through relative hypovolaemia whereas excessive reversal of the fluid shifts will cause cardiac failure and death from fluid overload. Dehydration can affect both.

Supporting Clinical Evidence

(a) There is a marked similarity between the cardiovascular changes observed in the spontaneously rewarming sheep (Lloyd, 1986) and the clinical observation that a bradycardia occurs during spontaneous rewarming (Burton and Edholm, 1955) and the fact that many patients admitted to hospital with a reasonable blood pressure develop a variable degree of hypotension after admission during a time they are beginning to rewarm spontaneously (Fell *et al.*, 1968; Lloyd, 1972, 1986; Pugh, 1967).

(b) It is well recognised that hypothermic casualties being brought off a mountain must not be carried in a 'head-up' position because of the danger of hypotension and brain damage. In one particular rescue whenever the people carrying the head of the stretcher were higher than those at the foot the patient became unconscious, to recover again when the stretcher was horizontal or head down (Jones in Marcus, 1979a). The patient had obviously been conscious when found and had been wrapped in surface insulation thus reducing the vasoconstrictor tone without any increase in circulating volume. The volume was sufficient to produce a blood pressure that could maintain a flow to the brain but not when gravity pooled the blood in the deconstricted vessels in the legs (orthostatic hypotension). The situation would be aggravated by the fact that autonomic function is impaired by hypothermia (Achar and Agarawala, 1972).

(c) Moderate surface warming is usually condemned as being dangerous as compared with rapid rewarming in a hot bath or slow spontaneous rewarming (Burton and Edholm, 1955), though this has been based on survival results and has been disputed (Fernandez *et al.*, 1970), again on case results. Some of the controversy may be due to ignorance of the role of fluid shifts. Warmth to the skin would provide perceived warmth and therefore a greater reduction in the cold-induced vasoconstriction (Duguid *et al.*, 1961) than would simple insulation and the outcome would therefore depend on the degree of reversal of the fluid shifts. Warm blankets would provide a large sensory input of warmth with a very small quantity of heat transfer to the tissues and therefore there would be very little fluid return to the intravascular space accompanied by a large drop in peripheral resistance and the outcome would be hypovolaemic hypotension. It is interesting that the worst mortality in cases of profound accidental hypothermia occurs when treatment is by exposure in a warm room (Lilja, 1983) because warm air would provide the maximum sensation of warmth with the minimum of actual heat supplied. A hot-water-circulating blanket, on the other hand (Fernandez *et al.*, 1970), might provide sufficient heat transfer to the superficial tissues to cause significant fluid shifts and maintain the circulating blood volume in spite of the drop in peripheral resistance. Warm packs (Neureuther, 1979) placed over areas of maximum heat loss — groin, axilla and neck (Hayward *et al.*, 1973) — will have a minimal effect on increasing the sensation of warmth but might provide some heat to the core and are probably therefore safer than warm blankets.

(d) The usual reason for advocating immersion in a hot bath in the early post-rescue period (Keatinge, 1969) is that this will decrease or shorten the after-drop of body temperature (Golden and Hervey, 1981). However, it has been shown that this after-drop of core temperature does not occur in the pulmonary vein (Golden, 1979; Hayward *et al.*, 1984a; Lloyd *et al.*, 1976a) and this reason is therefore not valid. The fact that the reverse fluid shift only happens when the cells are warm could explain the findings of a reduced rectal after-drop plus an increased pulmonary artery after-drop during rewarming in a hot bath (Hayward *et al.*, 1984a).

Hypotension is rare during recovery from acute immersion hypothermia whereas hypotension is common during recovery from the exhaustion hypothermia which occurs in mountains (Keatinge in Marcus, 1979a). During acute immersion hypothermia cooling is very rapid and there is insufficient time for dehydration to develop. On the other hand, in exhaustion hypothermia cooling has developed over a much longer time-scale and the associated exercise will have maintained the intravascular volume, even in the presence of total body dehydration (Tappan *et al.*, 1984), thus allowing the cold-induced diuresis to produce a larger fluid loss. These factors have probably been aggravated by sweating, respiratory fluid loss and lack of fluid intake. In experimental dogs, cooled and rewarmed in water, there was no rewarming shock in those animals rewarmed after having been cooled for eight hours or less, whereas those rewarmed after being cooled for twelve hours or more had a 50 per cent mortality after rewarming (Fedor *et al.*, 1958). The pre-death findings of a raised pulse rate and low ventricular pressure are suggestive of hypovolaemia (Fedor *et al.*, 1958). Again one possible explanation is provided by the time necessary for the development of dehydration.

The observation (Davies, 1975a) that immersion in a hot bath has revived many patients who were unconscious and pulseless when brought off the mountains was attributed to the rapid raising of the total body temperature. However, the initial moribund state could have been due to hypovolaemic hypotension following surface insulation plus some additional effect from the movement of the casualty during transport. Immersion in a hot bath would cause a rapid reversal of the hypothermic fluid shifts (auto-transfusion) and the effect would be more rapid because the fall in peripheral resistance had already occurred. The imposition of a small hydrostatic squeeze plus the rapid rise in body temperature would have additional benefits.

The beneficial effects on the fluid balance will be present if the hot bath is used but if after rescue the casualty has already adjusted to the loss of vasoconstrictor tone and has an adequate blood pressure the fluid shifts caused by the hot bath could be dangerous.

(e) If patients have been exposed to cold or are mildly hypothermic for prolonged periods the intercompartmental fluid shifts of the body fluids will have had longer to develop and might therefore be expected to be greater than in acute hypothermia. During rewarming there is a greater potential for reversal and the more rapid the rewarming the greater the surge of fluid into the vascular system and the risk of fluid overload with pulmonary oedema. The additional factor is that if the exposure to cold has been prolonged, it is unlikely that the severity of the cold stress has been very severe. Therefore there may not have been much vasoconstriction to cause increased central venous pressure which seems to be a factor in cold-induced diuresis, which causes a reduction in total blood volume.

It was observed that many patients being rewarmed from prolonged induced hypothermia developed pulmonary and/or cerebral oedema and the incidence was related to the speed of rewarming (Bloch, 1965). Recooling resolved the problem, presumably by reversing or slowing the fluid shifts. In some patients the excessive rewarming rate could occur spontaneously without added heat. If the elderly rewarm too rapidly many die and since many elderly patients live in cold houses they will have been exposed to moderate cold stress for a prolonged period before the final episode. If the rewarming is too rapid even if spontaneous, the fluid overload could be lethal and any method which accelerates rewarming will be dangerous (Duguid *et al.*, 1961; Lloyd, 1973) unless intensive care facilities are available to control the changes (Lloyd, 1972).

(f) It is interesting to consider one of the early deaths which occurred during rewarming from induced hypothermia (Talbot *et al.*, 1941). The patient suffered profound circulatory collapse and the authors suggested that 'the mechanisms of vasomotor collapse are different in rewarming from hypothermia as compared with those in surgical or medical shock' and concluded that 'in retrospect it is thought that sudden vasodilation was responsible for the cardiovascular breakdown'. This statement suggested that there would be increased circulation in the skin but when it was seen that the skin of hypothermia patients remained white and vasoconstricted until they had rewarmed (even in a hot bath) (Webb, 1973b) the idea was discarded and ventricular fibrillation as a result of the after-drop became the accepted mechanism of death. (Recent evidence has confirmed that there is no initial increase in limb and extremity blood flow during the initial rewarming in a hot bath (Savard *et al.*, 1984).) However, the case described by Talbot *et al.* (1941) had been one of prolonged hypothermia for therapeutic reasons and the description of the death with cough, frothy sputum and cyanosis with gasping and shallow respiration was more like that of cardiac failure with pulmonary oedema from fluid overload. Postmortem showed pulmonary congestion.

(g) The situations in which the 'diving reflex' hypothermia (rapid submersion hypothermia) occurs involve severe cold stimulus to the skin and there should therefore be a very high level of skin-cold-induced vasoconstrictor tone. Following removal from the cold stress the potential for a drop in vasoconstriction will probably be greater than in normal situations. If in addition the bradycardia which occurs during spontaneous rewarming (Burton and Edholm, 1955; Lloyd *et al.*, 1976b) is superimposed on the marked bradycardia already existing in the diving reflex, death would be inevitable from the combination of hypovolaemic shock and bradycardia. The victims who have survived this type of hypothermia have all had resuscitative treatment started as soon as the patient was removed from the water.

(h) The role of sleep and alcohol in post-rescue deaths. Captain Downie of the SS *Empire Howard* (Lee and Lee, 1971) described how nine men died after being rescued from −2 °C water even though they had been able to climb on to the rescue ship. All nine died while asleep. When normothermic people first fall asleep there is an initial vasodilatation shown by a rise of skin temperature with a slight fall in core temperature (Buguet *et al.*, 1979a; Lunn, 1969). When Captain Downie's men were rescued the vasoconstrictor tone due to cold sensation on the skin was removed and this effect would have been aggravated by the sensation of warmth in the trawler. When the men fell asleep the further vasodilatation could have proved fatal.

Captain Downie also stated that a small mouthful of spirits made them sleepy. It is traditionally taught that the use of alcohol is dangerous in the immediate post-rescue period because it causes vasodilatation. However, though it has been disputed that the increased facial redness increases heat loss (Vanggaard, 1978), alcohol intake suppresses shivering in the post-rescue period (Vanggaard, 1978). This in itself is not dangerous though it will lead to a longer rewarming period and the dangerous reputation it has acquired when given after rescue may be merely due to the fact that it is a sedative and has a tendency to make the person sleep. The old St Bernard dogs may not in fact have done much harm with their brandy since not only was the brandy diluted in a sugar solution (Collins, 1983b) but it was unlikely that any of their clients would fall asleep and the skin-cold-induced vasoconstrictor tone would be retained. The sugar solution could have been useful in its own right.

Conclusion

In discussing the after-drop the specific site at which the core temperature is being measured must be stated. In the undisturbed animal and man the temperature changes obey the normal principles of physical laws governing conduction of heat, modified to a very small degree by the presence of an intact circulation, and the drop in core temperature should be called the 'primary after-drop'. However, if some particular treatment or manoeuvre causes a drop in core temperature after the primary after-drop has been completed or causes an increase in the depth or duration of the normal primary after-drop, this change should probably be called a 'secondary after-drop'.

The after-drop undoubtedly occurs but that by itself does not mean that the after-drop is the cause of ventricular fibrillation and the evidence is against the idea. Ventricular fibrillation may be precipitated by any factor which depresses the normal subendocardial transmission, and these factors include any temperature changes which produce a gradient across the myocardium with the endocardium being colder than the muscle. It should not be forgotten however that death can still occur from ventricular fibrillation due to mechanical irritation of the heart. This may be caused by external cardiac massage or even by rough handling of the patient and the colder the heart the more vulnerable.

Death following rescue is most commonly due either to inadequate venous return or to fluid overload. The situation in any individual case will be the result of an interaction of several factors — loss of vasomotor tone, dehydration, fluid shifts and the efficiency and health of the heart. The only certain way of distinguishing between the two extremes of fluid balance is by monitoring the central venous pressure. This should be done routinely in hospitals but may be impossible for the rescue services, because vasoconstriction makes the veins very difficult to cannulate (Foray and Salon, 1985). However, knowledge of the circumstances surrounding the incident may give some indication but if doubt is still present as to the reason the blood pressure is dropping a rapid infusion of 300 to 500 ml of fluid (warm) should provide some guide. In hypovolaemia it will give an improvement in blood pressure though this may be temporary and the infusion may need to be continued. In fluid overload there will be no improvement but 300 to 500 ml will not be sufficient to worsen the prognosis.

PART 2: NON-HYPOTHERMIC EFFECTS OF COLD STRESS

8 GENERAL EFFECTS OF COLD

Cold or Dark?

There is difficulty in attributing all problems which occur in winter to cold alone because during the winter, nights are longer and days shorter and the light intensity is less, and there is evidence that plasma melatonin levels are affected by variations in ambient lighting, being highest in midwinter and lowest in midsummer. The further north, the colder the winter but also the greater summer/winter variation in hours and intensity of daylight. For example in the far north there is an increase in the incidence of non-pregnancy-related amenorrhoea during the dark winter months even though pregnancy rates are the same throughout the year (Stewart and Graham, 1984), and the suggested mechanism for the amenorrhoea is through an increased secretion of anti-gonadotrophic hormone by the pineal gland as a result of the decreased amount of light (Stewart and Graham, 1984). Similarly the fact that depression has been successfully treated by increasing the duration of light during the darker days suggests that light is important in the aetiology of depression. However, depression is associated with neurochemical changes in the brain (van Praag, 1983b) and in Finland, the peak incidence of depression occurs in late winter and early spring (Nayha, 1984b) which tends to match the winter period with the severest cold rather than the shortest daylight. It is known that suicide often occurs sometime after the deepest point of a depression (Nayha, 1984b) and the historical peak incidence of suicide is in the spring (Leppaluoto, 1984; Nayha, 1984b). There is also a suggestion that there are specific cerebral neurochemical changes associated with suicide (van Praag, 1983a; Stanley and Mann, 1983) and it is possible that both cold and light can singly or together produce the neurochemical changes in the brain leading to depression and suicide.

Death Rate

Even though many doctors have the clinical certainty that some conditions may be aggravated or caused by cold damp conditions, the

DHSS does not register the deaths of children or the elderly from these diseases as cold related (Phillips, 1982). In fact the true figure for cold-related deaths may be impossible to determine because of certification regulations (Adelstein, 1973) but possibly also because of official policy (Taylor, 1981). There is, however, no doubt that death rates rise in winter (Taylor, 1978) and a specific period of freezing weather was followed by a 10 per cent rise in deaths (BMJ, 1980). In Finland there is an excess mortality of 1,000 to 2,000 cases each winter as compared with summer, though it is interesting that the seasonal variation has decreased with improvements in housing (Nayha, 1984a). This might help to explain why the death rates for circulatory and respiratory disorders in Scotland in the years 1950 to 1980 have markedly deteriorated in relation to the rate in Finland for both males and females in the age group 55 to 64 (Catford and Ford, 1984) because there has been no improvement in housing in Scotland over those years. For ischaemic heart disease (IHD) the death rate in December is 24 per cent greater than in August, and for cerebrovascular accident the increase is 30 per cent (Nayha, 1984a). In the UK the high winter mortality for IHD and stroke varies between 20 and 70 per cent depending on the weather (Bull and Morton, 1978; Rose, 1966). For respiratory disease there is a 91 per cent increase in mortality in winter (Nayha, 1984a) and the fact that for all these causes the excess mortality is more marked in the lower social classes where more people work in outdoor occupations (Nayha, 1984a) suggests that the phenomenon is cold related and not affected by the duration or intensity of light. The increase in IHD mortality could be affected by a number of factors, e.g. a respiratory infection could result in increased stress on the heart or the cold could increase the cardiac work. It could also be secondary to the seasonal variation in blood pressure or because of the seasonal variation in living habits, e.g. walking in snow, shovelling snow or inadequate clothing (Nayha, 1984a). Throughout society there is a marked seasonal and climatic variation in death rates from ischaemic heart disease (IHD) with socioeconomic factors and rainfall increasing the risk, but the closest association is an inverse relationship between temperature and IHD deaths (West *et al.*, 1973a, b; West and Lowe, 1976). Deaths from IHD in the elderly also rise in winter (Bainton *et al.*, 1977), and there is an association between low temperature environments and sudden infant deaths (Bonser *et al.*, 1978).

In East Greenland the infant mortality has been reduced by improvements in hygiene and the presence of midwives (Robert-

Lamblin, 1984) but there are still many infant deaths during the first month of life and it has been postulated that there must be a genetic cause to explain the deaths which occur before the age of one year (Robert-Lamblin, 1984). However, though the neonatal mortality among the James Bay Cree Indians is the same as the neonatal mortality in Quebec city, the post-neonatal death rate for the Cree is eight times greater than in Quebec and the main cause is respiratory infection (Robinson, 1984), which suggests an environmental rather than a genetic cause of the higher death rate. In Alaska it has been shown that the factors which give rise to high infant mortality are a birth weight of 2,500 grams or less and mothers who are under 19 or less experienced (Pelto, 1984), which are very similar to the factors found in the UK.

In Greenland it has been observed that high housing standards and social groupings result in a low incidence of respiratory infection and a low rate of hospital admissions (Bjerregaard, 1984a). However, poor socioeconomic status as measured by housing density and income (Bjerregaard, 1984b) results in a high incidence of respiratory infection and hospital admissions (Bjerregaard, 1984a) and there is a linear association between socioeconomic status and mortality (Bjerregaard, 1984b).

Other Effects

Among construction workers winter sees an increased accident rate with decreased productivity, and an increase in the incidence of bronchitis and myocardial infarction (Taylor, 1978). In the elderly there is a rise of 80 per cent in the incidence of fractures of the neck of femur occurring outdoors in midwinter as compared with mid-summer, and this could be blamed on wind or icy surfaces. However, there is an astonishing 350 per cent rise in fractures of the neck of femur occurring indoors and this rise occurs within days of a fall in temperature (Allison and Bastow, 1983).

There is a significant correlation between cold weather and the incidence of testicular torsion (Shukla *et al.*, 1982; Williamson, 1983) and cold air has a very clear trigger effect on trigeminal neuralgia (Nystrom and Heikkinen, 1984).

There is an increased risk of lymphoproliferative cancer during the winter months in Finland and it has been suggested that this may be the result of the increase in serum adrenocortical hormones which occurs during the cold winter months (Leppaluoto, 1984). However, it is also known that stress and an altered environment, including hypogravity and hypergravity, can produce an effect on the immunologic responsiveness of the body (Barone and Caren, 1984; Bradley *et al.*, 1984). The long dark nights may therefore have some direct effect.

Cold does not have any aetiological significance in the causation of osteoarthritis and since the prevalence of seropositive polyarthritis is the same everywhere, cold does not increase the risk of rheumatoid arthritis. Nevertheless a cold or damp climate worsens the subjective pain symptoms and the same patient feels much better in a warm dry climate (Isomaki and Virsiheimo, 1982). This observation has implications for medical services in northern countries.

9 CUTANEOUS REACTIONS TO COLD

Subjective Effects

Man is very sensitive to differences and changes in temperature, especially changes downwards (Enander, 1984). The sensation of cold is related to the lowered average skin temperature and the sensation of local cold becomes more intense with increasing exposure (Enander, 1984). A peripheral temperature stimulus is considered pleasant when it tends to restore body temperature towards normal and unpleasant if it has the reverse tendency, e.g. cold applied to the skin is pleasant if the core temperature is raised but unpleasant if the core temperature is lowered (Enander, 1984). The fact that a person may feel warm if he moves from the cold into the warmth, even if the body temperature is still low (Enander, 1984), illustrates the point and suggests that the discomfort caused by cold may be the result of the vasoconstriction (Enander, 1984). Subjective discomfort caused by cold is greater if certain areas, e.g. forehead or feet, are cold, and the discomfort is increased by shivering (Enander, 1984).

Cold Allergy

Some people have an allergic response to cold (Back and Larsen, 1978; Horton and Brown, 1929; Wanderer, 1979) and the types of response have been classified (Kaplan, 1984; Webster *et al.*, 1942). In some individuals this allergy is manifested by a malaise with shivering, aching joints and generalised urticaria, and the susceptibility is transmitted as a genetic dominant (BMJ, 1975; Eady *et al.*, 1978; Tindall *et al.*, 1969; Ting, 1984). In cold urticaria there are sensitised mast cells in the skin. The exposure of the skin to cold causes degranulation of these cells with the release of hypersensitivity mediators both locally and into the systemic circulation (Wasserman *et al.*, 1977). It is interesting that in a review of the effects associated with mast cells in the skin (Daly *et al.*, 1984) no mention was made of cold urticaria. The local effects may include wheals at the site of local cooling and even cold drinks may produce lesions in the mouth and on the lips (BMJ, 1985). It is important that the diagnosis of familial cold urticaria should not be missed since it may occur even in an indoor swimming pool (Ting, 1984) and proper counselling and prevention of exposure to cold may save the life of a susceptible person (Ting, 1984). It has been suggested (BMJ, 1975) that some of the cases of death occurring within a few minutes of entering cold water are due to anaphylaxis in a person with previously unsuspected cold urticaria. It may be possible to provide some treatment for the condition using doxentrazole (Bentley-Phillips *et al.*, 1978) or a H_1-receptor histamine antagonist of which cyproheptadine is an example (Ting, 1984).

Raynaud's Syndrome

Another form of allergy is Raynaud's phenomenon (BMJ, 1975) which involves an over-reactive arterial vasoconstriction in response to a cold stress whose severity does not affect normal people (Burch and Giles, 1974). The normal reactive hyperaemia following arterial occlusion is virtually absent (Holti, 1985) and there is also a loss of the normal 'hunting' phenomenon of intermittent vasodilatation (BMJ, 1975). Even in the warm, people with Raynaud's phenomenon have an altered pulse contour because of an altered digital arterial viscoelasticity (Sumner and Strandness, 1972). There is a difference between Raynaud's disease and Raynaud's phenomenon as for example in scleroderma. The vasospastic attacks of Raynaud's disease are precipated by either cold or emotional stress or both together, whereas almost all attacks of Raynaud's phenomenon in scleroderma are precipitated by cold provocation alone (Freedman and Ianni, 1983). Raynaud's phenomenon is more readily induced if the core temperature is below 36 °C (Holti, 1985). It has been suggested that the term 'Raynaud's syndrome' be used as a term to cover both Raynaud's disease and Raynaud's phenomenon (Surwit *et al.*, 1983). A large percentage of patients have detectable anti-nuclear antibodies without any other evidence of auto-immune disease (Surwit *et al.*, 1983) but those without anti-nuclear antibodies had higher cortisol levels and lower noradrenaline levels than controls. One possible explanation for this is that the presence of glucocorticoids increases vasomotor reactivity (Surwit *et al.*, 1983). Raynaud's syndrome may be caused by light to moderate exposure to arsenic in mining (Linderholm and Lagerkvist, 1984) and may result in difficulties in working in the cold with uncovered hands. There is a similar increased sensitivity to cold in association with the hand vibration syndrome which may be caused by pneumatic drill usage, or by driving snowmobiles (Hassi *et al.*, 1984).

Biofeedback training might be worth considering in Raynaud's syndrome (Kappes and Mills, 1984), especially in the group without anti-nuclear antibodies, since there seems to be a hormonal element in these sufferers. If the attacks of digital ischaemia are incapacitating, the patients may consider the use of portable electrically heated gloves (Kempson *et al.*, 1983).

Acrocyanosis

Acrocyanosis is a symmetrical permanent cyanosis (in Raynaud's syndrome there is paroxysmal acrocyanosis) as a result of an increased sensitivity of the vasoconstrictor response to cold (Lahti, 1982). The aetiology is unknown, there are no complications and no treatment is needed (Lahti, 1982).

Other Syndromes

Cryoglobulinaemias, livedo reticularis and paroxysmal cold haemoglobinuria (Lahti, 1982) are problems which usually have an underlying medical pathology. The treatment should ideally be aimed at the underlying cause but may sometimes be symptomatic.

The most common skin problem in winter is winter itch (asteototic eczma). The cause appears to be a low relative humidity which causes decreased sweating and sebum secretion, and the skin becomes dry and itchy. The position is obviously worsened by central heating especially if the temperature is kept high, and treatment involves humidification of the room, emulsifying skin ointments and the avoidance of too much washing (Lahti, 1982). In the 'sick building syndrome' (Finnegan *et al.*, 1984) this condition should be kept in mind.

Chilblains

Chilblains are local inflammatory lesions which develop as a result of exposure to cold. They are more frequent in the humid climate of Great Britain than in the cold dry climate of the Nordic countries (Lahti, 1982), possibly because humidity increases thermal conductivity. Women are more often affected than men (Lahti, 1982). Inadequate clothing is an important predisposing factor (BMJ, 1975; Lahti, 1982) in the cooling and water loss which makes the skin brittle, which in turn leads to the symptoms of chapping and winter itch (BMJ, 1975). It is interesting that the provision of central heating in houses has reduced the incidence of chilblains (Lahti, 1982).

Frostbite

Local severe cold may cause the skin to freeze (Keatinge and Cannon, 1960) and this may progress to frostbite, which though it is most commonly associated with northern latitudes may also occur in unexpected parts of the world, e.g. in the Sahara desert at night (Barber, 1978). The subject of frostbite has been extensively reviewed (Foray *et al.*, 1979; Killian, 1981; Maclean and Emslie-Smith, 1977; Malhotra and Mathew, 1978; Malmros, 1977; Mills, 1966, 1968, 1973a, b and c, 1977, 1980, 1983b; Murazian *et al.*, 1978; Pelizzo and Franchi, 1978; Ward, 1974, 1975b; Welch, 1974).

Precipitating Factors

Frostbite is true tissue-freezing and occurs when there is sufficient heat loss in the local area to allow ice crystals to form in the extracellular spaces and extract cellular water (Mills, 1983b). There is also a vasomotor component (Foray and Salon, 1985; Schmid-Schonbein and Neumann, 1985). The cold-induced vasoconstriction produces stagnation, and the cold itself causes increased cellular aggregation and sludging (Schmid-Schonbein and Neumann, 1985). In normal cold exposure there is a decrease in local haematocrit (Schmid-Schonbein and Neumann, 1985), but if there is local vasodilatation, e.g. because of histamine release, the part will be perfused with blood containing a high concentration of red cells. This will increase the risk of red cell aggregation and stasis, and result in problems during rewarming (Schmid-Schonbein and Neumann, 1985). Lowering the core temperature increases the sensitivity to cold, i.e. a small cold skin stimulus, which normally has no effect, will cause an intense vasoconstriction in the fingers and feet if the body temperature is lowered (Grayson and Kuehn, 1979). This phenomenon may be important in the aetiology of frostbite (Grayson and Kuehn, 1979), especially if the blood volume is already depleted by dehydration which is a risk factor itself (Foray and Salon, 1985; Mills, 1983b; Schmid-Schonbein and Neumann, 1985). The likelihood is also increased by alcohol and excess tiredness (Hassi, 1982; Lahti, 1982).

The regions most commonly affected are the ears and nose (Hassi, 1982; Mills, 1983b) and the distal extremities of the limbs. Fashion can affect incidence. For example the incidence of frostbite of the ears varies depending on whether short or long hairstyles are in vogue (Mills, 1983b), and the physical immobility associated with the use of snowmobiles has also increased the number of cases (Hassi *et al.*, 1984). The clothing can also aggravate the situation. For example training shoes are dangerous especially if too tightly laced (Fraser and Loftus, 1979a; Mills, 1983b) and snow boots have felt liners which shrink and freeze if they become wet. The end result is that the compression stops or restricts the blood flow, and a similar compression can occur if neoprene boots are worn during ascent to altitude (Mills, 1983b). A restricted circulation increases the risk of frostbite and worsens the outcome (Mills, 1983b).

Since sensory and motor nerve activity is abolished at 7 to 9 °C, the disappearance of pain is an early warning of incipient cold injury (Vanggaard, 1985). To try to reduce the risk of developing frostbite there should be adequate fluid intake to prevent dehydration, and, where practicable, the feet and hands should be warmed at intervals, especially if there is total anaesthesia on attempting to move the fingers and toes.

Frostbite can be classified into a number of different grades of severity (Foray and Salon, 1985; Lahti, 1982; Maclean and Emslie-Smith, 1977; Ninneman *et al.*, 1984; Ward, 1974; Welch, 1974) but for practical purposes it is enough to divide frostbite into superficial and deep (Lahti, 1982; Mills, 1983b). However, since the part is hard, cold, white and anaesthetic and appears solidly frozen through even if the damage is only superficial, the initial assessment of the severity of the damage is often found to be inaccurate (Flora, 1985; Mills, 1973b) and there is no evidence that decisions about treatment are best determined by the severity of the damage (Mills, 1973b). The treatment regimen to be adopted should therefore be applicable for all degrees of frostbite.

Thawing

Thawing should not be attempted if there is the likelihood of the part being refrozen (Mills, 1983b) because repeated freezing causes much more damage than continuous freezing (Keatinge and Cannon, 1960; Mills, 1983b). It is possible to walk on frozen feet and people have done just that for 1 to 74 hours (Mills and Rau, 1983).

There are a number of methods of thawing the affected part and there seems to be differing prognosis. At present rapid rewarming in warm water (37.1 to 41.1 °C) appears to result in the greatest degree of tissue preservation and the most adequate early function especially in deep injury (Foray and Salon, 1985; Mills, 1983b). Gradual spontaneous thawing is probably satisfactory for superficial frostbite but not for deep injury (Mills, 1983b) while delayed thawing or using ice or snow rubbing often results in marked tissue loss (Mills, 1983b). The worst results undoubtedly follow thawing with excessive heat, especially dry heat at 60 °C or above (Flora, 1985; Foray and Salon, 1985; Mills, 1983b). These temperatures will be produced by diesel exhausts, stoves or wood fires (Mills, 1983b) and this is undoubtedly the reason for the very poor results achieved by Baron de Larrey during Napoleon's retreat from Moscow (Mills, 1973b). It has been suggested that rapid internal rewarming would result in better results but intra-arterial lines might cause more damage than they prevent, and warmed intravenous fluids are part of the standard management of the patient (Mills, 1983b).

The current management in Alaska (Mills, 1983b) is to immerse the part or the whole person in a whirlpool bath (41 °C) until the distal tip of the thawed part flushes. In Chamonix in the French Alps (Foray and Salon, 1985), the limb is placed in a 38 to 40 °C bath for 30 minutes with the whirlpool effect being produced by bubbling oxygen through the water. This thawing is not started till 15 to 20 minutes after the intravenous injection of a vasodilator (Foray and Salon, 1985). If there is no chance of tissue recovery, the part remains cyanotic and cold and blebs do not develop. (Rapid rewarming should not be used if the part has been thawed previously or if there is a danger of refreezing.) Sedatives or analgesics may be needed. After thawing the extremities are elevated (Flora, 1985; Foray and Salon, 1985; Mills, 1983b) and kept exposed on sterile sheets with cradles to avoid damage. Treatment is continued with whirlpool baths (35 °C) twice daily for 20 minutes with an antiseptic, e.g. hexachlorophene or betadine, added to the water (Foray and Salon, 1985; Mills, 1983b). The whirlpool has the effect of removing necrotic and infected tissue without causing damage to healthy tissue.

Surgery

Blebs are left intact unless they are infected. Escharotomy is performed when the eschar is dry and causing splinting of the digits (Mills, 1983b). After thawing, the formation of oedema may result in a compartment pressure syndrome and *fasciotomy* is then essential to avoid extensive tissue necrosis (Franz *et al.*, 1978; Mills, 1983b). Debridement or amputation should be delayed till mummification and tissue demarcation is complete (often 30 to 90 days) (Mills, 1983b). This is a profound change from the days when amputation was performed early (Cohen, 1968).

Other Measures

Most patients with frostbite, and/or hypothermia, are suffering from dehydration, and *rehydration* is a very important part of management and any fluids should be warmed (Mills, 1983b). There is a case for rehydrating with *low molecular weight Dextran* (Foray and Salon, 1985; Mills, 1983b; Schmid-Schonbein and Neumann, 1985) to try to reduce the cellular aggregation and sludging through haemodilution (Schmid-Schonbein and Neumann, 1985), and it may be worth continuing low molecular weight Dextran for ten to twelve days in the post-rewarming phase (Foray and Salon, 1985).

Sympathectomy produces a reduction in pain, a decrease in oedema and there is much less infection, either superficial or deep (Flora, 1985; Mills, 1983b). The observation that there is more rapid tissue demarcation may be the result of more rapid healing. However, the fact that the demarcation is more proximal may mean that the sympathectomy has caused more vascular shunting and therefore more rapid necrosis. Sympathectomy does not result in increased tissue preservation and sometimes a non-sympathectomised limb has had better results than the treated one despite apparently equal bilateral injury (Mills, 1973b; 1983b). The apparently variable results may have been due to failure to appreciate the effects of compartment syndromes and dehydration (Mills, 1983b) and current management includes alpha-adrenergic blockade using phenoxybenzamine hydrochloride 10 mg daily, increasing to 20 to 60 mg depending on effect and need (Mills, 1983b). The patient must be well hydrated after sympathetic blockade (Mills, 1983b).

Silver nitrate may be used either as 0.5 per cent solution lavaged over the area of frostbite after the whirlpool treatment or as 1 per cent to counteract severe drying, splitting and separation of the eschar

(Mills, 1983b). *Antibiotics* may be given intravenously, prophylactically for ten to twelve days (Foray and Salon, 1985), or only used in the presence of known infection (Mills, 1983b).

Thrombolytic enzymes are being evaluated (Flora, 1985; Mills, 1983b), including Arwin, which is a snake venom. This is claimed to be more specific than other kinases, and it may cuase the demarcation line to form more distally and more quickly (Flora, 1985). However, there is a risk in using these agents in the presence of other injuries, especially if there is the possibility of a head injury (Mills, 1983b). *Anticoagulants* and *vasodilators* are used in the post-thawing period (Foray and Salon, 1985) but there is disagreement as to their effectiveness (Mills, 1983b). *Tobacco* is prohibited because of its vasoconstrictor effect (Foray and Salon, 1985; Mills, 1983b). *Hyperbaric oxygen* was reckoned to be ineffective in the treatment of frostbite (Cohen, 1968) but may be of value in the post-thaw treatment (Mills, 1983b). *Biofeedback* training (Kappes and Mills, 1984; Mills, 1983b; Mills and Rau, 1983) may also prove to be a technique of value for the future.

The assessment of *tissue viability* may be assisted by using Doppler ultrasound or by measuring the temperature difference between the frostbitten area and a reference unaffected area, and comparing the differential before and after thawing (Foray and Salon, 1985). Technetium 99m isotopes have been injected and perfusion assessed radiologically (Mills, 1983b). This technique has been found to be more accurate than Doppler ultrasound for assessing viability (Mills, 1983b) and can give some indication of compartment pressures. However, clinical judgement should not be overruled by sophisticated technology in deciding whether or not a fasciotomy is necessary (Mills, 1983b).

The patient should be nursed in a pleasant environment and fed with a high-protein and high-calorie *diet*. Dislocations should be reduced immediately the part has been rewarmed but fractures are treated conservatively (Mills, 1983b). Digital exercises are encouraged throughout the day and, for the lower limbs, Buerger's exercises should be carried out four times daily (Mills, 1983b).

It should be remembered that hypothermia is often present along with frostbite, and treatment of the hypothermia takes precedence (Foray and Salon, 1985; Mills, 1983b). There may also be other injuries in addition to frostbite (Mills, 1983b), and frostbite can occur on top of thermal burns (Shimizu and Alton, 1982). These other points must be remembered in the total management of the patient.

Trench Foot (NFCI)

Cold can also cause tissue damage without freezing — 'trench foot', 'immersion injury', 'peripheral vasoneuropathy after chilling' (Ungley *et al.*, 1945), 'non-freezing cold injury' (NFCI) (Keatinge, 1969), 'tropical immersion foot', 'paddy foot' (Francis, 1984). It requires a different management from frostbite, though there is sometimes disagreement as to whether a particular case is one of frostbite (Fraser and Loftus, 1979b) or NFCI (McDonald, 1979; Marcus, 1979b). The historical background (Francis, 1984) and the pathogenesis (Francis and Golden, 1985) of NFCI have recently been reviewed.

NFCI develops when the legs are exposed to the wet and cold above 0 °C (Francis, 1984; Lahti, 1982) and, though wet conditions are not absolutely necessary (Maclean and Emslie-Smith, 1977), the development of NFCI requires longer exposure than does frostbite (Mills, 1973b). It was frequent during the wars, among soldiers living in wet trenches and sailors after long periods spent in lifeboats (Francis, 1984; Lahti, 1982; Maclean and Emslie-Smith, 1977). Even in the Falklands campaign in 1982, NFCI accounted for 20 per cent of the men received on the hospital ship *Uganda* (Francis, 1984). If the footwear has been soaked in sea water the incidence of NFCI is higher because the salt crystals attract water. In the mountains, NFCI can develop if the boots are impervious to water because the build-up of sweat inside the boot is the equivalent to immersion. Dehydration appears to be another important predisposing factor as in frostbite and hypothermia, and, as in frostbite, if the limb is dependent, immobile or is constricted by footwear (Francis and Golden, 1985; Fraser and Loftus, 1979a; Maclean and Emslie-Smith, 1977), damage is more likely to occur and be more extensive. Inadequate nutrition, fatigue, stress, intercurrent illness or injury are other predisposing factors (Francis and Golden, 1985). NFCI, or tissue damage with a similar pathogenesis and pathology (Francis, 1984), may occur even if the skin temperature does not drop below 16 °C (Maclean and Emslie-Smith, 1977), and cases have been recorded up to 29 °C (Francis, 1984).

The symptoms experienced by the troops in the Falklands were described as follows (Golden in Payne, 1984):

> Numbness began to develop after about 7 to 10 days. At night in their sleeping bags, the numbness would be replaced by paraesthesia or pain, or both — described by some as being like electric shocks

> running up the legs from their toes. In some cases the pain was enough to keep them awake. On weight-bearing in the morning the pain was sometimes almost unbearable for the initial 5 or 10 minutes, but would gradually wane and once again be replaced by numbness on re-exposure to cold. Some — particularly those with very severe nocturnal pain — found their feet had swollen to such a degree in the morning that they had difficulty in putting on their boots; or if it had been necessary for them to sleep with their boots on, they had difficulty in tying their laces.

When first examined the typical case has cold, swollen and blanched feet which feel heavy and numb. There is a sensation of 'walking on cotton wool'. This stage is rapidly succeeded by one of hyperaemia, in which the feet are hot and red, with swelling and pain which may be severe, and this phase may last for days or weeks (Marcus, 1979b; Mills, 1973b). The treatment involves removing the person from the hostile environment but whole body warming has also been recommended (Lahti, 1982) probably because of the possibility of associated hypothermia, though others recommend that rapid rewarming should be avoided (Maclean and Emslie-Smith, 1977). Apart from this, treatment consists of bed rest, with analgesics for the pain, and some advocate sympathectomy (Lahti, 1982), but opposition to sympathectomy is more widespread (Golden, F. StC, personal communication, 1985). Blisters may develop as in frostbite and may progress to gangrene.

Demyelination of nerves (Francis and Golden, 1985), and muscle necrosis and atrophy (Francis and Golden, 1985; Marcus, 1979b; Maclean and Emslie-Smith, 1977) may occur. Even after recovery there may be persistent after-effects with vasomotor paralysis, analgesia and paraesthesia, which may be permanent (Francis, 1984; Marcus, 1979b; Mills, 1973b), and early anhydrosis (Francis and Golden, 1985; Marcus, 1979b) or late hyperhydrosis (Francis and Golden, 1985; Mills, 1973b). There may be problems with toe rigidity and fallen arches (Francis and Golden, 1985), and osteoporosis may occur (Francis and Golden, 1985). In addition, the feet tend to develop a marked and persistent vasospasm when presented with cold stimuli (Francis and Golden, 1985; Mills, 1973b), and the vasospasm persists long after the cold stimulus has been removed (Francis and Golden, 1985). Re-exposure to cold is very liable to cause relapse (Francis, 1984). Some victims suffer permanently from intermittent local ulceration of the skin with fissuring and chronic infection (Francis and Golden, 1985; Mills, 1973b).

At present there is 'no satisfactory treatment for the many manifestations of NFCI' (Francis and Golden, 1985). Therefore prevention should be aimed for, especially since the cold hypersensitivity of the feet may persist for years or even be permanent (Francis, 1984; Francis and Golden, 1985; Mills, 1973b). Footwear is obviously very important in prevention, but shoes and boots have to perform many functions in addition to the prevention of cold injury, and the different requirements cause conflict in the design of footwear (Oakley, 1984). At the moment there is no boot or shoe which will prevent NFCI or frostbite (Oakley, 1984), and the way forward may be to design footwear on the modular pattern with a variety of inner, middle and outer components to be combined as required to fulfil the needs of any particular situation (Oakley, 1984). The most useful preventive measures (Francis, 1984) are (1) to limit the time the person is exposed to the hazardous environment; (2) taking a hot drink whenever possible — of thermal and hydration benefits; (3) adequate foot care to keep the feet as dry and abrasion free as possible. This system was used in the Second World War by the British troops but not by the American troops, and the result was that, even under identical conditions, the US troops suffered ten times the incidence of cold injuries incurred by the British (Francis, 1984). Unfortunately the exigencies of modern warfare, as experienced in the Falklands war, are such that the preventive measures are not always possible in practice (Francis, 1984). It is therefore important for the future to look at ways of breaking the vicious pathogenetic circle of cooling and vasoconstriction accompanied by a high level of sympathetic tone (Francis and Golden, 1985).

10 EFFECTS OF COLD ON LIMB FUNCTION

The effects of cold on limb function are not necessarily accompanied by a lowering of body temperature, especially if it is only the limbs that are exposed to the cold; in fact limb function may be impaired without shivering being induced. In fingers immersed in water at 0 °C to 4 °C there is a very steep temperature gradient from the skin, which is at a temperature only a few degrees above that of the water, to the internal finger temperature of about 20 to 25 °C (Greenfield *et al.*, 1950), though this latter temperature range is itself very low when compared with the normal core temperature of 37 °C. When the skin temperature drops to +20 °C the skin receptors are only 1/7 as effective in sensing movement as at normal temperatures. At 5 °C the skin receptors do not sense movement at all (Hassi, 1982). When the skin temperature drops to somewhere in the range +16 to +10 °C this causes pain (Enander, 1984; Hassi, 1982).

Among the more important effects of cold in the outdoor stuation are the effects on the hands, and cold certainly reduces manual performance and dexterity (Clark and Jones, 1962; Fox, 1961; Hirvonen, 1982), even when the rest of the body is kept warm (Enander, 1984; Hassi, 1982; Lockhart, 1960). This may be looked at under several headings.

Effect on Nerves

As nerves are cooled conduction slows progressively (Vanggaard, 1975) until at 4 °C reversible paralysis occurs (Holdcroft, 1981). However, prolonged exposure of nerves below 10 °C causes sensory and motor damage (Paton, 1983b). Exposure of the hands to a very cold environment may impair the function of the nerves after as short a time as 15 minutes even though there may have been no freezing of the skin. This impairment is not reversed by immediate rewarming of the hands in hot water but may occasionally persist for periods in excess of four days (Marshall and Goldman, 1976).

There is also a prolongation of the synaptic delay time when the neuromuscular junction is cooled (Katz and Miledi, 1965). The presynaptic nerve block is complete by 28 °C but above that temperature, the contractile ability of the muscle itself is impaired (Thornton *et al.*, 1976).

Effect on Joints

Joint stiffness is a common complaint in incipient hypothermia (Danzl, 1983) and in fact on exposure to cold the temperature in the joints falls faster than the temperature in the muscles (Hunter *et al.*, 1952) and cold joints are stiff joints (Coppin *et al.*, 1978). Cold increases joint stiffness and therefore resistance to movement by increasing the viscosity of synovial fluid (Hunter *et al.*, 1952) and this would increase the risk of tearing muscles or tendons if the person has to make a sudden movement.

Effect on Muscles

Cold muscles are notoriously liable to tears and this is the reason that athletes have to have a 'warm-up' before they take part in an event (Jensen, 1977; Krejci and Koch, 1980); the more explosive the event, e.g. 100-metre sprint, the greater the danger and therefore the more vital the warm-up.

Cold decreases the power and duration of muscle contraction (Clarke *et al.*, 1958; Foldes *et al.*, 1978; Fox, 1961; Horvath, 1981), e.g. handgrip strength is reduced by immersion of the forearm in 10 °C water (Coppin *et al.*, 1978) and this seems to be a direct effect on the muscle fibres (Guttman and Gross, 1956) since there is no decrease in blood flow (Coppin *et al.*, 1978). When the muscle temperature drops below 25 °C continuing physical activity becomes impossible (Freeman and Pugh, 1969). This impairment is temporary and full recovery can occur within 40 minutes of removal from the cold (Coppin *et al.*, 1978). This failure of muscle function may be due to failure of nerve conduction (Hayward, 1983; Hirvonen, 1982) and/or neuromuscular transmission (Feldman, 1971, 1979; Foldes *et al.*, 1978; Katz and Miledi, 1965) and/or impairment of muscle receptor activity (Hassi, 1982) as well as from a direct effect of cold on the muscle fibres (Hassi, 1982; Hirvonen, 1982).

The converse is also true in that raising the temperature of muscles improves the performance (Foldes *et al.*, 1978; Horvath, 1981), and this is one of the reasons athletes 'warm up' before an event.

Tactile Sensitivity

This can be affected by a number of factors at different levels of cooling (Enander, 1984), e.g. the mechanical properties of the skin at different temperatures, the chemical processes at nerves and receptors, and changes in local circulation, have an effect which is shown by the fact that sensitivity improves during cold-induced vasodilatation (Enander, 1984). The fact that results are better during cooling than during warming suggests that results are partly related to deeper tissue temperatures (Enander, 1984). The effects can be summarised as follows:

(1) The loss of sensitivity increases as skin temperature falls from 20 to 15 °C and becomes definite and obvious between 15 and 10 °C (Enander, 1984).
(2) There is disagreement as to whether there is an exponential loss of function as the skin temperature drops from 30 to 0 °C or if there is a critical temperature at 12 or 4 °C below which there is a sharp deterioration (Enander, 1984).
(3) Vibratory sense is maximum at a skin temperature of 37 °C with deterioration as the temperature changes in either direction (Enander, 1984).
(4) Punctate pressure sense becomes worse at temperatures below 25 °C but deteriorates rapidly below 10 °C (Enander, 1984).
(5) Detection of the impact of a small object is only 1/6 as efficient at 20 °C as at 37 °C (Enander, 1984), and the sensing of roughness is impaired below a skin temperature of 32 °C (Enander, 1984).

Manual Performance

There are difficulties in measuring all the factors involved in tests of manual performance. For example lowering the temperature of the joints increases the viscosity of synovial fluid (Hunter *et al.*, 1952) which diminishes the freedom of movement of the fingers, and therefore tests involving much joint movement are very susceptible to cooling of the fingers and hand (Enander, 1984). However, cooling the arm alone can produce a decrease in finger dexterity, and cooling of the whole body which causes shivering will also produce a decrement in the performance of some tests. The effect on manual performance of cooling the body including hand is greater than the effect of cooling the hand alone which in turn is greater than the effect of cooling the body alone (Enander, 1984).

The effects of cold on nerves, joints and muscles are factors which are all liable to cause clumsiness, loss of manual dexterity and impairment of co-ordination and therefore increase the risk of accidents.

With people who are not acclimatised, exposure to severe or even moderate cold stress results firstly in a numbing of cutaneous sensation and a reduction in sensitivity followed by an attenuated manual dexterity. Fox (1967) after reviewing the literature gives the figure of +8 °C as being the critical skin temperature in air for tactile sensitivity, and +12 °C as being critical for maximum manual dexterity, though it has been suggested that these figures are of little practical applicability (Enander, 1984). Above these temperatures although the hands may feel cold performance is little affected, while at lower temperatures there is a precipitous decline in performance affecting the muscle spindle mechanism, proprioceptors or the joints of the hand and wrist. However, people who are used to cold conditions or to working in the cold become to some extent acclimatised and unless the cold stress is severe their abilities may not be affected to any significant extent. Though cold has a great effect on blood flow in the hands (Hsieh *et al.*, 1965), cold acclimatisation is not due to any increase in blood flow (Hellstrom and Andersen, 1960). However, hands and arms do develop a thin but significant subdermal layer of insulating fat which lessens cold penetration, reduces heat loss and results in better muscle function (Petrofsky and Lind, 1975).

Not all tasks are equally affected by cold exposure, and slow cooling may impair function at a higher temperature than does rapid cooling (Enander, 1984), probably because the deeper tissues are more affected by slow cooling than by rapid cooling. After slow cooling this impairment persists after the hands are rewarmed to normal (Enander, 1984; Lockhart, 1960). While conditioning, training and familiarity with particular tasks will certainly enable those tasks to be performed at a low level of hand and finger sensitivity, they will only do so to a certain level of ability (Clark and Jones, 1962). The progressive effects of the cold on muscle function and control prevent the maintenance of full efficiency and result in a significant deterioration in motor performance (Biersner, 1976). The duration of the cold stress as well as its magnitude is of prime importance in determining reaction to cold. This was shown by Allan *et al.* (1974) in experiments to assess the ability of cold subjects to perform the survival escape procedures from aircraft. The escape procedure time was found to double after exposure at temperatures from −30 °C to +10 °C and for times varying from 15 minutes to an hour. The skin temperature inside the gloves registered between 4 °C and 12 °C and all elements of the escape procedure were affected. In such situations, however, or where only thin protective covering of the hands is possible, the use of limited auxiliary heating to raise the temperature around the cold exposed part can minimise or even eliminate the incapacitating effects of cold on hand and finger dexterity and improve the strength and speed of movement (Lockhart and Keiss, 1971). Physical exercise, at 40 to 60 per cent of maximum aerobic capacity, can increase the temperature of covered hands and feet even in the cold, though rewarming is delayed in unprotected limbs, and toes are more difficult to warm than fingers (Hellstrom *et al.*, 1966). From personal experience, it often seems to be that the extremities actually warm most in the first few minutes after the exercise has stopped. Another point is that equipment intended for use in the cold should be designed so that all controls can be handled with thick gloves (Provins and Clarke, 1960) since the hands will remain warmer and therefore more efficient but the use of gloves will also avoid the risk of frostbite or freeze/burn which may occur if the equipment has to be handled with bare hands in extreme cold. However, adequate gloves impair manual performance (Enander, 1984).

Psychological Factors

Motivation may affect performance in tests and subjective reactions (Teichner, 1958) and the state of arousal and the emotional state of the subject will also affect results (Enander, 1984). Large, slow swings of temperature may improve performance, i.e. some environmental stress may be necessary (Enander, 1984). There is a psychological adaptation to cold (Enander, 1984) and habituation to cold may merely be the result of a reduction in the distracting effect of cold (Teichner, 1958). The fact that acute exposure to cold under hypnosis can produce reactions similar to those produced by acclimatisation (Enander, 1984) shows the importance of psychological factors in trying to assess the effects of cold. Certainly performance under normal conditions is no guide to likely performance in the cold (Enander, 1984).

11 EFFECTS ON THE CARDIOVASCULAR SYSTEM

Exposure to cold causes a number of physiological thermoregulatory adjustments intended to reduce heat loss and these changes affect the cardiovascular system, with the cardiac output rising 64 per cent and the blood pressure and the heart rate rising 25 per cent (Hayward *et al.*, 1984a). Cold stress also causes catecholamine secretion (Danzl, 1983; Keatinge *et al.*, 1984; Mager and Francesconi, 1983; Weihl *et al.*, 1981) in order to increase heat production (Mager and Francesconi, 1983). However, though the catecholamine secretion is increased during the initial stages of cooling, it falls as the core temperature falls from 33 to 29 °C (Chernow *et al.*, 1983). These changes can obviously have an immediate effect but prolonged or repeated exposure to cold may have longer-term consequences for some medical problems and it has been observed that there is a continuing raised level of noradrenaline in winter (Brennan *et al.*, 1982).

Hypertension

In normal people the blood pressure (BP) is higher in the winter months than in the summer months (Brennan *et al.*, 1982; Leppaluoto, 1984; Nayha, 1984a) and similarly patients with untreated essential hypertension have a higher blood pressure in winter than in summer (Sato, 1978), both of which will obviously complicate the task of the physician trying to regulate antihypertensive agents (Hawthorne and Smalls, 1980). Cold stress causes a rise in blood pressure as a general effect (Alexander, 1979) and even a cold room may cause a rise in BP (Brennan *et al.*, 1982). Despite this, when it was noted that people had a higher BP at home than in hospital, the temperature factor was dismissed as unimportant even though hospitals are always much warmer than homes (Young *et al.*, 1983). The pressor effect of a cold outdoor temperature increases with age and in thinner people (Brennan *et al.*, 1982). Cold on the face and respiratory organs causes peripheral vasoconstriction and a rise of blood pressure (Hassi, 1982; Horvath, 1981). Increased blood pressure also correlates with increased rainfall (Brennan *et al.*, 1982), i.e. another factor which increases cold stress. However, the rise in pressure in response to cold is not the result of more effective vasoconstriction (Leppaluoto, 1984), but the cold-induced catecholamine secretion (Danzl, 1983; Keatinge *et al.*, 1984) may be relevant.

Exercise normally results in the diastolic pressure being lowered or remaining level but if the exercise is accompanied by the inhalation of cold air the diastolic pressure rises (Hartung *et al.*, 1980; Hattenhauer and Neill, 1975; Horvath, 1981; Leon *et al.*, 1970) and this may precipitate angina because as the ventricular pressure rises so does the myocardial oxygen requirement (Gorlin, 1966). Cold on the face itself can cause a vagal-induced bradycardia (Linderholm, 1982) and hypertension (Hassi,, 1982) and there is no ethnic difference between Eskimos and European whites (Le Blanc *et al.*, 1975). This response persists in spite of exercise (Le Blanc, 1976) and is actually enhanced by adaptation to cold in contrast to the sympathetic mediated cold pressor response which diminishes on adaptation. The cold pressor test causes a rise in BP and in circulating catecholamines (Caplan *et al.*, 1984) and plasma catecholamine levels are higher in winter (Brennan *et al.*, 1982). The effects of adrenaline resemble the haemodynamic abnormalities of essential hypertension and this is particularly evident during stress (Schalekamp *et al.*, 1983). After an infusion of adrenaline the BP remains raised for several hours after the infusion has been stopped (Schalekamp *et al.*, 1983), and one possibility is that raised adrenaline levels maintained over a period might result in chronic hypertension (*Lancet*, 1982). It has also been suggested that, in genetically predisposed individuals, acute surges in BP from environmental factors may produce the cardiovascular changes which perpetuate hypertension (*Lancet*, 1983). There is one additional factor in this problem. There is an increase in circulating adrenocortical hormones during the colder winter months (Leppaluoto, 1984) and the presence of glucocorticoids increases the vasomotor reactivity to noradrenaline (Surwit *et al.*, 1983). The fact that in normotensive people, of those who showed a hyperreactive response to the cold pressor test, 71 per cent later became hypertensive as compared with 19 per cent of those who had a normal response (Wood *et al.*, 1984), suggests that repeated exposure to cold may be an important factor in the development of essential hypertension. A prolonged steady exposure to cold would not have this effect because the sympathetic mediated cold pressor response diminishes on adaptation to cold and this is more likely to occur on prolonged exposure to cold.

Cerebro-vascular Disease

It is known that a rise in blood pressure is associated with an increased risk of cerebral haemorrhage (Leppaluoto, 1984) and an increased incidence of intracranial haemorrhage has been reported in winter in Minnesota (Ramirez-Lassepas *et al.*, 1980) and an increased incidence of stroke in winter and spring in England (Haberman *et al.*, 1981) and in Finland (Leppaluoto *et al.*, 1984). When three cases of intracranial haemorrhage which occurred after cold exposure were examined (Caplan *et al.*, 1984) they were attributed to the rise in blood pressure and circulating catecholamines caused by the cold, and it was suggested that intracranial haemorrhage after exposure to cold may be the first symptom in a person in whom persistent hypertension will subsequently develop. The changes in blood viscosity and coagulation factors may also be relevant in the causation of cerebral thrombosis (Keatinge *et al.*, 1984).

Ischaemic Heart Disease (IHD)

People with normal cardiovascular systems and functional reserve are unaffected by cold stress or the inhalation of cold air. However, the cold may be crippling for those with reduced cardiovascular reserve (Alexander, 1974; Hartung *et al.*, 1980; Linderholm, 1977, 1982), even if the person is warmly dressed (Hassi, 1982). Without warm clothing cold disables through an increase in angina but with warm clothes the disability is caused by dyspnoea not angina. If cold water is sprayed over the head it may produce ventricular ectopics (Balfour, 1983) and the inhalation of very cold air can cause ECG abnormalities in cardiac patients (Hattenhauer and Neill, 1975; Horvath, 1981; Murray, 1962). The effect of cold is so great that a post-coronary rehabilitation jogging programme could not continue in winter without some protection for the participants against breathing cold air (Kavanagh, 1976). It is not possible to predict, from tests performed in the warm, the reaction of patients with angina when they are exposed to cold (Backman and Linderholm, 1984; Watters *et al.*, 1983). Even in normal people, breathing cold air may produce benign changes in cardiovascular dynamics (Leon *et al.*, 1970) and coronary artery constriction (Hassi, 1982). Beta-receptor blocking drugs counteract the effect of cold by reducing the heart rate and the rate pressure product, and nitroglycerine by dilating the blood vessels (veins) and reducing the filling pressure of the heart and therefore the work load on the heart. If these drugs are used the exercise performance in the cold becomes comparable to that at room temperature (Hassi, 1982). The cold-related increase in catecholamines discussed earlier may be the factor which precipitates a myocardial infarction (MI).

The cold pressor test (immersion of the hand in cold water) causes a tachycardia and a rise in blood pressure (Le Blanc *et al.*, 1975; Mudge *et al.*, 1976) but while the response in normal people is to maintain a normal coronary blood flow, people with proven coronary artery disease show a decrease in coronary artery flow (Mudge *et al.*, 1976). People who suffer clinically from angina but have radiographically normal coronary arteries behave in the same way as normal people (Mudge *et al.*, 1976).

There are recognised risk factors for IHD, though there is disagreement over some of the individual factors. The risk of IHD and MI is certainly increased by *cigarette smoking* (Hansen, 1977b; *Lancet*, 1981a). A *raised blood pressure* is also a risk factor (Hansen, 1977; Karvonen, 1977; *Lancet*, 1981a; Leppaluoto, 1984), and as discussed earlier, cold may be an aetiological factor. *Lack of exercise* is also a factor but the risk of MI is only affected by the level of leisure time physical activity and fitness and not by the level of physical activity at work (Gyntelberg, 1977). The advantage of exercise training may be that improved fitness allows an increased heat production on exposure to cold and therefore the tolerance to cold is improved and the blood pressure rises less (Moriya, 1984). However, because of the increased oxygen requirement in the cold, any particular level of exercise may only cause angina if the exercise is done in the cold (Horvath, 1981; Linderholm, 1982). A recent report suggests that a high ratio of waist to hip circumference is associated with an increased risk of IHD in men (Larsson *et al.*, 1984) and in women (Lapidus *et al.*, 1984) and this finding may also be related to exercise levels.

The role of *cholesterol* in the aetiology of IHD is problematical. It was claimed that mortality from IHD was very low in the native population in Greenland (Dyerberg and Bang, 1982), and that this was due to the observed low levels of serum cholesterol, triglycerides and low-density and very-low-density lipoproteins (Dyerberg and Bang, 1982). However, the statistics are based on material which includes few autopsies, and often even inadequate clinical examination (Helweg-Larsen, 1984). As a result it has been suggested that the incidence of IHD deaths is likely to be much higher than actually reported (Helweg-Larsen, 1984). This contention is supported by the case of a 35-year-old native Greenlander who died suddenly in police custody, and a forensic post-mortem examination revealed evidence of an acute MI with severe coronary and aortic atherosclerosis (Helweg-Larsen, 1984). Though the deaths from IHD rise as the social class falls (*Lancet*, 1981a), the cholesterol levels are higher in the higher social classes than in the lower (*Lancet*, 1981a) and there was no difference between the social classes with regard to fat intake or vegetable consumption (Marmot *et al.*, 1978). After a period between 1974 and 1978 when the death rates from IHD were static, the IHD death rate for England and Wales fell between 1979 and 1983 despite an increased fat intake and a rise in serum cholesterol levels (Burch, 1984). Though the level of serum cholesterol was of some predictive value within each social class, the magnitude was much less than the mortality differences between the social classes. At least one authority now recommends that only very high levels of cholesterol should be treated (Oliver, 1983). It is of interest that the death rate from heart disease per 100,000 was 350 in 1910 and 340 in 1920. By 1930 it was 380 but there was a steady fall thereafter till it reached 220 in 1975 (Harper, 1983). Throughout this period fat consumption rose steadily and the highest figure for deaths was at the lowest point of the pre-war depression. During the depression the money available for food and fuel would be severely limited for a large section of the population and it is interesting that, during the era in which active steps were taken to improve the housing for the less wealthy and the social services backup, the death rate fell. After 1945 a special classification was made to cover arteriosclerotic heart disease and IHD. The figure for this rose from 180/100,000 in 1950 to 230 in 1968 and then fell to 180 by 1980. It may be coincidence but the fall in IHD figures occurred at the time that more people were insulating their houses and installing central heating.

Climatic factors look as if they have a role in the causation of MI. In northern Sweden there is a higher incidence of chest pain as compared with the two southern regions of the country, and since the incidence of smoking is similar in all regions the only remaining factor is the colder climate in the north (Englund *et al.*, 1977). In Finland the death rate from IHD in winter corresponds with the mean January temperature (Valkonen and Notkola, 1977) and mortality from IHD increases in direct relation to the fall in environmental temperature (BMJ, 1980; Keatinge *et al.*, 1984; West *et al.*, 1973a, b; West and

Lowe, 1976) and the rates rise at once after a few cold days (Keatinge *et al.*, 1984; Leppaluoto, 1984), especially in the elderly (Bainton *et al.*, 1977; BMJ, 1980). The increased death rate after a snowstorm, even if the temperature is not very low (Leppaluoto, 1984), may be due to increased stress, either physical, because of the difficulty of moving through the snow, or mental, possibly due to fear of falling, and both physical and mental stress cause a rise in blood pressure which is not blocked by B-blocking drugs (Francois *et al.*, 1984). In the snow these stresses may be added to the stress of the cold, and wiping the snow with bare hands is equivalent to a cold pressor test (Caplan *et al.*,1984). A wet climate increases the cold stress and the incidence and mortality from IHD also rise as the rainfall increases (BMJ, 1980; West *et al.*, 1973a, b; West and Lowe, 1976). In the UK, there is an increasing gradient of IHD from the south-east to the north-west of the country, i.e. as the climate changes from warm to cool, and from dry to wet (BMJ, 1980), and in Finland the lowest IHD mortality is in the milder south-west and highest in the colder east (Pyorala *et al.*, 1977), closely mimicking the distribution of hypertension in Finland (Aromaa *et al.*, 1977). However, the IHD incidence is not genetically linked, since when the Helsinki police, who employ people from all parts of the country, were studied, it was found that those from the east had a slightly lower incidence of IHD deaths than those from the south-west despite those from the east having slightly higher cholesterol levels (Pyorala *et al.*, 1977).

IHD mortality also increases as the socioeconomic factors decline (BMJ, 1980; *Lancet*, 1981a; West *et al.*, 1973a, b; West and Lowe, 1976), including lower educational attainment (Mitchell, 1984), and in Finland the IHD death rate also corresponds closely with the density of housing (Valkonen and Notkola, 1977). It is interesting that pre-war, the death rate in social class 1 from IHD was greater than in social class 5 whereas now the rate for social classes 4 and 5 exceeds the rate for social classes 1 and 2 (*Lancet*, 1981a). There is no evidence that the traditional risk factors for IHD have shown a similar change between the social classes. One thing which has changed over this period is that the housing occupied by social classes 1 and 2 has steadily improved on a thermal assessment with central heating, insulation, double glazing, etc. becoming more and more generally installed, whereas this was not the case for social classes 4 and 5. In people over the age of 60 the death rate from IHD is greater in the UK than in New York but central heating is less common in the UK especially for the older generation (Bull and Morton, 1978). In

Edinburgh the risk of MI is three times greater than in Stockholm (Oliver *et al.*, 1975; Olsson *et al.*, 1977) and it was found that people in Edinburgh smoked more, had higher blood pressure and were less fit (Logan *et al.*, 1978; Olsson *et al.*, 1977) but differences in climate and housing were not examined.

Cardiac Failure

Exposure to cold causes a peripheral vasoconstriction with the result that large volumes of blood are shunted into the capacitance veins in the chest (Coniam, 1979; Horvath, 1981) and may be seen on an X-ray. During the first three days of exposure to cold there is a temporary continuous increase in venous pressure (Wood *et al.*, 1958) and this sudden surge of blood may cause overloading and failure of a vulnerable heart. Cold therefore increases the cardiac work by increasing the oxygen need, the preload is increased by the fluid shunting and the afterload by the hypertension and vasoconstriction. Elderly people may therefore be precipitated into cardiac failure by a sudden cold snap.

Recent research has suggested one mechanism by which cold can cause MI and cerebral thrombosis (Keatinge *et al.*, 1984). Subjects exposed to cold for six hours showed, in addition to the expected rise in blood pressure, an increase in the packed cell volume, an increase in the circulating platelets and an increased viscosity of the blood. Exercise is accompanied by an increase in the circulating level of adrenaline and this produces a release of sequestered platelets, and the effect is also produced by the sympathetic stimulus produced by exposure to cold. The increase in viscosity and the increase in circulating platelets increases the risk of thrombosis. The increased incidence of MI which occurs within 24 hours of the onset of a cold spell could be explained by this mechanism since it would probably take about that time for a house to cool sufficiently to produce the changes in the blood. The later increase in deaths from cerebral thrombosis is explained by the fact that death occurs some time after the occurrence of the thrombotic episode.

It has been suggested (Wells, 1977) that the phenomenon of sudden death while cranking a car on a cold morning (McMichael, 1974) or while shovelling snow (Whittington, 1977) could be due to ventricular fibrillation triggered by a stream of cold air in the respiratory tract passing close to the heart. This is unlikely since it has been shown with hot air (Moritz *et al.*, 1945) and with cold air (Dery, 1973b) that even in intubated animals the inspired air temperature is equilibrated with the core temperature before the air has reached the first bronchial bifurcation beyond the trachea. Only in subfreezing arctic air coupled with hyperventilation is it possible to produce low temperatures in the more distal airways (McFadden, 1983). In fact these deaths are probably the result of a combination of factors:

(1) Unsuspected coronary vascular disease.
(2) Hypertension from the isometric exercise (Committee on Exercise, 1972).
(3) An increase in circulating catecholamines from the cold (Mager and Francesconi, 1983; Weihl *et al.*, 1981), the stress (Rosch, 1983; Taggart *et al.*, 1972), mental and/or physical (Francois *et al.*, 1984) though not from isometric exercise (Robson and Fluck, 1977). The stress response to exercise is increased by facial cooling (Riggs *et al.*, 1983).
(4) An unaccustomed increase in oxygen requirements.
(5) A cold pressor test effect caused by wiping the snow with bare hands (Caplan *et al.*, 1984).
(6) All these factors superimposed on the effects caused by cold — hypertension, vascular spasm and wind-induced bradycardia.

If people with myocardial insufficiency undertake isometric exercise in the cold the wonder is not that cases of myocardial infarction occur but that infarction is not invariable.

Ventricular extrasystoles are common during the first two minutes of immersion in cold water (Keatinge and Evans, 1961) and may be a trigger for ventricular fibrillation when superimposed on the increased arterial and venous pressure secondary to the vasoconstriction following cold immersion (Keatinge and Evans, 1961; Wood *et al.*, 1958) and the increase in catecholamines (Weihl *et al.*, 1981). These effects of cold are reduced by repetition of the exposure and by clothing (Keatinge and Evans, 1961; Martin *et al.*, 1978).

The body does not have to be fully immersed for cold water to have a profound effect. Immersion of the face alone in cold water causes a bradycardia (Gooden, 1982), though there is disagreement as to whether during this manoeuvre there is any difference caused by the breath being held in inspiration or expiration (Elsner and Gooden, 1983; Kawakami *et al.*, 1967), but the phenomenon persists in spite of exercise (Stromme and Ingjer, 1978). The severity of the bradycardia is influenced by a number of factors (see 'Diving reflex', pages 298 to 302) but is not altered by physical fitness. There is an associated vasoconstriction which results in decreased limb blood flow even though the limbs are not exposed to the cold stress (Stromme and Ingjer, 1978). Because a similar bradycardia is found in diving mammals the phenomenon has been called the 'diving reflex' (Folinsbee, 1974) and it has been suggested that the survival of people, especially children, following prolonged submersion in very cold water is due to this 'diving reflex' (Nemiroff *et al.*, 1977). This 'diving reflex', i.e. bradycardia on immersing the face in cold water, has been used as a means of terminating episodes of paroxysmal ventricular tachycardia (Gooden, 1982; *Lancet*, 1981b; Wayne, 1976; Wildenthal *et al.*, 1975) though the treatment is not without danger and should only be attempted when there are appropriate resuscitation skills and support equipment available (Elsner and Gooden, 1983; Gooden, 1982; *Lancet*, 1981b). The test can also be used to investigate the autonomic nervous system (Gooden, 1982).

12 RESPIRATORY EFFECTS OF ENVIRONMENTAL COLD

Reflex Responses

Immersion in cold water causes an increased respiratory rate with a resulting hypocapnoea (Cooper *et al.*, 1976; Golden and Hervey, 1972; Keatinge and Evans, 1961) and, at least in the experimental situation, tetany can develop (Golden and Hervey, 1972). Very vigorous exercise can overcome the hypocapnoea and the response is also reduced by preheating the person in a sauna (Cooper *et al.*, 1976). This may be a factor preventing a high mortality associated with the cold water plunge which follows a sauna.

When cold air is blown across the backs of patients with lung disease there is a reflex bronchoconstriction even though the person is breathing warm air. Similarly ice applied to the face of normal subjects will cause a rise of airway resistance. This is a reflex mechanism produced by the stimulation of thermally sensitive receptors in the skin or mucosa (McFadden, 1983) and the effects cease as soon as the stimulus is removed.

Direct Damage

Though nasal breathing is uncomfortable in very cold environments (Horvath, 1981) it is generally believed that the very efficient mechanism that the upper respiratory tract has for warming cold inspired air precludes the possibility of cold injury to lung tissues (Maclean and Emslie-Smith, 1977), and certainly there was no evidence of respiratory damage among winter joggers and cross-country skiers (Buskirk, 1977), even though in one ski race the temperature was −28 °C with a wind-chill equivalent to −55 °C (Faulkner *et al.*, 1980). However, the breathing of cold air during rest or at light work can cause benign changes in pulmonary function (Guleria *et al.*, 1969; Hsieh *et al.*, 1968) and the inhalation of very cold air damaged the epithelial lining of the upper respiratory tract in normal men and dogs (Houk, 1959; Moritz and Weisiger, 1945). It is therefore necessary to examine any evidence that may suggest that environmental cold can cause either acute or chronic respiratory problems.

Physiology

The respiratory tract is not merely a passage through which oxygen is transported to the alveoli. It also has a protective function with the cough mechanism and mucociliary clearance preventing foreign material from reaching the lung parenchyma. Another protective feature is providing the alveoli with a constant environment of air at a constant temperature with 100 per cent humidity. This necessity may be a relic of terrestrial man's development from an aquatic origin. The subject of respiratory heat and water exchange has been well reviewed by McFadden (1983) and is summarised below.

The inspired air is warmed and humidified during its passage to the alveoli. As the temperature of the air rises, its water-holding capacity also rises, and 100 per cent humidity is achieved through evaporation from the fluid layer lining the airways, and, because of the very low thermal capacity of air, this evaporation accounts for the greatest proportion of total respiratory heat loss (Burton and Edholm, 1955). The respiratory mucosa cools because of the convective and conductive heat loss to the air plus the evaporative loss and this means that, when the air is being exhaled, heat is returned to the mucosa by conduction, convection and by condensation of the water vapour. When the air is finally exhaled it is still fully saturated though, because it is much cooler than alveolar air, it has a much lower water content. There is, however, a net moisture loss and heat loss because environmental air is never fully saturated. As much as 50 to 66 per cent of the heat transferred to the air during inspiration is lost to the body on expiration. It used to be believed that the inspired air had equilibrated with body temperature and had achieved full saturation by the time it had reached the tracheal bifurcation, and this is certainly true if the subject is breathing quietly and at rest. However, there is now evidence that the temperature in the airways can drop below normal 'core' temperature. Not only is the temperature of the respiratory tract, as measured in the retrotracheal portion of the oesophagus, lowered in proportion to ventilation (Hartung *et al.*, 1980; McFadden, 1983) but the severity of the temperature drop is increased by lowering the temperature and/or the humidity of the inspired air (McFadden, 1983). In fact under very severe experimental conditions, using isocapnic hyperventilation of 60 l/min with −17 °C air, the tracheal temperature could fall to 20 °C with the temperature of the air still being only 27 °C deep in the right lower lobe (McFadden, 1983). It is therefore obvious that the conditioning of the inspired air, which starts as soon as the air enters the body through the nose or mouth, is a continuous process which continues as far down the respiratory tract as is necessary to produce completely conditioned air for the alveoli (McFadden, 1983). One safety factor is that the most distal airways are supplied by blood from the pulmonary circulation and not from the bronchial artery and this would be a new heat source. The degree to which the tracheobronchial tree cools during respiration is therefore determined in practice by the temperature and humidity of the climate and the physical activity of the individual.

The bronchial circulation is part of the systemic circulation and, like the circulation to the skin, it can be exposed to wide fluctuations in temperature and supplies an organ which plays a part in thermoregulation. It is therefore reasonable to examine the evidence of any vasoconstrictive response of the bronchial vasculature to cold. If vasoconstriction did not occur the bronchial blood circulating through the larger air passages could be cooled to very low temperatures and this should be reflected in a lower temperature of the blood in the heart and great vessels than in the pulmonary artery, but in normal situations this does not happen (McFadden, 1983). In normal man there is no evidence that any heat loss occurs in the alveoli because the extremely small temperature differences which can be detected between the pulmonary artery and systemic circulation can be accounted for by the endothermic and exothermic reactions which occur as part of the transfer of oxygen and carbon dioxide to and from haemoglobin (McFadden, 1983). However, in experiments with sheep (Lloyd *et al.*, 1976a) the aortic temperature, as measured in the thoracic descending aorta, was lower than the pulmonary artery temperature before and during the induction of hypothermia and during spontaneous rewarming and rewarming in a hot bath (Figure 12.1). This suggests that there was in fact cooling of the blood during its passage through the lungs, and this is supported by the fact that when airway warming (the provision of warm humidified air) was introduced, the aortic temperature rose above the pulmonary artery temperature. These experiments were not the normal situation in that the animals were anaesthetised, which affects peripheral vasoconstriction, and had an endotracheal tube, which transfers the

Figure 12.1: A Comparison of Sites of Heat Uptake in Sheep During Cooling and Three Rewarming Procedures

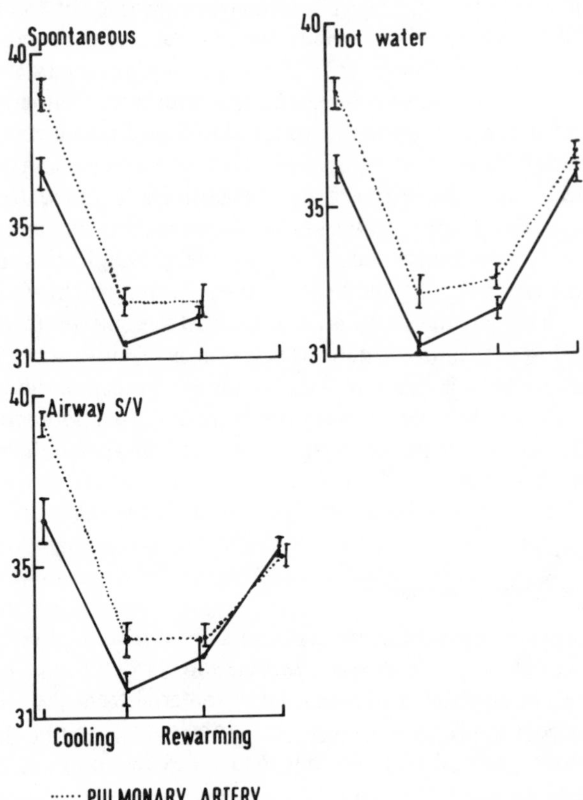

conditioning of the air further down the respiratory tract. However, if there was no vasoconstriction, the blood circulating in the trachea during exercise or hyperventilation would be at body temperature and there would be no explanation for the fall in the oesophageal temperature which accompanies exercise and hyperventilation (McFadden, 1983) and it has been observed, by direct visualisation of the trachea in normal subjects, that, as the tracheal temperature falls during hyperventilation, the mucosa shrinks and becomes pale (McFadden, 1983) in what appears to be a response which is exactly the same as that shown by skin when subjected to a greatly increased heat loss. This mechanism could be of great value by preventing the temperature of the upper airways from rising and thus would provide the optimal thermal gradient for the recovery of heat and moisture during expiration (McFadden, 1983).

The fluid lining the airways is a thin layer composed of 95 per cent water and 5 per cent glycoproteins, the latter secreted by goblet and serous cells and mucus glands. The water layer is maintained by active ion transport across the epithelium with water following as a result of the osmotic gradient produced. When first formed at the airway surface the secretions are nearly isotonic with plasma but with respiration they become hypertonic, suggesting a loss of water to the inspired air. If the airways have been cooled excessively, there will be an increased possibility of condensation during expiration and, on theoretical grounds, this might collect as excess fluid in the trachea. If that were the case, the osmolarity of the surface fluid in the trachea would be lower than in the deeper air passages. This is not in fact so (McFadden, 1983). With mouth breathing the osmolarity of the surface liquid in the trachea rises even more as the evaporative loss is increased as a result of by-passing the nasal humidification (McFadden, 1983).

Acute Effects

Bronchospasm (Exercise Asthma)

The weather can affect the incidence of asthma in a number of ways (*Lancet*, 1985), e.g. a particular combination of rainfall and humidity may result in an antigen-rich aerosol of material from the pollen of the short ragweed (*Lancet*, 1985). Nevertheless, for most asthmatic subjects, the onset of cold weather means a reduction in symptoms because of a reduction in the environmental allergens (Aas, 1975; Rees, 1984). However, for some people winter is a time of increased problems. In some asthmatics airway resistance is increased by exercise either immediately (Deal *et al.*, 1979a, b; McFadden, 1981; Miller *et al.*, 1965; Wells *et al.*, 1960) or in the post-exercise period (Strauss *et al.*, 1978) and the mechanism seems to be through removal of heat and moisture from the respiratory tract. As further support for this idea it has been noted that the bronchospasm induced by exercise is in fact unrelated to exercise except in so far as exercise causes an increase in ventilation and an identical picture can be produced by the same degree of respiratory heat loss as a result of isocapnic ventilation increased voluntarily at rest (McFadden, 1981). The heat loss mechanism is suggested because the bronchospasm can be abolished by the inhalation of air humidified and warmed to body temperature. As further proof that the bronchospasm is due to heat loss, the inhalation of warm air gives very little benefit whereas humidified cold air gives some improvement (Strauss *et al.*, 1978) i.e. the anti-bronchospasm effect of the inhaled gas is proportional to the heat carried. In fact when air, which is warmed and humidified to alveolar values, is inhaled it is impossible to induce bronchospasm however vigorous the exercise or hyperventilation (McFadden, 1983). This helps to explain why, in exercise-induced asthma, swimming is a better means of improving fitness than running or cycling (Rees, 1984) since the swimmer will be inhaling air with a high level of humidity above relatively warm water (McFadden, 1981).

Bronchorrhoea

When divers breathe cold oxyhelium at depth the loss of heat from the respiratory tract becomes colossal. If the rate of respiratory heat loss exceeds 172 kcal/hour the diver experiences a tightness in his chest and difficulty in breathing (Hayes, 1985). After breathing very cold gas for five to ten minutes there is a tendency for the divers to develop bronchorrhoea (Hayes, 1985; Hayes *et al.*, 1982). Warming and humidifying the gas postpones the bronchorrhoea to a later time or greater depth (Hayes *et al.*, 1982) and when the divers breathe dry gas the bronchorrhoea is worse than when the gas is humidified (Hayes, P.A., personal communication, 1984). This suggests that the bronchorrhoea is due to respiratory heat loss and that condensation of water vapour plays no part in its aetiology.

In one interesting experiment with two divers one developed bronchspasm while the other, at the same thermal load, developed bronchorrhoea (Hoke *et al.*, 1976). The divers, who were in a thermoneutral environment (30 °C), developed their respiratory problems when breathing cold (0 to 7 °C) oxyhelium gas at a depth of 800 feet of sea water. The problem was relieved by breathing warm (23 to 32 °C) oxyhelium gas but recurred whenever the cold oxyhelium was reintroduced. Both problems were therefore the direct effect of cold (respiratory heat loss) on the respiratory system. This suggests that bronchospasm and bronchorrhoea are two facets of the same clinical problem caused by respiratory heat loss.

Mechanisms

The mechanism for the bronchospasm remains uncertain. It is sometimes said that bronchospasm can be induced in asthmatic people by stress or suggestion and in fact saline injected into the trachea caused bronchoconstriction in asthmatics, whereas it had no effect in normal subjects (Lewis *et al.*, 1984). However, the bronchoconstriction was related to the volume and temperature of the saline, and there was no bronchoconstriction when air was being breathed at 37 °C and 100 per cent relative humidity. The effect was therefore a result of airway cooling and not suggestion (Lewis *et al.*, 1984) and it seems likely that anxiety and stress, by causing hyperventilation, produce cooling of the airways and thus bronchoconstriction (Lewis *et al.*, 1984).

It has been suggested that the reduction in temperature or the changes in hydration of the bronchial mucosa may stimulate the release of inflammatory mediators, histamine and neutrophil chemotactic factor, from the mast cells (Lee *et al.*, 1983). However, the oral use of a histamine H1 receptor antagonist only gives partial protection against exercise asthma, and only in some people (Patel, 1984).

Since a major part of respiratory heat loss occurs through evaporation of moisture from the respiratory tract to humidify the inspired air (Burton and Edholm, 1955), the body must respond by increasing the secretion of fluid to replace that which is lost. Evaporation of moisture will result in drying and cooling of the underlying mucosal cells which will then respond by increasing the secretion of fluid and, in the ideal situation, the volume of fluid produced will exactly match the volume lost through evaporation but under extreme or abnormal conditions an imbalance may occur between the volume secreted and the volume evaporated. If the volume produced is excessive the fluid will collect in the major airways (bronchorrhoea), whereas, if the volume of the secretions produced is inadequate, the secondary defence response may be bronchospasm to decrease the flow of air to the bronchi.

Hypothesis

Cooling and/or drying of respiratory mucosa triggers the release of a chemical mediator to increase the secretion of fluid. This is an active process involving absorption of water into the cells and then excretion into the respiratory passages. The process may be accompanied by swelling of the cells, and the degree of swelling may be related to the volume of water that needs to be transported across the cells. It is possible that at least some of the elements of clinical bronchoconstriction may not be due to muscle contraction but to swelling of the cells lining the airways, since this would also reduce the diameter of the airways. It is interesting that the use of a hypotonic vehicle for the intratracheal administration of ipratropium caused marked bronchoconstriction, whereas ipratropium in an isotonic vehicle, or normal saline alone, caused very much less (Mann *et al.*, 1984). The hypotonic solution would be rapidly absorbed into the cells lining the airways and, if not released further, would cause the cells to swell and reduce the calibre of the airways. It may therefore be that the defect in exercise asthma is that, while the cells lining the airway have a normal water uptake capacity, there is an inability of the cells to secrete the ions which are necessary to produce the osmotic gradient for the transport of water.

There is a close association between hay fever and allergic asthma which is often associated with rhinitis (Rees, 1984), and hay fever is characterised by nasal congestion and a rhinorrhoea, another suggestive link between swelling of the cells lining the respiratory tract and excessive secretion into the respiratory tract. The fact that divers with a large respiratory heat loss experience tightness in the chest and difficulty in breathing early while the bronchorrhoea takes five to ten minutes to develop (Hayes, 1985) provides further support.

Parasympathetic neural activity has been suggested as the mechanism causing the bronchospasm (Lee *et al.*, 1983; McFadden, 1981), and in diabetic autonomic neuropathy there is a diminished bronchial reactivity to cold, possibly mediated through the vagus (Heaton *et al.*, 1984). If this was the case atropine, a parasympathetic blocker, would prevent the attacks, but it has been observed that atropine in fact interacts with the obstructive stimulus caused by exercise and moves the site of the obstruction from the large to the small airways (Deal *et al.*, 1978; McFadden, 1981). In addition, though the nocturnal increase in vagal tone has been suggested as a cause of nocturnal asthma (Barnes, 1984), vagal blocking had no effect on the overnight reduction in peak expiratory flow (Rhind *et al.*, 1985). However, atropine may have some effect in reducing the transport of fluid across the cells, and the decreased surface water thus caused would reduce the humidificating capabilities of the upper airways and transfer the evaporative heat loss to the smaller airways.

Since the secretion of fluid is an active process it is likely that there would be a delay in the onset of the increased fluid output in response to the cold stress and/or an overrun of increased fluid secretion after the increased respiratory heat loss had stopped. Certainly the productive cough following exercise in cold air precedes bronchospasm by many minutes (Juniper, 1980), and in exercise asthma, though the temperature of the airways returns to normal within five minutes of stopping exercise, the respiratory obstruction steadily worsens during this five minutes and takes 30 to 60 minutes to abate (McFadden, 1981). Similarly in divers breathing cold oxyhelium it was noted that though the pain and discomfort, caused by breathing the very cold gases, stopped as soon as the temperature of breathing mixture was raised, the bronchorrhoea persisted for 15 to 20 minutes (Hayes *et al.*, 1982). The facts suggest that bronchospasm and bronchorrhoea are both triggered by chemical mediators which can be secreted immediately the stimulus occurs but, because once secreted they are present in the tissues, the effect continues for some time after the stimulus has been removed until their degradation has taken place.

An interesting phenomenon is that after repeated bouts of exercise there is a refractory period during which further exercise fails to cause bronchospasm (Lee *et al.*, 1983; McFadden, 1981). Since Intal, sodium cromoglyolate, a mast cell stabiliser, usually abolishes exercise-induced asthma (Rees, 1984), it has been suggested that the post-exercise refractory period is due to mediator exhaustion (Lee *et al.*, 1983), but this explanation seems unlikely since repeated isocapnic hyperventilation does not produce a refractory period (McFadden, 1981) whereas repeated exercise, breathing warm humidified air, does result in a refractory period (Lee *et al.*, 1983). In other words, exercise is necessary for the development of the refractory period. The flow of fluid to the lining of the airways can be greatly enhanced by vagal stimulation and exposure to catecholamines and exercise produces cholinergic and sympathetic stimuli (Hartung *et al.*, 1984; Keatinge *et al.*, 1984; McFadden, 1983). Repeated exercise may therefore result in the pre-existing presence of such a high level of cholinergic and sympathetic activity that the fluid secretion increases immediately the next bout of exercise starts and the improved moisture exchange could prevent airway cooling.

Most bronchodilators are sympathomimetic agents and, though the traditional explanation for their mechanism of action is through relaxation of the bronchial smooth muscle, at least some of their effect may be through facilitation of the ion excretion from the cells lining the air passages with shrinkage of the cells as the water follows the ions into the air passages.

The disaster in Bhopal in India in 1984 may lead to some understanding of the chemical mediators involved. The victims of the methyl isocyanide gas developed dyspnoea first followed by a hypersecretion of bronchial secretions and people could drown in their own secretions. This could be due to the chemical triggering the tracheobronchial secretions with the dyspnoea caused by the initial swelling of the cells lining the airways. The clinical picture is remarkably similar to that described in divers when the rate of respiratory heat loss becomes excessive (Hayes, 1985).

Clinical Conditions

Asthma. When normal and asthmatic subjects perform the same tasks the calculated respiratory heat loss appears to be the same (Hodgson *et al.*, 1984) but there may be differences in response in the presence of acute or chronic inflammation or between various diseases (McFadden, 1983). Infection or inflammation is associated with swelling of the cells and, if the suggested hypothesis is correct, it becomes obvious that infection will worsen the clinical picture in asthma. This may explain why asthmatics become more sensitive to thermal stimuli as the underlying disease process worsens, with bronchospasm being caused by lesser degrees of cooling. Though it requires isocapnic hyperventilation with subfreezing air to produce a small but significant airflow obstruction in normal subjects (Deal *et al.*, 1980; McFadden, 1983; O'Cain *et al.*, 1980), if the person has an upper respiratory tract infection, the breathing of very cold air can cause respiratory obstruction but this response disappears as the infection clears (Horvath, 1981; McFadden, 1983; Rees, 1984).

The air temperature drops at night and most people keep the bedroom temperature lower than the rest of the house, and this, plus the fact that breathing warm humidified gas reduces nocturnal wheeze (Barnes, 1984), suggests that at least part of the problem in nocturnal asthma is due to respiratory heat loss.

Divers' Bronchorrhoea. Helium under pressure has a heat transfer capacity similar to that of water and, in divers breathing oxyhelium under pressure, the respiratory heat loss may at times exceed the heat loss from the body surface. Breathing oxyhelium therefore removes large quantities of heat from the respiratory tract and the physiological response to increased respiratory heat loss is the increased secretion of fluid into the airways. Unfortunately, in the case of oxyhelium, the major portion of the heat is lost through the direct warming of the cold helium with the evaporative heat loss being a much smaller proportion than under normal conditions. Because the respiratory mucosa is unable to differentiate between cooling due to evaporation and cooling due to direct heat loss, it responds to both with an increased secretion of tracheal fluid. Since the volume secreted is appropriate for the same total respiratory heat loss occurring under normobaric conditions, it is excessive for the particular situation found under hyperbaric conditions and therefore results in bronchorrhoea.

Other Phenomena. There are a number of clinical phenomena which can be understood in the light of the above hypothesis.

Exposure to a cold atmosphere sometimes causes a persistent dripping from the nose and this cold-weather rhinorrhoea is most noticeable when the person first comes into a warm room after having been out in the cold. A similar rhinorrhoea may occur in runners mouth breathing during a race in cold weather.

Some people develop a cough which can persist for an hour or more in the period immediately following vigorous exercise out of doors and this is more obvious in cold weather.

When a person is admitted to hospital he often complains of a dry stuffy nose, and sometimes patients also develop a dry cough. However, the air in a hospital is usually centrally heated and is therefore warmer than the outside or home environment and as it is warmed the relative humidity drops. Some of the clinical observations in the 'sick building syndrome' (Finnegan *et al.*, 1984) may also be related to this hypothesis.

Sub-acute Effects

Pulmonary Oedema (Excess Fluid in the Respiratory Tract)

Oedema has been considered one of the complications of hypothermia (Harnett *et al.*, 1983a) but though pulmonary oedema is a frequent complication in elderly individuals found in the hypothermic state, it is not clear whether pulmonary oedema is a consistent finding in acute immersion hypothermia.

Walther (1862) described oedema in the lungs of rabbits dying from hypothermia, and in experiments using dogs one out of eleven showed acute pulmonary oedema (Woodruff, 1941). In the Dachau experiments (Alexander, 1945) a great number of subjects showed a profuse oversecretion of mucus with vesicular foam at the mouth reminiscent of that seen in pulmonary oedema. However, there were no other definite clinical signs of pulmonary oedema and auscultation showed merely sharpening and impurity of breath sounds. This foaming at the mouth sometimes appeared as an early symptom at 32 to 35 °C body temperature and had no prognostic significance with regard to the fatal or non-fatal outcome of any one experiment. The terminal symptoms of a hypothermia victim on Mount Adams in 1966 included laboured breathing which produced a frothing foam at the mouth characteristic of pulmonary oedema and a pathologist found evidence of pulmonary haemorrhage and oedema in each of ten fatal cases of accidental hypothermia (Lathrop, 1972).

The diagnosis of pulmonary oedema is often made on very imprecise criteria and in fact is often used to denote fluid in the respiratory tract. It is, however, possible for there to be excess fluid through a number of mechanisms, as follows:

(1) Bronchorrhoea, i.e. an inappropriate excess production of bronchial secretions, has been discussed earlier but the clinical presentation may be misinterpreted and diagnosed as pulmonary oedema, or infection.

(2) There is another possible factor in the development of pulmonary oedema. The cilia lining the airways beat at a rate of approximately 1,000 to 1,500 times each minute and this causes the mucus to flow towards the glottis at the rate of approximately 10 to 20 mm/min (Cherniak *et al.*, 1972). The cilia are not influenced by nerve impulses but are very susceptible to chemical changes in the blood and ciliary action is depressed by cold (Best and Taylor, 1966), e.g. in a 0.2 mm diameter rat airway beat frequency was 13/s at 35 °C and 2/s at 20 °C (Irravni, 1967), and in the rabbit trachea 20/s at 37 °C and 7/s at 20 °C (Hakansson and Toremalm, 1965). Ciliary activity is also depressed if the temperature of the inspired air is below 30 °C (McDonald and Stocks, 1965; Watts, 1963) and the lower the core temperature the more likely that the air passing over the cilia will be below 30 °C.

The cilia are also affected by the humidity of the air. In rats, ciliary activity ceased completely when the humidity was reduced to 50 per cent (Dalhamm, 1956) and excised rabbit respiratory ciliary activity slowed to 8 per cent of normal in five to ten minutes after exposure to room air (Toremalm, 1901). In subjects breathing dry anaesthetic gas there were significant alterations in the ciliated respiratory epithelium after as short an interval as one hour whereas groups breathing 60 per cent humidified gas at room temperature and 100 per cent humidified gas at body temperature suffered no ill effects (Chalon *et al.*, 1972).

In the rescue situation the normal inspired air is cold and therefore also has a low relative humidity when warmed to body temperature and therefore the cilial activity is likely to be doubly depressed by the inspired air being both cold and dry. Therefore slowing of ciliary activity through cooling and/or drying of the respiratory mucosa could allow an accumulation of mucous secretions in the respiratory tree, presenting a clinical picture resembling pulmonary oedema.

(3) There is also a possible circulatory element. While an increase in pulmonary blood flow does not produce pulmonary oedema, nor does an increase in left atrial pressure cause pulmonary oedema at low flow rates, pulmonary oedema does occur if there is an increase in both left atrial pressure and an increase in pulmonary blood flow. The two factors are interrelated in that pulmonary oedema can be caused by either a moderately low flow rate if the atrial pressure is high or at a lower atrial pressure if the flow rate rises (Sniderman *et al.*, 1984). In normal circumstances, an increased left atrial pressure will be accompanied by an increased pulmonary blood volume, and it may be that the oedema is due primarily to the increased blood volume and not the left atrial pressure.

The pulmonary blood flow is increased by exercise (Sutton and Lassen, 1979), and, since cold exposure results in an increased oxygen demand similar to that caused by exercise, the same increase in pulmonary blood flow could be expected in cold exposure. Hypoxia, even if not severe, will also require increased flow rates. Hypoxia may occur if the environmental oxygen is low, as for example at altitude. However, a lack of oxygen-carrying capacity in the blood would have the same effect. This diminished capacity could be produced by anaemia or by a raised level of carbon monoxide in the blood, as is found in smokers (Harding and Mills, 1983), in exposure to heavy traffic fumes (Wright and Shephard, 1979) or if non-flued gas appliances are used in inadequately ventilated rooms.

Cold exposure causes peripheral vasoconstriction and the blood is accommodated in the pulmonary capacitance vessels (Harnett *et al.*, 1983a; Maclean and Emslie-Smith, 1977; Sutton and Lassen, 1979) and this would increase the pulmonary blood volume. Hypoxia also causes catecholamine release and an increased pulmonary blood volume (Sutton and Lassen, 1979; Mognoni and Lafortuna, 1985), and there is also an increase in the left ventricular afterload (Olsen *et al.*, 1983; Sutton and Lassen, 1979).

There are several clinical situations in which conditions could be such that an increase in pulmonary blood flow and increased pulmonary blood volume would occur together and produce 'pulmonary oedema'.

(4) Pulmonary oedema can also occur in cardiac failure.

Clinical Problems

High Altitude Pulmonary Oedema (HAPO). The risk factors for HAPO are a too rapid ascent to relatively hypoxic altitudes, indulgence in strenuous physical exercise at altitude, youth (Heath and Williams, 1981) (possibly because children are always active?), cold and anxiety (Coudert, 1985). Cold has the potential for causing, or contributing to, HAPO either through the circulatory or the respiratory mechanism.

In the circumstances of HAPO, exercise and hypoxia are present, and the resultant increase in pulmonary blood flow would be accentuated by the increased oxygen demand of any cold stress. The pulmonary blood volume would be increased by the vasoconstrictor response to cold, and the catecholamine release caused by cold (Maclean and Emslie-Smith, 1977; Weihl *et al.*, 1981), by hypoxia (Mognoni and Lafortuna, 1985) and by exercise (Coudert, 1985; Hartung *et al.*, 1984). (Interestingly norepinephrine is the only proven factor causing pulmonary vasoconstriction (Coudert, 1985).) The fact that HAPO occurs at lower altitudes (even less than 2,000 metres) if there is a unilateral absence of a pulmonary artery, and it occurs in the lung with the pulmonary artery (Hacket *et al.*, 1980), is further suggestive evidence of the flow/volume relationship in the causation of HAPO in that all the blood has to pass through only half the normal vascular volume.

In HAPO the pulmonary artery pressure rises before there is any oedema (Coudert, 1985). The fact that the inhalation of oxygen reverses the pulmonary arteriolar vasoconstriction at altitude (Coudert, 1985; Heath and Williams, 1981) does not eliminate the possible contribution from cold exposure (see later). Some cases of HAPO occur at night and this may be because sleep accentuates hypoxia (Coudert, 1985), but it should not be forgotten that the environment is usually colder at night and metabolic heat production is reduced while heat loss is increased.

There is also the possibility of a respiratory element in HAPO. Both hypoxia and exercise will markedly increase minute ventilation volumes and, since the humidity of the air is low at altitude and there is a drop in temperature (1 °C per 150 metres) (Heath and Williams, 1981) which will further reduce the moisture content of the air, the respiratory heat loss will be greatly increased. The person at high altitude is in fact faced with the three factors which will increase cooling of the respiratory tract, viz. cold air, dry air and hyperventilation (McFadden, 1983) and therefore the risk of excessive tracheobronchial secretions in susceptible people is increased. The dry, cold air will also be liable to impair ciliary activity, especially when associated with hyperventilation.

The typical symmetrical butterfly distribution of pulmonary oedema, seen frequently on X-ray in uraemia and left ventricular failure, are not seen in HAPO and basal horizontal lines and pleural effusion are rare, whereas in HAPO the appearances are of a coarse mottling which may occur in any area of either lung, though there are suggestions that it may appear first in the upper and middle lobe areas (Heath and Williams, 1981). The lung bases are usually unaffected on X-ray (Coudert, 1985). A further complicating factor is the observation that the reduction of the lung surfactant phospholipids produced by acute hypoxia is aggravated by the superimposition of cold. In addition the utilisation of surfactant is increased by hyperventilation (Kumar *et al.*, 1980). This might be a factor in producing the characteristic X-ray distribution of HAPO.

Freezing the Lungs. In severe exercise in extreme arctic conditions horses can develop 'frosting' of the lungs (Burton and Edholm, 1955; Schaefer *et al.*, 1980) and sled dogs can die showing signs of acute lung oedema (Schaefer *et al.*, 1980). Similarly many arctic hunters report having had episodes of 'freezing the lungs' which never occurred at rest but only when engaged in physical activity so demanding that the men would have to pant with open mouths because of air hunger (Schaefer *et al.*, 1980). The winter arctic air is very cold and is therefore very dry and any moisture will be present as microscopic ice crystals. In addition to warming and humidifying the inspired air the tracheobronchial tree will have the extra heat loss caused by the latent heat of the thawing of the ice crystals. The normal warming and humidifying system of the nasopharynx having been by-passed, the site of respiratory heat loss is moved into the major air passages and beyond. The most severe degree of airway cooling will occur when frigid, therefore dry, air is inhaled at high minute volumes (McFadden, 1983). In the special circumstances of the arctic winter, the hyperventilation of vigorous exercise might increase the heat loss to the level of 172 kcal/hour at which bronchorrhoea occurs (Hayes, 1985), providing a possible explanation for 'freezing the lungs'. The subjective sensations may have been similar to those experienced by the divers (Hayes *et al.*, 1982) and may have given rise to the name for the human condition. If a similar bronchorrhoea occurred in overdriven horses, the fluid reaching the pharynx might, in the very severe conditions in which it occurred, have frozen, hence 'frosting' of the lungs. Cold, hypoxia and exercise may also contribute to the pulmonary oedema through the pulmonary blood flow/volume interrelationship.

Respiratory Infection. Upper respiratory tract infections (URTI), bronchiolitis, sinusitis and otitis media are commonly found together in varying combinations and are likely to have similar aetiologies and all are more common in winter. It is usually assumed that the cause is an increased incidence and transmission of viral infections and this would be facilitated by the increased secretion of adrenocortical hormones during the winter months (Leppaluoto, 1984). Despite this increase in adrenocortical hormones, cold stress does not increase the risk of viral infection under controlled experimental transmission (Penttinen, 1982). However, the increased isolation of viruses in winter (Williams *et al.*, 1984) may be secondary to the cold-stimulated increase in circulating adrenocortical hormones. When a severe cold spell is prolonged for months the death rates falls and this is ascribed to a decrease in influenza infections (BMJ, 1980), though it is never explained how outdoor cold will kill viruses transmitted indoors by droplets. In fact most clinical cases are diagnosed as viral infection because of the lack of purulence in the secretions from the respiratory tract. There may therefore be other factors.

There is an increased incidence of the URTI disorders in the lower socioeconomic groups, even in the Mediterranean region (Gundersen and Havag, 1975). It is, however, unlikely that the three-fold greater incidence of infections in Greenland as compared with Denmark (Zachau-Christiansen, 1975) can be accounted for purely by the differences in the proportion of poor socioeconomic circumstances between the two countries and therefore cold must itself be a factor. In the epidemiology of URTI, it has been noticed that there is a geographic variation with the incidence rising in association with the cooling power of the climate as calculated from temperature and windspeed (Balsvik and Strass, 1975; Gundersen and Havag, 1975). In addition the incidence increases with increased environmental humidity (Gundersen and Havag, 1975), i.e. there is a direct relationship between the environmental cold stress and the incidence of URTI. Similarly the relationship with the low socioeconomic groups is possibly because they are the very groups who are likely to have housing problems, as discussed earlier, which cause increased cold stress in the home. The symptoms of acute URTI may therefore be due, at least in part, to the responses of the body to cold. If there is increased inappropriate respiratory secretions and swelling of the cells, this could mimic sinusitis and some of the bronchial signs and there could be a contribution from pulmonary oedema precipitated by a hyperdynamic, hypervolaemic pulmonary circulation as in HAPO. The fact that antibiotics are often given for URTI and the symptoms clear within a few days, as they may also do without antibiotics, may be totally unrelated to controlling infection or developing immunity but may be related to the time it takes the body to adjust to the circulatory and respiratory changes produced by sudden cold stress. It is relevant that it is during the first three days of exposure to cold that the venous pressure is raised (Wood *et al.*, 1958). Therefore the rate of change of cold stress may be more important in the aetiology of URTI than any absolute figures of temperature and the critical period may be three days.

There are a number of clinical observations which may support this idea:

(1) It has been said that if a viral respiratory infection does occur in winter the harmful effects are increased, especially in the old and the sick (Penttinen, 1982) but this would also be true if the 'viral infection' was merely the respiratory effects of cold as described above.
(2) Bronchopneumonia is a common finding in elderly people in cold circumstances and this may be due to a combination of cold-depressed ciliary activity or bronchorrhoea with or without a contribution from a hyperdynamic pulmonary circulation. Secondary opportunist infection may then occur.
(3) The mechanisms discussed above may have some bearing on the observations that even low-tar cigarettes caused respiratory symptoms in young smokers (Rimpela and Rimpela, 1985), and that infant respiratory morbidity was related to parental smoking and, to a lesser degree, to the use of gas for cooking and domestic heating (Ogston *et al.*, 1985).

There are important implications if indeed cold stress causes a large proportion of so-called 'respiratory infections' because recurrent respiratory infections and bronchiolitis result in reduced pulmonary function (Carson *et al.*, 1984), and reduced pulmonary function, a morning cough and decrease in social class are all risk factors for increased mortality (Hansen, 1977b). In one northern study the high proportion of young people with obstructive airways syndrome, i.e. a productive cough and a reduced FEV_1, could not be explained by smoking, and exposure to very low temperatures was considered to be a very important factor (Belleau *et al.*, 1984). The suggested similarity of mechanism between 'viral respiratory infection' and HAPO raises the possibility that 'viral respiratory infection' may also be accompanied by pulmonary hypertension which could be relevant in the aetiology of chronic bronchitis (see later).

The 'old wives' tale' that you will get a cold if you sit around in wet clothing or with wet feet, may be reflection that wet clothes or wet feet will increase the heat loss and, when houses are unheated in winter, this extra cold stress may trigger the cardiovascular and respiratory changes discussed above. Similarly it is part of folklore that a prolonged cold snap is needed to kill off the viruses. Since a severe cold spell is usually combined with calm, dry conditions, the cold stress will actually be less than in milder, wet and windy conditions. Another factor is that the human body adjusts to changes and therefore a prolonged cold spell would allow any circulatory/respiratory factors to become compensated. Rapid change affects the body more than slow change over the same absolute range — witness the fact that HAPO occurs not at an absolute altitude but in association with a too rapid ascent and too much exercise too soon, and similarly it is possible to cool a person to hypothermia without the person being aware or shivering, if this is done slowly.

Chronic Effects

A rise in pulmonary artery pressure (PAP) may be caused by hypoxia (Heath and Williams, 1981; Reeves *et al.*, 1979) but it may also be produced by cold stress (Bligh and Chauca, 1982) and the effects of the two stresses are additive (Coudert, 1985), even though the effector mechanisms are different (Bligh and Chauca, 1982). It has been suggested that the effect of hypoxia on PAP is through a local effect of oxygen partial pressure on the pulmonary vasculature, whereas the effect of cold involves peripheral sensor stimulation, the central nervous system and the efferent innervation of the pulmonary vasculature (Bligh and Chauca, 1978). The fact that cattle can develop pulmonary hypertension in winter at an altitude which has no effect on the PAP in summer, and this winter rise of PAP is reversed by the inhalation of oxygen (Bligh and Chauca, 1982; Will *et al.*,

1978) provides further support for the link between the two stresses. The rise in PAP caused by hypoxia is augmented by acidosis (Reeves *et al.*, 1979) and also by hypothermia (Benumof and Wahrenbrock, 1977). Exercise also accentuates the pulmonary vasoconstrictor effect of hypoxia (Coudert, 1985). In the light of the above observations, it is interesting that it has been claimed that noradrenaline is the only proven factor causing pulmonary vasoconstriction (Coudert, 1985), and noradrenaline secretion is raised by hypoxia (Mognoni and Lafortuna, 1985),in cold exposure (Goode and McDonald, 1982; Maclean and Emslie-Smith, 1977; Mager and Francesconi, 1983) and by exercise (Coudert, 1985; Hartung *et al.*, 1984).

From the evidence of the aetiology of systemic hypertension, where it is suggested that repeated or prolonged rises in pressure may eventually lead to a permanent hypertension (*Lancet*, 1982), it may be that repeated exposure to episodes of cold may have as much effect on PAP as continuous exposure to a greater severity of cold. There has, however, been no investigation into this question. It is of interest that the rise of PAP produced by acute hypoxia is promptly reversed by the relief of the hypoxia in contrast with the chronic picture. The difference is perhaps explained by the fact that the pulmonary arterioles become narrowed during acute hypoxia but become hypertrophied during chronic hypoxia (Reeves *et al.*, 1979).

Clinical Conditions

Monge's Disease or High Altitude Pulmonary Hypertension (HAPH). Though hypoxia is the prime precipitating factor in HAPH, 35 per cent oxygen given at altitude does not restore the PAP to normal despite providing an inspired oxygen tension equivalent almost to that at sea level (Heath *et al.*, 1968). However, on returning to sea level there is a logarithmic fall in PAP (Reeves and Grover, 1975), reaching normality after two years (Heath *et al.*, 1968). This may be due to increased barometric pressure, though one factor which has not been considered is the drop of temperature with altitude (Heath and Williams, 1981; Ward, 1975a); at 4,500 metres the temperature could be 30 °C lower than at sea level. The great diurnal variation in tropical mountains produces night temperatures significantly lower than the low daytime temperature in the shade, though there may be considerable heat input from the sun (Heath and Williams, 1981). These factors together with the likelihood of wind at altitude may result in an unexpectedly high rate of heat loss. Because of the lower temperatures and lower barometric pressures at altitude the water vapour content of the air is very low (Heath and Williams, 1981) and this along with the hyperventilation at altitude causes a very high respiratory water, and therefore heat, loss. In fact the respiratory moisture loss at altitude may be sufficient to cause dehydration (Heath and Williams, 1981). Any factor which increases cold stress increases oxygen needs and will therefore act indirectly by aggravating any existing hypoxia. Vigorous anaerobic exercise will normally cause a metabolic acidosis and the lower the oxygen tension of the air the lower the intensity at which exercise will be anaerobic. Up to an altitude of 5,000 metres the quantity of lactate produced after maximum exertion is the same as at sea level (Cerretelli and di Prampero, 1985). However, the hyperventilation caused by hypoxia causes a severe respiratory alkalosis which is still present on exercise (Heath and Williams, 1981). Though the amount of lactate produced in response to maximal exertion at altitudes over 5,000 metres is reduced in proportion to the reduction in buffer capacity (Cerretelli and di Prampero, 1985), there is a long delay (8 to 20 minutes) after the exertion before the lactate levels start dropping (Cerretelli and di Prampero, 1985). Despite the initial relatively low levels of lactate after exercise, the delayed metabolism might cause as much problem with the PAP as higher levels present for shorter durations. There is the added complicating factor that at extremely high altitudes the renal excretion of bicarbonate is slowed and therefore the reduction in base excess is much less than predicted (West, 1984). The homeostatic mechanisms of the body try to produce compensatory changes for any alteration in acid/base status and, at moderate altitudes, there is therefore likely to be a build-up of acid metabolites which, because of the degree of respiratory alkalosis, may be at a higher absolute level than during the metabolic acidosis induced by moderate exercise at sea level. Any vigorous exertion at altitude will almost of necessity require anaerobic metabolism and therefore a further accumulation of the metabolic (fixed) acids. At altitude therefore hypoxia, exercise, cold stress and a variable, but consistently raised, level of fixed acids might all contribute to the raised PAP, and the contribution from increased noradrenaline secretions must also be considered. The hypoventilation present at the onset of sleep will aggravate the hypoxia of altitude and can produce a marked arterial desaturation during sleep at altitude (Coudert, 1985; Sutton and Lassen, 1979). Return to sea level might act through the reduction in the environmental cold stress and the respiratory heat loss as well as through the restoration of oxygenation. The lower diurnal variation of temperature at sea level may also be important. Return to sea level will also restore the acid/base status to normal with a reduction in the circulating level of the fixed acids, and the higher ambient oxygen tension will mean that more vigorous exercise can be undertaken without a metabolic acidosis developing.

Eskimo Lung. In the Arctic many middle-aged and elderly Inuit develop progressive pulmonary hypertension with a progressive decrease in maximum mid-expiratory flow and the end result of 'Eskimo lung' is death from right-sided heart failure (Schaefer *et al.*, 1980). Since most Eskimos live at or near sea level there is no question of high altitude hypoxia being a contributory cause. TB, bronchiectasis and inhaled dust from soapstone carving were eliminated as being prime predisposing factors (Schaefer *et al.*, 1980). Repeated viral respiratory tract infections in infancy and early childhood have been suggested as a cause (Rode and Shephard, 1984) and though this point was examined and considered not to be a factor (Schaefer *et al.*, 1980), both views may be correct if the relationship between cold stress and 'viral respiratory infections' considered earlier is correct. Smoking certainly caused respiratory impairment but poor respiratory function cannot be attributed purely to smoking (Rode and Shephard, 1984) and the worst ventilatory function was amongst the north-eastern arctic Inuit aged 40 to 80 years who did not smoke or only smoked lightly (Schaefer *et al.*, 1980). These Inuit had been hunters and trappers when young and the work had involved repeated episodes of hard physical work even during the severe cold of winter. Similar respiratory problems were noted among elderly white trappers, whose mode of work when young had been similar to that of the Inuit trappers, and among native and immigrant Russian workers engaged for long periods in hard physical work while exposed to extreme temperatures in Siberia (Schaefer *et al.*, 1980). The fact that Inuit women and Inuit men who did little hunting in winter were relatively free of Eskimo lung confirmed the causative effect of severe cold and heavy exercise (Schaefer *et al.*, 1980).

The environment for winter hunting in the Arctic will inevitably include severe cold and in these circumstances, even without muscular work, there is a tendency towards acidosis (Alexander, 1979), which would augment any rise in PAP due to the cold (Bligh and Chauca, 1982). If the cold exposure is very severe the oxygen available in the air may be marginally sufficient for the needs of heat production (mimicking the situation at high altitude), and vigorous muscular exercise, as would occur during hunting, by taking priority over the needs of heat production, could lead to unexpected and unsuspected lowering of the body temperature (Hirvonen, 1982), in addition to a metabolic acidosis. Both factors would aggravate any rise of PAP and it is likely from the circumstances that the hunter would be exposed to the severe systemic and respiratory cold stress for some time after the severe exertion. Recurrent episodes of exertion by repeatedly boosting the cold-induced pulmonary hypertension may result in a permanent elevation of the PAP. It is interesting that patients with Eskimo lung claimed that they were very much more sensitive to cold after one or more specific events (Schaefer *et al.*, 1980). The high PAP once present may be steadily progressive or may be boosted by subsequent winter hunting expeditions but whatever the mechanism Eskimo lung becomes established. The raised levels of noradrenaline during cold exposure would tend to cause the problem to persist. Many, but not all, arctic hunters related their respiratory problems to distinctly remembered episodes of 'freezing the lungs' while out hunting and, if 'freezing the lungs' is a type of cold-induced bronchorrhoea, there would be an almost inevitable secondary hypoxaemia and this would accelerate the onset of Eskimo lung.

One case, in which severe pulmonary damage was attributed to cold (Houk, 1959), occurred in the Antarctic with a temperature lower than −55 °C but, since it occurred at an altitude of 3,000 metres, the cause of the pulmonary damage was disputed and blamed on HAPO (Miller, 1974). From the evidence given above, altitude and cold may both have played a part.

Chronic Bronchitis. Though patients, homozygous for the gene producing the enzyme Alpha-1-protease inhibitor, have a 70 to 80 per cent chance of developing chronic bronchitis and emphysema, these only account for 1 per cent of patients presenting with chronic bronchitis at clinics (Snider, 1981). Nor can infection be the complete answer since in one study neither viral nor bacterial infections were identified in approximately 50 per cent of exacerbations (McHardy *et al.*, 1980).

It has been noted that the pulmonary vascular pathology in chronic bronchitis and emphysema is identical to that in Monge's disease (HAPH) and all differ from the pathological changes of pulmonary hypertension associated with cardiac shunts or left atrial hypertrophy

(Heath *et al.*, 1968). Therefore the pulmonary vascular changes in chronic bronchitis and emphysema appear to fit those of a disease produced by hypoxia though, since the pathological changes in Eskimo lung are also similar, the contribution of cold should not be overlooked.

Smoking causes hypoxia through increased carboxyhaemoglobin (COHb) levels (Calverley *et al.*, 1982) and this may affect non-smokers in inadequately ventilated rooms (Wright and Shephard, 1979). In fact the established heavy smoker is living with a hypoxia equivalent to that found at an altitude of several thousand feet (Harding and Mills, 1983). Similarly a high car density increases the COHb levels affecting particularly males who work in or drive through polluted areas (Wright and Shephard, 1979) and this association with the resulting hypoxic stimulus may partially account for the major areas of mortality from chronic bronchitis in the UK being in large conurbations (Howe, 1972). In the established condition long-continued supplementary oxygen improves survival and may slow the rise (MRC, 1981; Rees, 1984) or may sometimes lower the PAP, i.e. improved oxygenation lowers but rarely completely reverses the raised PAP. Long-term oxygen may also act on the main pulmonary artery by reducing the high circulating level of noradrenaline (Haneda *et al.*, 1983). This is an interesting suggestion in the light of the many factors discussed earlier which increase noradrenaline secretion, and the claim that noradrenaline is the only proven factor causing pulmonary vasoconstriction (Coudert, 1985).

During sleep even normal people can have periods of apnoea of at least ten seconds up to ten times a night and, in some, these periods may be longer and more frequent, producing severe hypoxia and a rise in PAP (Apps, 1983; *Lancet*, 1979). In addition the onset of sleep is normally associated with slight alveolar hypoventilation and carbon dioxide retention (Phillipson, 1978) and therefore respiratory acidosis (Trilapur, 1984), and in fact the greatest number of nocturnal deaths among patients with chronic bronchitis and emphysema occur in the first hour of the night (McNicholas and Fitzgerald, 1984). This nocturnal increase in deaths could, however, be prevented by low flow oxygen (McNicholas and Fitzgerald, 1984).

However, hypoxia alone cannot explain the increased incidence of acute exacerbations of chronic bronchitis which occur during the winter as compared with the summer months. This must be related to increased cold stress despite there being no observed association between exacerbations of chronic bronchitis and outside air temperature or wind velocity (McHardy *et al.*, 1980). Because the rate of heat loss is more dependent on wind and humidity than on absolute temperature, there is often a dangerous degree of heat loss on relatively mild winter days. The respiratory heat loss is also increased in winter because, despite the high relative humidity, the total volume of water in vapour form is lower than in summer (Howe, 1972). The mechanism of an exacerbation in winter may in fact be related to the respiratory or circulatory factors discussed earlier under the heading 'Respiratory Infections' (see page 121).

The bedroom is usually the coldest room in the house and in poor-quality housing it may not only be very cold but damp as well. Temperature receptors in the upper airways and perinasal area produce an inhibition of ventilation which is more marked at low ambient temperatures and they also decrease the subjective sense of dyspnoea in the cold (Burgess and Whitelaw, 1984). Therefore in a cold bedroom there is a decreased respiratory drive at a time when there is an increased oxygen requirement. Cold on the face may produce apnoea (Horvath, 1981) and this will accentuate the problem. During the first onset of sleep even the bed is at its coldest which unfortunately coincides with the period of hypoventilation. This would add the pulmonary vasoconstrictive effect of cold stress to that of sleep apnoeic hypoxia. Unfortunately the bronchitics who have the lowest arterial oxygen tensions during the day have the greatest drop in arterial oxygen tension at night (Stradling and Lane, 1983). Between 1 and 5 a.m. there is evidence of arrhythmogenic ECG changes in patients with chronic bronchitis and emphysema (Tirlapur, 1984) and therefore some of the deaths may be due to a cardiac arrhythmia. However, any factor which increases oxygen demand or depresses the respiratory drive will increase the risk of hypoxia and arrhythmias, and environmental cold itself increases oxygen demand (Burton and Edholm, 1955; Harding and Mills, 1983).

The marked increases in mortality from bronchitis with decreasing social class (DHSS, 1976) may be partly due to differences in the domestic and working environment, e.g. social class 5 especially in large towns are more likely than class 1 to have inadequately heated and damp houses, to work in colder environments even if indoors and to be doing work physically hard enough to produce a metabolic acidosis. Exercise and exposure to cold both cause an increased oxygen requirement (Harding and Mills, 1983; Horvath, 1981), and exercise will accentuate any hypoxia-induced rise in PAP (Coudert, 1985).

In the social and geographic epidemiology of chronic bronchitis there are many factors which could contribute to hypoxia through an increased oxygen demand or a depressed respiratory drive, and there is also a marked possibility of cold stress and respiratory or metabolic acidosis. In the aetiology of any individual case of chronic bronchitis it might therefore be worth evaluating the possible contributions from hypoxia (smoking, traffic fumes or sleep apnoea), environmental cold stress, at home or work, and exertion-induced acidosis. By doing this an explanation may be found for the social class difference in urban mortality from chronic bronchitis and the low incidence in farm workers and it may be possible to tailor therapy more closely to the individual.

Sudden Infant Death Syndrome (SIDS). The definition of SIDS is 'the sudden death of an infant which is unexpected by history, and in which a thorough post mortem examination reveals no adequate cause of death' (Beckwith, 1970, cited in Deacon and Williams, 1982). The old name for SIDS was 'smothering' which suggested that the child had been suffocated accidentally or deliberately by the mother, but this does not fit the facts in any but an infinitesimal minority. If the baby was found dead in bed beside its mother it was reckoned that the mother had 'overlaid' her baby during her movements during sleep. There is absolutely no evidence to support this, and in fact it is known that, when a child is in bed with the mother, the sleeping movements of the mother are minimal.

Many explanations have been advanced for SIDS and it is now becoming clear that there is no one aetiology. In fact, with improvements in pathological diagnosis, many cases which were previously considered to be SIDS now have other diagnoses attached. Suggested aetiologies for SIDS have included Legionellosis (Nigro *et al.*, 1983), malignant hyperthermia (Harriman and Ellis, 1983) and overheating (Stanton, 1982).

It has also been suggested that SIDS is a result of viral respiratory infection (Deacon and Williams, 1982). This, however, cannot be the whole answer since there are very low rates of SIDS reported from Stockholm, Copenhagen, the Netherlands and Middle Bohemia (Deacon and Williams, 1982) and there is no evidence of a reduced risk of respiratory infection in these areas. In fact viruses were found in only 200 of 763 cases of SIDS and there was a similar distribution in live controls (Williams *et al.*, 1984). Even when there is positive bacteriological or viral isolation there may be no histological evidence of even minor infection (Bain and Bartholemew, 1985).

Neonates often have periods of apnoea during sleep, and it is therefore tempting to suggest that SIDS may be due to the apnoeic episode being so prolonged as to precipitate cardiac asystole. Certainly prolonged apnoea is the most favoured aetiological cause, and it has been suggested that the apnoea may be precipitated by epilepsy, stridor, aspiration or heart disease (Stanton, 1982), or by infection, especially with respiratory syncitial virus and the influenza and para influenza viruses (Williams *et al.*, 1984). Another possible mechanism for precipitating apnoea is from gastro-oesophageal reflux, common in babies, which may trigger laryngospasm and apnoea (Barrie, 1983). However, even positive evidence of inhalation is not proof since this may occur during resuscitation (Bain and Bartholemew, 1985). It has been postulated that the mechanism is a manifestation of the 'diving reflex' (Elsner and Gooden, 1983; *Lancet*, 1981) in which the laryngeal stimulation may trigger a reflex apnoea and bradycardia which may be prolonged enough to cause death. It has also been suggested that repeated episodes of sleep apnoea, or apnoea from other causes, by producing repeated alveolar hypoxia, could, through repeated stimulation of pulmonary vasoconstriction, gradually result in hyperplasia of the pulmonary vascular smooth muscle, and in fact pulmonary vascular hyperplasia is reported at necropsy in many cases (Powell *et al.*, 1983; Shannon and Kelly, 1982). It is not possible to be sure how much of this hyperplasia is a remnant of the neonatal state, though the repeated alveolar hypoxia might cause the hyperplasia to persist and even become more marked.

Despite the presumed aetiological importance of apnoeic episodes, the occurrence of SIDS could not be predicted by the measurement of the longest episode of central apnoea. Nor have predictive results been found from monitoring the EEG (Lacey, 1983), ECG patterns (Southall *et al.*, 1983), or respiratory or heart rate patterns (Wilson *et al.*, 1985). In fact, though apnoea monitors are supplied for home use, the indications for their use are very imprecise, and while their presence will comfort some parents, it has not yet been shown that they save lives (Bain and Bartholemew, 1985; Simpson, 1983). Episodes of prolonged apnoea are sometimes detected after a near-miss episode of SIDS and may be a consequence of the episode rather than the cause (Southall *et al.*, 1983), though the fright of the episode may result in note being taken of previously ignored apnoeic episodes.

The fact that some twins, homozygous and dizygous, died on the same day (Powell *et al.*, 1983) suggests that environmental factors may be important, though the twin sibling is sometimes unaffected (Bain and Bartholemew, 1985). One point, which none of the above theories can explain, is the seasonal variation in the occurrence of SIDS with an increased incidence in premature babies and during the winter months (Bain and Bartholemew, 1985; Elsner and Gooden, 1983; Froggat *et al.*, 1971; Powell *et al.*, 1983; Stanton, 1982). The one fact about winter is that temperatures are at their lowest of the year and there is an association between low temperature environments and SIDS (Bonser *et al.*, 1978; Deacon and Williams, 1982). However, the seasonal increase in winter is not related to temperature alone. It was found that there is a greater incidence in cold-wet weather than in cold-dry weather and this relationship was true for Australia, New Zealand, Canada and the UK (Deacon and Williams, 1982). Therefore the relationship is with the severity of the total cold stress. Babies have a low body weight, a large body surface/body weight ratio and their heads are large in proportion to the rest of the body and will therefore be a more significant route for heat loss than in an adult. Babies also tend to be inactive during the first few months and spend a lot of time asleep. Therefore an environment which may be comfortable for an adult may in fact be causing cold stress for the baby.

In the neonate, exposure to cold may result in an increased metabolic acidosis (Gandy *et al.*, 1964), increased oxygen consumption (Darnall and Ariagno, 1978) and sometimes a lower arterial oxygen tension (Stephenson *et al.*, 1970), and these effects may persist beyond the immediate neonatal period. In winter therefore the neonate and small baby may be subjected to the same three stress factors — environmental cold, alveolar hypoxia and metabolic acidosis — which have been shown to be associated with pulmonary hypertension in adult disorders.

There is a syndrome called persistent pulmonary hypertension of the newborn (PPHN) and this is associated with a high mortality (50 per cent) and morbidity. If the child can be successfully treated the pulmonary vascular abnormality regresses with time and there is no residual cardiac abnormality (Bernbaum *et al.*, 1984). The recommended treatment is to ventilate the baby with 100 per cent oxygen at high ventilatory rates and high pressures, sufficient to produce a hypocarbic alkalosis (Bernbaum *et al.*, 1984). These measures would reverse hypoxia and compensate for any metabolic acidosis and, because the treatment would have to be done in hospital, the environment would be warm and the oxygen would be warmed and humidified, thus counteracting the three factors known to cause a rise in PAP. It may be that some cases of SIDS are the same syndrome as PPHN which have not been recognised, and it is interesting that the only feature found to have a predictive value for SIDS death was a higher than normal pulse rate (Wilson *et al.*, 1985), which may be a reflection of pulmonary hypertension.

There are a number of risk factors which have been shown to be associated with SIDS though none appear to be absolute:

(1) The majority of cases of SIDS occurred among infants who were normal at birth with regard to weight and gestation (Bain and Bartholemew, 1985). Pre-term delivery or low birth weight (Powell *et al.*, 1983), however, appears to result in increased risk. In these infants the subcutaneous layer of fat is usually undeveloped and there is a greater surface area to body weight ratio than in the normal baby. Both of these points will increase the tendency to heat loss and will raise the temperature necessary for thermoneutrality. These infants may be suffering from cold stress at temperatures which do not affect adults or normal children.

(2) The babies who showed a poor weight gain and were therefore considered to have average or poor nutrition had an increased risk (Powell *et al.*, 1983). The poor weight gain may indeed be due to inadequate nutrition and in adults (Howitt, 1971) and children (Paton, 1983) malnutrition is known to increase the risk of hypothermia even in relatively mild climates (Paton, 1983b; Sadikali and Owor, 1974) and therefore undernourished babies would again have an increased susceptibility to cold stress. The failure to gain weight may, however, be a secondary phenomenon. If the baby is exposed to increased cold stress, a higher than normal proportion of an adequate food intake may have to be catabolised to maintain thermal equilibrium, and therefore failure to gain weight may be an indicator of excessive cold stress (Briend and de Schampheleire, 1981). It is of interest that, though epidemiological studies suggested an association between child abuse and SIDS, a study found that not only was there no increase in the incidence of psychiatric or emotional disturbances or problems among the mothers of SIDS victims, but the only risk factor recognisable at birth for child abuse which was also a risk factor for SIDS was a concern about the maternal ability to care for and especially feed the baby (Roberts *et al.*, 1984). In most cases there was a good standard of mothering and there is no detectable

differences in families to suggest who might suffer SIDS until the tragedy strikes (Bain and Bartholemew, 1985).

(3) Though SIDS can affect all social classes (Bain and Bartholemew, 1985), there is an association with socioeconomic factors (Powell *et al.*, 1983; Williams *et al.*, 1984). The social factors which increase the risk include poverty, an unmarried mother, parent under 20 and social class 5, and in all these cases finance is almost certainly a problem. One solution is likely to be to reduce the level of heating in the house and, though an adult may not suffer, a small child may unintentionally be exposed to cold stress. The fact that the child is probably in the bedroom (traditionally the coldest room along with the bathroom) for a greater proportion of the 24 hours than is an adult merely compounds the problem. As discussed for chronic bronchitis, a cold room decreases ventilatory drive through receptors in the upper airways and perinasal region (Burgess and Whitelaw, 1984) while increasing the oxygen requirement and cold on the face may cause apnoea (Horvath, 1981), thus possibly exaggerating apnoeic episodes. Cold may also act by stimulating receptors in the nose and on the face which exaggerate any bradycardia produced through the 'diving reflex', and this response is most noticeable in premature babies who also have a diminished response to carbon dioxide (Elsner and Gooden, 1983). It is therefore possible that the very low incidence of SIDS in Stockholm, Copenhagen, Middle Bohemia and the Netherlands (Deacon and Williams, 1982) may be because housing and tradition keep the baby warmer.

(4) There is an association with respiratory infection (Deacon and Williams, 1982; Williams *et al.*, 1984). This was suggested on the grounds that (a) there is an increased incidence of both SIDS and respiratory infections in winter; (b) there is an increase in SIDS during outbreaks of influenza; (c) there is an associated increased incidence of SIDS at the same time as there is an increased isolation of respiratory syncitial virus and attacks of bronchiolitis; (d) there is an increased incidence of respiratory infection in problem families which also have an increased incidence of SIDS; (e) 53 per cent of families thought that the baby had suffered colds or snuffles in the period up to three weeks before the death, 27 per cent reported these symptoms in the last two days of life and 25 per cent in the interval between three weeks and two days (Bain and Bartholemew, 1985). However, 21 per cent of families reported no respiratory symptoms (Bain and Bartholemew, 1985), and, in a direct comparison with age-matched live infants, no differences were noted in the health of

the two groups (Bain and Bartholemew, 1985). As discussed earlier, a cold stress environment may increase the risk of apparent respiratory infection, i.e. when a clinical diagnosis is made of acute respiratory infection or bronchiolitis, the symptoms may in fact be due to physiological/pathological changes produced by cold stress. The increased isolation of viruses may be due to the increased circulating level of adrenocortical hormones found in winter (Leppaluoto, 1984).

Hypothermia is another possible cause of SIDS because in infants the colour usually remains a healthy pink during the development of hypothermia. Many, if not all, of the environmental factors discussed as possibly contributing to SIDS through pulmonary hypertension would obviously also apply to the development of hypothermia and possible 'cot death', and it is of interest that hypothermia itself also causes a rise in pulmonary artery pressure (Benumof and Wahrenbrock, 1977).

If hypothermia or cold-induced pulmonary hypertension are indeed common causes of SIDS, it is easy to understand the observation that previous near-miss SIDS rarely continue to definite SIDS (Stanton, 1982) since the family is likely to keep the environment warmer, even if accidentally, e.g. by having the baby in the same room as the adults for most or all of the 24 hours. The early epidemiological finding that many of these cases occurred in babies who were in bed with their mothers can be understood because the mothers had taken them into bed for warmth in a cold bedroom — a solution advocated for small babies on cold nights in Africa (Briend and de Schampheleire, 1981).

13 EFFECTS OF COLD STRESS ON CEREBRAL FUNCTION

General

There is an ideal environment of temperature and humidity for the performance of mental tasks, and an increase in cold stress causes a decrease in performance (Enander, 1984). There is also an inverse relationship between cold discomfort and work rate (Enander, 1984).

Experimental data on the effects of cold are limited but there are a number of factors which make assessment of experimental work difficult. Cold causes apathy (Enander, 1984) and distracts the person from the test (Teichner, 1958; Vaughan, 1977). Cold on the skin also produces discomfort but this has an arousal effect which is sensitive to the interaction between core and skin temperatures. However, the end effect is to impair the results in certain tests (Enander, 1984). Performance in the cold is task dependent and is also affected by familiarity with the cold (?acclimation) and by the level of anxiety (Enander, 1984), and finally, well-motivated subjects can remain cognitively unimpaired even though the core temperature has dropped (Baddeley *et al.*, 1975).

Cold (hypothermia) causes a decrease in word recognition ability (Davis *et al.*, 1975) and if the cold stress is by immersion there is also an impairment in other tests (Davis *et al.*, 1975) as well as an impairment of memory, especially recent (Coleshaw *et al.*, 1983). The speed of reasoning is slowed by a low body temperature but remains accurate (Coleshaw *et al.*, 1983). Powers of judgement are also affeted by cold stress (Baddeley, 1966).

Early work with target-finding tests suggested that the speed of mental reaction is markedly affected by cold with considerable and progressive impairment of efficiency. The immediate major impairment is followed by a gradual recovery of efficiency with the passage of time but, if the cold stress is continued, the final level of performance is lower than in a non-cold environment (Teichner and Kobrich, 1955). However, other studies indicated that reaction times were little affected down to ambient temperatures of −37 °C (Enander, 1984; Teichner, 1958). The discrepancy may be due to the distracting effect of the pain and stress caused by the cold (Enander,

1984), to the fact that rapid cooling produces effects which are not seen with slow cooling (Ellis *et al.*, 1985), or possibly because in the first studies there was some degree of whole body cooling.

Poulton *et al.* (1965) studied the effects of cold, particularly wet cold, on the vigilance of lookouts and after exposure for periods as short as half an hour to temperature conditions approximating to those of the Arctic (−2 °C to 0 °C) visual perception efficiency was adversely affected by 25 to 30 per cent. The additional chill factor of wind (20 to 30 knots) and wet from rain or spray reduced visual efficiency by as much as 50 per cent even at higher ambient temperatures (2 °C to 5 °C). Some of this effect may have been due to the cold-induced apathy (Enander, 1984). Even sleeping in the cold caused a decrease in vigilance performance. Reaction times were also impaired by sleeping in the cold, and remained impaired, whereas detection performance after the initial impairment showed some improvement with time. It has been suggested that the impairment is due to a decrease in the proportion of Rapid Eye Movement (REM) sleep (Buguet *et al.*, 1979b) and certainly performances were worse after a very cold night, during which the REM sleep deprivation increased (Angus *et al.*, 1979).

If the mean skin temperature falls, as well as causing discomfort, it has the effect of affecting the estimation of the passage of time (Fox, 1967; Lockhart, 1960), and Baddeley (1966), studying time estimation in cold immersion work with scuba divers, showed that the ability to judge or estimate the passage of time was significantly affected by cold, resulting in slow time counts and underestimates of elapsed time.

Obviously the extent of the insidious effects of cold on the powers of judgement and other mental functions must be of vital importance in all situations where cold environment and mental reactions are both of significance as for example in diving. It is, however, difficult to establish the relationship between deep body cooling and performance (Baddeley *et al.*, 1975; Biersner, 1976; Davis *et al.*, 1975; Fox, 1967; Vaughan, 1977). Despite this, it has been claimed that cold is the most important factor in North Sea diving accidents (Rawlins, 1981) and, even in a relatively warm sea off the American coast, the death of a diver in the Sealab 3 experiment has been assessed as being due to cold having impaired the vigilance and performance of the diver (Booda, 1973; Rawlins, 1981).

Mistakes Due to Cold Stress

As long ago as 1939 it was observed in factories that the incidence of injury due to accidents was less at an environmental temperature of 18 °C than at higher or lower temperatures (Vernon, 1939) and the increase at lower temperatures was attributed to loss of manual dexterity (Goldsmith and Minard, 1976). In the construction industry as well, cold weather causes an increased incidence of accidents and a drop in work output (Taylor, 1975). However, when 100 fatal accidents in the construction industry were examined and analysed (Health and Safety Executive, 1978) no attempt was made to include a consideration of cold as a factor and not even the time of year was given.

Among workers in a cold store Andrew (1963) has detected low-grade euphoria, personal irritability and a reduction in the ability to concentrate, and in a similar environment silly errors, clerical, verbal and mechanical, have also been observed (Watt, J., personal communication). Errors certainly increase during cold exposure (Enander, 1984; Teichner, 1958). There are many tests of mental function, and a test has been developed (Ellis, 1982) specifically for assessing mental function during mild cooling, but it may be difficult to apply this in severe cold environments, such as cold stores, which produce particular technical problems. A typical cold room is kept at −30 °C to −40 °C and there is an additional cold stress of a wind produced by a fan circulating the air. Tests requiring prolonged writing are not possible due to the risk of frostbite, and verbal tests suffer from the disadvantage that if the subject is affected by the cold the tester is likely to be similarly affected. To overcome this problem the tests can be recorded on tape and transcribed for study in thermal comfort. In an unpublished pilot study this system was used to try to identify tests which could be used later in a definitive study, though the noise from the fan interfered with the recording. The only test which gave reproducible results was for the subject to name as many different objects as possible from a selected group in a time limit of 30 seconds. The groups used were flowers, towns, countries, surnames, trees and rivers, each given 30 seconds. If an object was repeated during the 30 seconds this was considered an error as was dysarthria and an obviously wrong object, e.g. New York for a flower. It was found that the number of errors increased in the cold stress as compared with control values in ambient conditions, the impairment becoming obvious in the range of total body heat debt of −3.5 per cent to −7 per cent of the pre-test total body heat values. The subject was unaware of the drop in performance, often thinking that he had done particularly well when in fact the results showed the greatest impairment. It is recognised that a person developing hypothermia is unaware of the development of mental impairment (Hamilton, 1980).

Hallucinations in Cold Stress

Introduction

Exposure to cold produces indications of psychological stress (Armstrong, 1936; Armstrong and Heim, 1940; Payne, 1959) and it is recognised that changes in personality and hallucinations are a sign of incipient hypothermia among climbers (Ogilvie, 1977) and may be a sign of hypothermia in the elderly (Kurtz, 1982). If hallucinations are an important effect of pre-hypothermic cold stress, there should be case reports from cold environments.

Mountain regions are often cold but cold exposure can be a problem even when the mountains are neither very high nor very northerly. For example the hills of Scotland are low and in a temperate zone of the world. Nevertheless the tree line is lower in Scotland than in Norway and the presence of arctic vegetation and wildlife on many of the hills suggests that there is more cold stress on the Scottish hills than would be expected from their low absolute altitude.

Cold water immersion is another cold stressor but, unless the person is in a warm part of the world, he is likely to succumb to hypothermia before rescuers arrive and therefore any hallucinations would remain unreported. However, people in small boats or on life rafts are liable to cold stress from spray and wind-chill but are likely to survive longer and therefore have a better chance of rescue alive, with the possibility of reporting any hallucinations which may have occurred.

Case Report

Case 1. (Clarke, 1976). On 24th September, 1975, after a 14 hour climb to the summit of Everest, Doug Scott and Dougal Haston had to make an unplanned bivouac on the way down in a snow hole at 28,600 feet with a still air temperature of −35 °C. During the night they both hallucinated that there was a third person in the snow hole and this was the supplies officer at base camp, the one person who would have had available the equipment such as sleeping bags, food and oxygen needed to make the night safer and more bearable.

Case 2. (Steele, 1972). Also on Mount Everest, Bill Kurban, inadequately dressed, climbed in a hurry to Camp 3 and repaired a radio aerial before being taken into a tent suffering from the cold. After being settled for a while, he said, 'I want a pee', and, though he was advised to do it through the tent flap, he insisted on going outside and nearly fell down 1,000 feet of ice. During the night Kurban's behaviour and conversation were irrational, possibly the result of hallucinations as to where he was. In the morning on the way down he did not use his safety wire and he also claimed that he could see men lying in the *bergschrund*.

Case 3. (Schell, 1978). Two people, dressed only for a day's skiing, fell into a crevasse on the Matterhorn in February 1976. During the second night the man, who was the less well clad of the two, began to hallucinate — 'Look! There is a lift with people going up. Let's take it!' On the third night the woman hallucinated that a cable-car attendant was flashing a light into their hole telling her that rescue would come in the morning, though rescue did not come until the fifth day.

The low hills of Scotland abound in tales of 'sightings' (McOwan, 1979) and in fact many place names incorporate the Gaelic word for fairy (*sidh*, pronounced see), e.g. Glen Shee, Ben Tee, Ben Shee. Over the centuries, sightings or hallucinations have been reported by people in the Cairngorm mountains (McOwan, 1985) but probably the most famous tale from this area is the legend of the Big Grey Man of Ben Macdhui.

Case 4. (Gray, 1970; McOwan, 1979). In 1891 an experienced mountaineer Professor Collie (Organic Chemistry, University of London) was returning in a mist from the summit of Ben Macdhui when he heard the crunch of footsteps behind him. These only occurred when he was walking and one for every three or four steps of his own. He looked around but could see no-one and this caused such a terror that he ran four or five miles in panic. When he told this story the legend of the Big Grey Man of Ben Macdhui was born.

Case 5. (Gray, 1970). A man investigating the phenomenon of the Grey Man was spending a very cold January night alone beside Ben

Macdhui's cairn. Immediately after going to bed he had a strange state of mind, being aware of the cold and feeling some sense of terror. He fell asleep and then woke up with a sense of very severe fear. When something brown blurred the edge of a moon beam, panic reactions took over but when these passed he got up and looked outside. He saw a great brown hairy creature which he estimated to be at least 20 feet in height. In the morning there were no footprints.

Case 6. (Vanggaard, L., personal communication, 1982). Two members of the Danish military sledge patrol, 'Sirius', in north-east Greenland were pinned down by a storm in a small valley. The storm was very severe (wind 100 to 120 knots, temperature −30 °C) and their tent and outer sleeping bags were torn off by the wind and lost. Both men suffered severe third-degree frostbite of the feet. On the second day of the storm they hallucinated that they were taking part in an experiment and discussed how long it should last. They convinced themselves that Dr Vanggaard would soon call it off. After reaching safety they claimed that their hallucination had helped them through the stressful situation.

Case 7. (Lee and Lee, 1971). Paul Shook was an airman who ditched into the Gulf of Mexico. On the second day he reported that he again felt the cold and misery and once more drifted off into fantasy. That night he had a feeling of total dissociation, though he was aware, and he imagined that a small boat had found him. He started to tell the man to go to notify the coastguard of his position, but then decided that that was not a very good idea and that, since he could not last much longer, he had better go with the boatman. All seemed real and vivid at the time.

Case 8. (Lee and Lee, 1971). The USS *Indianapolis* was sunk in the North Pacific by enemy action and on the third day the survivors had hallucinations that the ship had not sunk or that there was an island close by. This latter hallucination was so real that some took off their life-jackets and died while trying to swim to the island. That night (the third) the hallucinations took the form that the enemy were still after them and trying to kill them, and this again was so real that some fought and killed each other.

Case 9. (*Lloyd, 1986*). A 77-year-old woman was admitted to hospital having fallen out of bed. She was unable to communicate.

Her rectal temperature was 25 °C, her blood pressure and pulse unrecordable and her heart rate of 19/min was only recordable on an ECG. She eventually rewarmed, recovered and returned home 37 days after admission. It was discovered through talking to neighbours that she had had a two-week history of hallucinations prior to admission.

Case 10. (McHarg, 1980) One cold January night in north-east Scotland a lady had to abandon her car and walk eight miles home. At about 2 a.m. she neared Dunnichen Hill and saw figures carrying flaming torches in different parts of the area. They looked as if they were checking a large number of dead bodies, and were acting as if they were skirting water. The clothing worn was consistent with that worn by the Picts in the seventh century AD, and there were other details. The coincidence is that this was the site of the Battle of Nechtansmere in 685 AD in which the Picts destroyed the invading army of the Northumbrian king in one of history's decisive battles, since it prevented England extending to the whole of Scotland and thrust the border south. The mere or lake is now drained but archaeologists have been able to trace its original size and position and the figures were walking round where the edge would have been. While the lady had heard of the battle, she had no knowledge of any historical details even of the exact site of the battle.

There are many other case reports of people seeing figures, talking to non-existent people, feeling fear or a presence, or seeing things or hearing sounds or irregular footsteps on land or in or on water (Gray, 1970; Item, 1976a; Lee and Lee, 1971; Lloyd, 1982, 1983a; McOwan, 1979) and in most of these incidents the description of the weather conditions suggests that cold stress was present. This raises the question as to why people hallucinate and what determines the content of the hallucination.

Why do People Hallucinate?

It is said that hallucinations occur when the *core temperature* drops below 32 °C (Hirvonen, 1982) but in many of the cases described above, if the core temperature was below 32 °C when the hallucination occurred, it is unlikely that the person would have survived.

Hallucinations occurring among climbers at high altitude are usually attributed to *hypoxia* (Herligkoffer, 1954; Pozner, 1969) but this cannot be the complete explanation since the hallucinations have not invariably occurred at the highest point of the climber's journey and similar hallucinations have occurred to people at much lower altitudes and even at sea level. Acute anoxic anoxia is not generally associated with hallucinations (Hatcher, 1965) and when acute hypoxia occurs in aircraft cabin decompression at altitude, whether rapid or slow, it is associated with unconsciousness or at least clouded consciousness and the pilot is able to recognise the symptoms of hypoxia and take appropriate action (Brooks, 1984). Even in one pilot whose emergency oxygen supply was faulty but who survived a sudden decompression at an altitude of over 54,000 feet (Brooks, 1984), hallucinations were not reported. Similarly in patients in hospital, hallucinations only seem to occur when cerebral hypoxia has been present for some time, suggesting that hallucinations are not primarily due to inadequate oxygenation of the cerebral neurones but may be the result of changes in cerebral biochemistry secondary to the hypoxia. Hypoxia in fact does cause a marked inhibition of dopamine release, the extent depending on the degree of hypoxia (Wustmann *et al.*, 1982), and the evidence that apomorphine, a dopamine agonist, reverses the behavioural effects of hypoxia adds support (Wustmann *et al.*, 1982). The dopamine release mechanism gradually adapts to hypoxia (Wustmann *et al.*, 1982).

A possible alternative mechanism is through hypoxia occurring as a result of *cerebral perfusion pressure* being lowered, as was the suggested mechanism for bizarre mental awareness during resuscitation from cardiac arrest (Gilston, 1978). However, cerebral blood flow is very carefully regulated over a wide range of conditions and a drop in inspired oxygen tension causes an increase in cerebral blood flow (Hernandez, 1983). The decrease in cerebral blood flow in hypothermia is because of the drop in metabolism associated with the lowered temperature (Hernandez, 1983). Therefore if the perfusion pressure was sufficiently low to cause hypoxia in association with hypothermia, there would also be impaired consciousness and from the case reports this is not so.

Another possibility is that the hallucinations occur as a form of *hypnosis*. Hypnosis (Mellet, 1980) is an unusual state of consciousness in which distortions of perception (possibly including those of place and time) occur as uncritical responses of the subject to notions from an objective source (usually the hypnotist) or a subjective source (his own memory) or both. Indeed, subjects may accept into their consciousness emotions and memories of events as if they were current realities. The induction of hypnosis is often performed by reducing all outside stimuli to a monotonous visual one, e.g. a pendulum, and a monotonous auditory one, the voice of the hypnotist. This is a form of *sensory deprivation* which has been known for many years to be a cause of hallucinations (*Encyclopaedia Brittanica*, 1973b). It is interesting that the hallucinogens dextroamphetamine and LSD not only facilitate the induction of hypnosis, but also produce psychological and EEG changes reminiscent of hypnotic phenomena (Mellett, 1980).

Spontaneously occurring states in which distortion of perception is apparent are commonplace in intervals between full consciousness and sleep (Mellett, 1980), and hallucinations at sea of other people being present have been reported as the patient was waking from a 'sleep' brought on by extreme weariness (Lee and Lee, 1971) and in situations where sensory stimuli are monotonous and rhythmical, e.g. a long-distance swimmer hallucinated when he came to a calm patch of water, a single-handed sailor found that he hallucinated voices especially when solitude and fatigue were accompanied by monotonous occupations (Lee and Lee, 1971), and on land a reduction of external stimuli through mist, darkness, solitude or sitting down to relax are all frequent associates of hallucinations (Gray, 1970; McOwan, 1979). The content of some of the hallucinations and the relevance to the environmental situation suggests the possibility of self-hypnosis.

Neuropharmacology

Dopamine agonists produce auditory hallucinations delusional ideas and changes in mood (Turner *et al.*, 1984), and *sympathomimetics*, even when being used as nasal decongestants, may cause nightmares (Bain, 1984; Miller, 1984) or visual hallucinations which the very young may be unable to describe (Drennan, 1984). When these facts are considered along with the evidence from hypoxia and hypnosis, the fact that the symptoms of alcoholic intoxication can be mimicked by hypobaric hypoxia (Harding and Mills, 1983), hypoglycaemia (MacInnes, 1979) and incipient hypothermia (Pugh, 1968), suggests that there may be a common factor in these phenomena. It is therefore worth considering the known neurochemical abnormalities discovered in other hallucinatory situations. Indeed, it has been suggested that some (Fischman, 1983) or all (Lloyd, 1983a) hallucinogenic states have a common neurochemical basis.

There are a number of known neurotransmitters and there is evidence that these agents act in a complex system of interlinked controls. The observation that the effect of dopamine on haloperidol-sensitive receptors can be blocked by methysergide (a specific 5-hydroxytryptamine (5HT) antagonist) suggests that 5HT synapses must be located downstream from the haloperidol-sensitive dopamine receptors (Frens, 1980) but 5HT has an inhibitory effect on noradrenergic and dopaminergic nerves (Eccleston, 1982; Fischman, 1983) and the dopamine system is controlled through a post-synaptic feedback loop (Nilsson and Carlsson, 1982; York, 1979) involving non-dopaminergic interneurones (Beart, 1982).

The noradrenergic system and the β-endorphin system have an extensive and reciprocal relationship and β-endorphin stimulates dopaminergic activity in the central nervous system (Berger and Barchas, 1981; Miller *et al.*, 1984) while dopamine inhibits β-endorphin (Holaday and Loh, 1981). An increase in cerebral catecholamines produces an increased analgesia whereas catecholamine depletion results in a diminution of analgesia and there is therefore the possibility that analgesia is mediated through dopaminergic and noradrenergic neurones (Smith and Loh, 1981) and not through the endorphin system alone. There are several positive feedback loops controlling β-endorphin release and dopamine and 5HT may have opposite effects in this control system (Holaday and Loh, 1981). In this feedback loop system a period of overactivity results in tolerance developing and later there is a shutdown of β-endorphin release (Holaday and Loh, 1981). Understanding of the complex interrelated system of inhibitory and excitatory controls is complicated by the fact that there are a number of different dopamine receptors (Beart, 1982; Cools, 1982; Cooper *et al.*, 1982; Nilsson and Carlsson, 1982; Offermeier and van Rooyen, 1982), different 5HT receptors (Lomax and Green, 1979) and different opioid receptors (Hill and Hughes, 1984; Jasinski, 1984; Smith and Loh, 1981).

Syndromes Associated with 'Hallucinations'

The classical disease associated with hallucinations is Type 1 (acute) *schizophrenia* (Crow, 1980), and since it has also been extensively studied, the mechanisms will be considered in some detail. The current treatment is with the neuroleptic drugs which act by blockade of the dopamine receptors with a secondary increase in dopamine turnover. Since depriving a receptor of its transmitter produces receptor supersensitivity through augmenting the number of receptor binding sites (Snyder, 1983), this may explain the increase in the number of dopamine receptors, which is the only change found consistently in the postmortems of type 1 schizophrenic brains (Crow, 1980), though there is the suggestion that the cause may be genetic or due to dopamine-receptor-stimulating antibodies (Knight, 1982).

However, neuroleptics also block 5HT transmission (Snyder, 1983) and, since 5HT inhibits dopamine neurotransmission, if there is a decrease in 5HT neurotransmission, this removes dopamine inhibition with a resulting increase in dopamine activity giving rise to the dopamine theory of schizophrenia (Fischman, 1983).

It has been stated that there is no evidence of a disrupted opioid system in schizophrenia (Berger and Barchas, 1981; Thompson, 1984). However, the neuroleptic drugs like haloperidol, while blocking dopamine receptors and 5HT transmission, also cause an increased release of β-endorphins (Holaday and Loh, 1981) and administered β-endorphins can cause an akinesia similar to that produced by neuroleptics, and may produce an improvement in the symptoms of schizophrenia (Berger and Barchas, 1981). In addition the opioid antagonist naloxone can produce an improvement in schizophrenia (Berger and Barchas, 1981; Miller *et al.*, 1984; Snyder, 1983).

There is therefore evidence of possible disturbances in the dopamine, 5HT and opioid systems in schizophrenia. The symptoms of type 2 (chronic) schizophrenia are unrelated to dopaminergic transmission and may be associated with structural brain damage (Crow, 1980).

Dreams were believed to occur only during rapid eye movement (REM) sleep (Oswald, 1975) but dreaming similar to and indistinguishable from those reported in REM sleep can occur in all other conventional natural states of consciousness, viz. relaxed wakefulness, sleep onset and non-REM sleep (Vogel, 1975). Dopamine agonism activates REM sleep, an effect which is blocked by dopamine antagonists (Trimble, 1981), but it is also suggested that dreams occur when certain cells become excitable because of a loss of 5HT and noradrenergic inhibition (Fischman, 1983). As a person drifts from being awake into non-REM into REM sleep there is a decrease in serotonin outflow and in REM sleep 5HT neurones are virtually silent (Fischman, 1983). Reserpine, which depletes the intraneural stores of 5HT and catecholamines, increases REM sleep and enhances the effects of hallucinogens. The tricyclic antidepressives and MOAI drugs suppress REM sleep (Fischman, 1983; Oswald, 1975) and eliminate the hypnogogic hallucinations of narcolepsy

(Fischman, 1983).

Prolonged *sleep deprivation* is associated with hallucinations (Wilkinson, 1965) and it has been shown in rats that REM sleep deprivation causes a supersensitivity of the dopaminergic receptors in the rat brain (Tufik *et al.*, 1978). REM sleep deprivation intensifies fantasy in fantasy-impoverished subjects (Vogel, 1975) and improves depression (Vogel, 1975).

Amphetamine overdose causes hallucinations indistinguishable from those in type 1 schizophrenia (Crow, 1980; Snyder, 1983). It is thought that the effets are due to increased dopamine release (Crow, 1980) and inhibition of re-uptake inactivation (Snyder, 1983). However, amphetamines may also act on 5HT receptors (Sellers *et al.*, 1979), and it is suggested that the onset of amphetamine psychosis coincides with dopamine depletion rather than with the period of increased dopamine availability (Fischman, 1983). Amphetamines cause a large decrease in 5HT and 5HIAA in all regions of the brain (Fischman, 1983), and amphetamine may enhance the therapeutic effect of phenothiazines and thus reduce the psychotic symptoms in schizophrenia (Fischman, 1983).

LSD psychosis also resembles schizophrenia and it appears to act through the 5HT system (Crow, 1980; Fischman, 1983; Jacob and Girault, 1979).

The hyperthermic effect of amines like LSD is related to their hallucinogenic potential (Jacob and Girault, 1979) and all drugs which cause hallucinations alter body temperature. In addition, every major hallucinogenic drug — LSD, psilocin, amphetamine, etc. — which give altered consciousness similar to dreams and schizophrenia inhibit the 5HT containing neurones of the dorsal raphe nucleus (Fischman, 1983). It is in fact suggested that the peculiar property of hallucinogens is the ability to inhibit 5HT cell firing without increasing 5HT synthesis (Fischman, 1983). In normal people REM sleep deprivation is followed by a rebound increase in REM sleep but not in schizophrenic patients (Fischman, 1983).

All potent analgesic agents, including *opiates*, may produce psychotomimetic side-effects (Jago and Restall, 1983) and the mechanism is suggested as being due to interaction with the opioid sigma receptor (Pleuvry, 1983). The symptoms of *morphine withdrawal* have been attributed to dopamine release (Cox, 1979) though the withdrawal will cause stress which will result in β-endorphin release (Holaday and Loh, 1981).

It has been suggested that the hallucinations and delirium which occur during the recovery from *ketamine* anaesthesia are a result of interaction with the sigma opioid receptor (Pleuvry, 1983). The incidence of these side-effects can be reduced by using a heavy opioid premedication (Jago *et al.*, 1984) and by a benzodiazepine (Currie and Currie, 1984).

During *benzodiazepine withdrawal* hallucinations, visual and auditory, can occur along with perceptual distortion, delusions, sensations of unreality and depersonalisation (Ashton, 1984) but there is still doubt as to whether this is through a 5HT, an adrenergic or an opioid mechanism (Ashton, 1984). Haloperidol reduces the hallucinations (Ashton, 1984) and propranolol and clonidine may produce some benefit (Tyrer, 1984).

The β-adrenergic blocker, *propranolol*, crosses the blood brain barrier and causes hallucinations and nightmares in some people (Cremona-Barbaro, 1983; Nickerson and Collier, 1975). It can also produce depression (Cremona-Barbaro, 1983), a condition in which there is a decrease in intracerebral 5HT (Curtius *et al.*, 1983; Eccleston, 1982; van Praag, 1982), though the noradrenergic and dopamine systems (Curtius *et al.*, 1983; Eccleston, 1982) and 5HT (Gaillard, 1983) are also involved in depression.

Alcohol intoxication is known to be associated with hallucinations and alcohol and hypnotics reduce the incidence of REM sleep and also the bizarreness of dreams (Oswald, 1975). However, *withdrawal* of these drugs after long-continued use is associated with nightmares (Sillanpaa, 1982), fear, restlessness and REM sleep that intrudes into wakefulness (Oswald, 1975). This is accompanied by bizarre dreams, i.e. the hallucinatory state of delirium tremens (Oswald, 1975).

Hallucinations have occurred in association with *high fever* and from the evidence of the cases described earlier, *prolonged cold* stress seems also to be associated with hallucinations. There is now a voluminous literature on the neurochemical transmitters controlling body temperature (Lomax and Schonbaum, 1979; Milton, 1982) and the same and other publications discuss the thermal effects of many drugs. It is certainly true that dopamine, noradrenaline, serotonin (5HT) and the opioid receptors are all concerned with temperature regulation and the involvement of the opioid system is illustrated by the observation that the rise in body temperature which occurs after exercise is abolished by the use of naloxone (de Meirleir *et al.*, 1985). It is therefore easy to understand how heat stress and cold stress could both produce hallucinogenic neurochemical changes. In fact since heat loss is activated through the release of 5HT (Cox, 1979), it is possible to speculate that prolonged cold stress might result in prolonged inhibition of 5HT release, thus producing effects similar to the hallucinogenic drugs.

Stress, both physical and mental, not only stimulates the dopaminergic system (Horita and Snow, 1980), but also results in β-endorphin release (Holaday and Loh, 1981; Miller *et al.*, 1984; Vidal *et al.*, 1983), though the effects can be mitigated by diazepam and GABA (Vidal *et al.*, 1983).

Premonitions are one form of *extra-sensory perception* (*ESP*) and proven premonitions have occurred in conditions in which, as shown above, there are neurochemical abnormalities, e.g. premonitions of the Aberfan disaster occurred in dreams (Greenhouse, 1972), a proven premonition of the assassination of President Kennedy occurred while a scientist was participating in an experiment with a hallucinogenic drug (Greenhouse, 1972), and one writer, who found that he could only write stories while in a trance or altered state of consciousness, wrote a story in 1895 which gave a very close prediction of the sinking of the *Titanic* even though the *Titanic* was not even planned at that time (Greenhouse, 1972). Other premonitions have occurred under hypnosis (Greenhouse, 1972). Total deprivation of all the normal sensory input is the standard procedure in any experiment on ESP which involves the transfer of thoughts from one room to another, and in a seance there is total silence and the room is kept dark. This is sensory deprivation, similar to but greater than used in hypnosis and it has been known for many years that sensory deprivation can cause hallucinations (*Encyclopaedia Brittanica*, 1973b). It is therefore at least possible that ESP is also mediated through the same neurochemical changes. The hallucination in Case 10 described above has similarities with the phenomena associated with ESP.

There is evidence that different factors known to cause hallucinations can *interact*. For example there is a supersensitivity of the dopaminergic receptors in sleep deprivation (Tufik *et al.*, 1978) and the effects of cannabis are increased by sleep deprivation (Carlini and Lindsey, 1974).

There are other phenomena which are known to be associated with neurochemical abnormalities similar to those in the above examples. For example the evidence suggests that the GABA, 5HT, noradrenaline and dopamine systems are involved in *anxiety* states (Braestrup and Nielsen, 1983) and there is a decrease in brain noradrenaline levels in *panic* attacks (Hamlin *et al.*, 1983). Also, not only is *depression* associated with low levels of intracerebral 5HT (van Praag, 1983a), but the lowest levels of 5HIAA, a 5HT metabolite, are found in those depressed patients who had attempted *suicide* (van Praag, 1983a) and there is an increase in the number of $5HT_2$ binding sites in the frontal cortex of suicide victims (Stanley and Mann, 1983).

The bulk of the evidence suggests that the hallucinations are biochemically induced, though in any individual case in the field the cause of this biochemical change is probably multifactorial. For example in situations of prolonged cold stress there is likely to be associated physical and/or mental stress and therefore sleep will be disturbed, leading to sleep deprivation. This could be in addition to fatigue and possibly hypoxia if the problem occurs at altitude. Any diminution of sensory input, e.g. night or mist, would accentuate the problem by mimicking hypnosis, and there are many drugs which could also contribute. On the same basis it is not surprising that, in the disaster situation at sea, dreams and hallucinations should have similar content (Lee and Lee, 1971).

There is a suggested *genetic predisposition* to schizophrenia (Crow, 1980). Some people are better hypnotic subjects than others and some people are better than others in obtaining predictions or 'contacts' during a seance (Greenhouse, 1972). Interestingly the same people have often had more than one episode of dissociation, hallucinations and visual or auditory misinterpretations (Lee and Lee, 1971; McOwan, 1979), e.g. the Everest climber Frank Smythe hallucinated not only a companion while on a lone climb on Everest but also 'kite balloons', and had an episode of dissociation (Smythe, 1956) and many years later he had another hallucination while climbing in Scotland (McOwan, 1979). The fact that some people in cold stress situations hallucinate, while others in the same or similar situations do not, supports the idea of a genetic predisposition to hallucinate.

Hallucinations tend to wear off after a few days (Lee and Lee, 1971) even though the cold or other stress has continued. The neurochemistry provides some explanation for this clinical observation in that the inhibition of dopamine release produced by hypoxia gradually adapts (Wustmann *et al.*, 1982), and in the control of β-endorphin release, tolerance develops in the feedback loop after a period of overactivity, and later there is a shutdown of β-endorphin release (Holaday and Loh, 1981).

What Determines the Content of the Hallucination?

Since the cerebral dopaminergic pathways interconnect with many parts of the brain (Trimble, 1981), there is a possible wide variation in the hallucinations produced, and the hallucination experienced by any individual depends on other factors.

Some hallucinations are obviously triggered off by misinterpretation of distance, natural objects or unusual natural sounds (Gray, 1970; Lee and Lee, 1971; McOwan, 1979), e.g. (1) some sightings of figures can be explained by the 'spectre of the Brocken', named after a mountain in Bavaria, which is simply the shadow of the observer, sometimes distorted or magnified, thrown by the low sun against an opaque wall of mist (Gray, 1970); and (2) even though snow may feel a uniform consistency underfoot, apparent irregular following footsteps may be due to variations in the snowfield which, however, will only be seen when the footsteps are examined later (Elliot, 1980). Misinterpretation is understandable in view of the impairment by cold exposure of the function of many of the higher senses.

Deep desires, physical or mental, may be revealed in dreams, e.g. the starving man dreams of food (Brent, 1974; Lee and Lee, 1971), and the urgent needs of people for food, rescue or company could be expressed in hallucinations as in some of the above cases, but the sensation of other beings is more than a psychological necessity for survival of people alone (Pozner, 1965) since it has occurred with several people together or to single people in a group. Yet other hallucinations are obviously closely related to a subject about which the person had been doing a lot of thinking, and some people were aware that they were in a peculiarly strange or receptive state of mind before a particular incident. The hypnotised subject 'hallucinates' from his own experience, though guided by the words of the hypnotist, and the phenomena of premonitions, seances and ESP may be the brain 'tuning in' to some as yet unknown influence. When a person gets to safety from a hypothermia situation the fact that he is often unable to give the exact location of the party (Jones in Marcus, 1979a; Pugh, 1964, 1966) is probably another manifestation of disordered mental function which may not have progressed to frank hallucinations.

Fear would compound any misinterpretation and subjects in an experiment on arctic survival developed malaise, apathy and a totally unreasoned fear that they would be abandoned by the researchers (Rogers, 1971). Even experimentally, apathy is known to accompany cold stress (Enander, 1984). It is interesting that in many of the case reports of hallucinations fear was also described (Gray, 1970; Lee and Lee, 1971; McOwan, 1979). Unmotivated fear is also common among Danish fishermen (Vanggaard, 1977) and fear was also present in the case of the *Notts County* crewman (Pugh, 1968). It is also interesting that explorers have a morbid fear of the arctic night (Simpson, 1972) and, while this may be due to disorganisation of the central nervous system biological rhythms (Simpson, 1972), this may be exacerbated by cold.

Clinical Implications

In some of the cases people have responded physically to an hallucination and, in the hazardous environments in which these incidents have occurred, an inappropriate response may be, and in some of the case reports has been, fatal. With this in mind other incidents can be understood:

(1) A diver, known to be cold before and during a dive, severed his own life-line (Rawlins, 1981).

(2) One of Peary's scientists went mad during an arctic winter (Simpson, 1972).

(3) Polar Eskimos recognise a hysterical mental condition which occurs in winter and which they call *pibloctoq*. In this the person suddenly goes beserk, rushing out of the house, throwing their arms in the air and doing a number of other irrational actions such as taking their clothes off, jumping in the sea or climbing icebergs (Simpson, 1972).

(4) (Brent, 1974). In Scott's fatal Antarctic expedition, when Titus Oates said: 'I am going outside and may be some time', it was assumed that this was an act of self-sacrifice to allow the remainder of the party the chance to survive. The factors which led to this assumption were: (a) before the journey started Oates said that anyone who broke down and became a hindrance to the party should sacrifice himself; and (b) when Oates was weakening and holding them up because of his slowness, he asked what he should do and Scott assumed he was thinking of self-sacrifice. However, there are facts which could cast doubt on this assumption: (i) In the diary, after Oates had asked what he should do, there is the strong underlying sense that Scott felt that Oates would be doing the right thing if he did sacrifice himself and Scott went so far as to order Wilson to hand over 30 Opium tablets apiece so that anyone who wished could end their life. Oates, however, did not use the Opium and it was six days later before Oates walked out of the tent. (ii) Scott wrote in his diary: 'We

did intend to finish ourselves when things proved like this, but we decided to die naturally in our tracks.' There is no reason why Oates may not have felt the same. (iii) Oates is reported as 'feeling cold and fatigue more than most' almost two months before he died and in the last two weeks he had frostbite and was so weak that he could not pull the sledge and was very slow. (iv) They all had a lack of sufficient food and had been losing weight steadily and therefore their vulnerability to cold would have increased. It is therefore almost certain that Oates would be at least mildly hypothermic and his last remark could be the polite Victorian gentleman's equivalent of Kurban's 'I want a pee' (Case 2 above). Oates's action may therefore have been the result of a hallucination or at least disordered cerebration rather than a gesture of self-sacrifice.

(5) It is always assumed that the madness exhibited by Mertz in Mawson's tragic Antarctic expedition in 1912 (Bickel, 1977) was due to hypervitaminosis A through eating the livers of the huskies but some of the symptomatology was different from the classical description of vitamin A toxicity and was very similar to the *pibloctoq* of the Eskimos and since Mertz had frostbite he was certainly suffering from the cold. The severest symptoms occurred during his last day during which he was being pulled on the sledge and therefore not producing heat through exercise and at the end he lapsed into a coma and died. Mawson also ate the husky livers and, though he also showed many of the signs of vitamin A toxicity, he survived and this in spite of being alone for three weeks in weather conditions similar to Scott's and falling into crevasses on more than one occasion. Mawson did, however, get the sense of a 'presence' accompanying him for some time after Mertz's death.

(6) The phenomenon of paradoxical undressing in the cold was first reported in 1952 and Wedin (1976) included this and other reported cases in his review which totalled 35 cases culled from the Swedish police records. Other cases were also reported (Wedin *et al.*, 1979). Once the possibility became known other cases were reported in the lay press (*Scotsman*, 1978) and a mountain rescue team found one dead victim by following a trail of cast-off clothing (Stewart, 1977). The importance of recognising that this phenomenon exists is because of possible misinterpretation of the cause, e.g. where a body is found partially undressed or with severely disordered clothing, especially if the body is that of a child or woman, the police are liable to interpret the death as resulting from a sexual attack (Wedin, 1976). This can also happen in the elderly, though it is liable to be

misdiagnosed as dementia or a cerebral episode. For example, an old woman of 82, who lived alone and had a previous history of cerebrovascular disease, was admitted to hospital after having been found wandering in her house confused and totally naked. Her rectal temperature on admission was 33.5 °C. She was successfully rewarmed and eventually transferred to an eventide home though her confusion did not clear immediately on reaching normothermia (Lloyd, 1986). Another patient, aged 91, who persistently switched off all the heating in his house even in winter, was found sitting naked on the floor having tried to light a fire. His confusional state also took several days to clear (unpublished observation). The cause of paradoxical undressing may be due to cold and/or drugs causing an hallucination about warmth or having reached home and shelter, or the particular neurochemical changes in the brain may be similar to those which are usually only present in conditions of extreme heat and the person will then misinterpret this cerebral biofeedback and respond by undressing.

When nine men in a lifeboat in December 1909 were found dead from hypothermia and there were the clothes of a tenth man who had apparently undressed and jumped into the icy water, insanity caused by the presence of interplanetory travellers (Gourlay, 1979) is rather a contrived explanation for what is more likely to be another case of paradoxical undressing.

It is interesting that in the tragic Scott Antarctic expedition of 1912 (Brent, 1974), Petty Officer Evans was the first to die and Scott's diary records the sequence of events. On 13th February, 'Evans has no power to assist with camping work.' On the 16th, 'Evans has nearly broken down in brain.' On the 17th, Evans had fallen behind and when they went back they found him 'on his knees with clothing disarranged, hands uncovered and frostbitten, and with a wild look in his eyes'. He was comatose by the time they had erected the tent and he died just after midnight. This is probably not only the first-recorded (if unrecognised) case of paradoxical undressing, but also one of the best observed.

(7) The observation that unemployment results in an increased risk of suicide (Platt and Kreitman, 1984) has been disputed on the grounds that unemployment did not cause stress (Shapiro and Parry, 1984). It is possible to postulate that since unemployment results in a reduced income, there is likely to be a lower level of heating in the house. The prolonged effects of cold stress, possibly in conjunction with other factors, might result in alterations of the cerebral

neurochemistry in such a way as to increase the risk of suicide.

Conclusion

Cold is a stress which may produce hallucinations and other mental changes before the person's physical abilities are impaired.

The mechanism has many similarities to hypnosis but there is probably an underlying neurochemical basis and it is suggested above that the specific abnormality may develop in the dopamine/5-hydroxytryptamine/opioid system. Cold may act synergistically with other hallucinogenic factors, e.g. hypoxia, drugs, sleep deprivation or fatigue, aggravated by mental or physical stress to produce the particular intracerebral neurochemical disturbance which makes the person susceptible to unusual influences. This may be manifested as hallucinations and the forms of the hallucination may be determined by inner thoughts or desires or by misinterpretation of external stimuli. Some of the phenomena recorded while in this neurochemical state are not understood and are therefore sometimes called Extra Sensory Perception. Minor variations in the neurochemical changes may produce changes in mood and possibly suicidal tendencies in susceptible individuals. Minor variations in the neurochemical changes may be the cause of depression, apathy, fear or panic — phenomena also observed in cases of cold exposure. It is also possible that suicide occurring in a cold environment may be precipitated by cold-induced neurochemical changes.

The importance of this hypothesis lies in the fact that, if a person responds to an hallucination, any actions will be inappropriate to the person's actual situation and may lead to the death of the individual or of others. In these circumstances the death has traditionally been attributed to 'pilot error' and the true cause, cold stress or hypothermia, has been overlooked. Even when it was noticed that some fishermen in the North Atlantic showed a change in character or behaviour before they were accidentally lost at sea, their deaths were ascribed to suicide (Richardson, 1981) and the possible contribution of cold stress was apparently not even considered. Even when a crewman of a fishing boat eventually died of hypothermia, his state of panic and apparent madness was attributed to him having had a leg deformed from a previous accident (Pugh, 1968).

Postscript

There is evidence that, in this field of hypothermia also, the general public were ahead of the medical profession in their knowledge of the effects of cold. For example in folk-lore or stories, whenever ghosts are seen, the writer always mentions that the room had an unnatural iciness or that a sense of chill came over the person.

Hans Andersen, who died in Copenhagen in 1875, wrote many fairy tales and, though some of the tales have a philosophical or social message, there is one, the story of the 'Little Match Girl', which may have been one of the earliest accounts of this physiological phenomenon. However, Charles Dickens was a contemporary of Andersen and *A Christmas Carol* written in 1860 may have preceded or followed the 'Little Match Girl'. It is interesting that Dicken's novels also criticised the social and moral evils of his time.

There are a number of versions of the story of the 'Little Match Girl', but the main points are common to them all. It was New Year's Eve and a very cold night. A little girl had lost her shoes and her thin ragged clothes were wet from the snow which had fallen all the previous day. She found a dry spot where she curled up and tried to keep warm for the night. She was also very tired and hungry and her hunger would have been aggravated by the smell of cooking coming from the houses. In a vain attempt to get some heat she struck one of the matches she had been trying to sell. In the flame of the first match she imagined that she saw a stove with a hot blazing fire and in the second a table spread with wonderful food which she could almost taste, but each time, as she tried to move closer, the match went out and the image disappeared. In the light of the third match she imagined a Christmas tree with candles and, when it disappeared as before, she looked up to where the candles had been and saw the stars. The flame of the fourth match grew very large and, in the circle of light she saw her recently dead grandmother, the only person who had loved and cared for her. The girl was so terrified of losing her grandmother that she struck match after match. Eventually the old lady took the girl in her arms and they soared up to heaven. The girl was found the next morning dead from hypothermia but with a gentle smile on her face.

The girl, in a situation lacking mental stimulation, i.e. huddled in a corner at night, was obviously suffering from cold stress, fatigue, loneliness and hunger, and while hypothermia was developing, she hallucinated. The hallucination about food, while related to her hunger, was probably triggered off by the smells of cooking coming from the houses and the hallucination about the Christmas tree and candles was a misinterpretation of the visual impulses caused by looking at the stars, though possibly also related to her loneliness. The other two hallucinations seem to be entirely related to her needs for heat and love. There was obviously also impairment of visual function because the flame of the fourth match seemed to grow very large.

In *A Christmas Carol* the setting is Christmas Eve and Dickens emphasises the cold and damp in such phrases as 'cold, bleak, biting weather', 'the cold became intense', 'it had been foggy all day', 'foggier yet and colder', 'piercing searching biting cold' and he even mentioned that running water was freezing. He also mentions the inadequate heating from coal fires both in the office and in the large house — 'had to sit over the fire to get any sensation of heat' — both because of miserliness. Scrooge has five hallucinations though Dickens has mentioned a suitable trigger incident earlier in the story. The first hallucination of the door knocker becoming the face of his dead partner Marley and the second where Marley appears in person were triggered by the charity collectors asking if he were Scrooge or Marley, by this reminding him that Marley had been buried seven (a mystical number) years earlier on Christmas Eve and by the fact that Scrooge was living in Marley's house. The ghost of Christmas past was triggered by being asked to Christmas dinner by his nephew, the son of his sister who had been the only person to be kind to Scrooge as a child, and by a boy singing a carol through the letter box. His memory of his days as a clerk with a kindly man was a stark contrast to the way he treated his own clerk, and other items led on from the earlier ones. The ghost of Christmas present was triggered by his earlier wondering how his non-wealthy nephew and his very poor clerk could still wish people a Merry Christmas. Tiny Tim and his crutch and the future vacant chair came from his earlier comment 'better if the poor and ill died soon to decrease the surplus population'. The ghost of Christmas yet to come was a realisation that he was unloved if not hated. There were two misinterpretations. The first was that a sound outside reminded him of chains dragging and this set off the memory that ghosts were supposed to drag chains. The second was the ghost of Christmas yet to come which eventually 'shrunk, collapsed and dwindled into a bed post'.

PART 3: METHODS OF TREATMENT

INTRODUCTION

With accidental hypothermia, prevention is obviously the ideal to aim for and much can and has been done by education, training and the use of correct equipment, which includes the domestic environment for the elderly. However, even good training cannot eliminate mischance, or the headstrong waywardness of human nature, and treatment will always be necessary. Once a person has developed hypothermia, treatment can be subdivided into (1) restoration of the body temperature to normal; and (2) measures intended to sustain life until normothermia is achieved.

Golden (1979, 1983) posed the question 'Why rewarm?' and suggested that the usual reasons given for actively encouraging rewarming were as follows:

(1) 'The incidence of complications is directly related to the duration of hypothermia.' It is probably true that the rate of complications during rewarming rises if the person has been hypothermic for more than eight hours (Braun, 1895; Nicolas and Desjars, 1979). However, it has been claimed that the incidence of complications and late mortality is related to the time victims remain at temperatures in the hypothermic range (Davies *et al.*, 1967; Exton-Smith, 1973). This is more difficult to accept since patients who had been kept hypothermic for several days for therapeutic reasons (Bloch, 1965; Talbot *et al.*, 1941) had no problems during the hypothermia, and problems during rewarming seemed to be related to the rate of rewarming. It is true that for superficial cold injury, e.g. frostbite, the longer the duration, the greater the damage. It is also true that at core temperatures below 28 °C the risk of ventricular fibrillation, either spontaneous or triggered by external factors, rises very rapidly and in the same temperature range electrical defibrillation is very difficult. It is probably therefore justified to suggest that the time a victim remains with a core temperature below 30 °C should be reduced to a minimum with the provisos that the treatment used does not increase the risk of ventricular fibrillation and that there are adequate facilities to treat cardiac arrest if it should occur (Golden, 1979; 1983).

(2) 'The hypothermic patient is unable to generate sufficient metabolic heat to rewarm spontaneously.' It is commonly believed

that as the body temperature drops below 35 °C metabolism declines proportionally or exponentially (Maclean and Emslie-Smith, 1977). The authority for this is usually given as Burton and Edholm (1955), and Golden (1979) believes that this was based on the work of Dill and Forbes (1941). Initially evidence from surgical and anaesthetic experience reviewed by Blair (1964) supported Dill and Forbes's suggestion but subsequent work (Blair, 1969) showed that despite anaesthesia and curare to control shivering, oxygen consumption at 27 to 26 °C was still 73 per cent of normal. After a close scrutiny of the paper (Dill and Forbes, 1941), Golden (1979) concluded that the figures did not provide evidence for a decrease in shivering but in fact suggested pulmonary shunting with ventilation/perfusion inequalities, which are common in immobilised patients, accompanied by a decreased oxygen extraction from the blood. The Q_{10} effect was also quoted as being used to provide supportive evidence (Golden, 1979). However, the Q_{10} was applied to the metabolic heat production of the body as a whole and no account was taken of the heat production of the individual tissues and organs. The vital organs of the body core, i.e. brain, heart, lungs, kidneys and hepato-portal system, only constitute 8 per cent of the body weight but, in a normothermic person at rest in a basal state, they contribute 56 per cent of the heat production whereas muscles and skin only contribute 25 per cent of the heat from 52 per cent of the body mass (Aschoff and Wever, 1958; Carlson and Hsieh, 1965). In the hypothermic situation the muscles and skin are at very low temperatures while the core organs are protected and are at a much higher temperature than the muscles and skin. Therefore the heat production of the core organs will be much less depressed than the heat production from the muscles. Lunn (1969) also noticed that, in patients recovering from induced hypothermia, the temperature rise was initiated in the non-muscular tissues with the temperature, even of the respiratory muscles, only rising after the return of spontaneous respiration.

The clinical evidence is that a person can rewarm spontaneously from very low temperatures, e.g. 24 °C (Braun, 1985), or 18 °C (Laufman, 1951), even if the environment is only normal room temperature. It is therefore probably safe to say that if all the heat loss from the body is prevented, and this must include the respiratory heat loss, the body will rewarm spontaneously from any temperature. The problem is in providing perfect insulation and if, as shown by a core temperature which fails to rise or continues to fall, the body's heat production is insufficient to overcome the minimal heat loss remaining in any particular clinical situation, active rewarming measures will be necessary.

(3) 'Active rewarming reduces the magnitude of the afterdrop and its associated complications.' As has been discussed earlier, the significance of the after-drop and its contribution to post-rescue deaths has been exaggerated, if not completely misconstrued.

It has been suggested that treatment should start as soon as the victim is found (Foray and Salon, 1985). Mills (1980), on the other hand, argues that a patient with severe hypothermia is in a 'metabolic ice-box' and his chances of survival are likely to be reduced by anything which disturbs the equilibrium, whether this is active rewarming or continued cooling (Mills, 1980, 1983a). There is, however, agreement that immediate measures should be taken to prevent, or at least slow, further cooling (Foray and Salon, 1985; Mills, 1980, 1983a). It is also considered important to start rewarming as soon as possible and therefore the delays involved in transporting a victim to a large hospital may be unacceptable, even with the use of helicopters (Foray and Salon, 1985).

Before deciding how to rewarm, the argument arises as to whether the rewarming should be slow or rapid and the views of the two sides have been widely discussed (Duguid *et al.*, 1961; Fernandez *et al.*, 1970; Golden, 1983; Gregory and Doolittle, 1973; Harnett *et al.*, 1983a; Ledingham and Mone, 1980; Marcus, 1978; Miller *et al.*, 1980). However, much of the controversy has resulted because hypothermia was considered a single entity which, as discussed earlier, it obviously is not and therefore like was not being compared with like. For example it is impossible realistically to compare the very thin Dachau prisoners rapidly cooled by immersion in cold water with elderly patients who have gradually become cold with all the accompanying problems caused by the shifts of body fluids. Even with methods of rewarming there does not seem to be agreement as to what constitutes rapid rewarming, e.g. airway warming, during which patients have rewarmed at 0.5 to 1 °C/hour (Lloyd, 1973), is considered to be slow rewarming, whereas a rate of rewarming of 0.5 to 1 °C/hour, achieved through the use of a heat cradle, was described as rapid external rewarming (Ledingham and Mone, 1972). Similarly Lash *et al.* (1967) described peritoneal dialysis as providing 'rapid' rewarming, though the rectal temperature only rose from 21 °C to 21.1 °C over the two hours peritoneal dialysis was being used. This controversy also ignores the difference between heat supplied through the core and surface reheating. Mills (1980, 1983a) has suggested that the rate of rewarming is irrelevant if the person is under 'total physiological control', i.e. is being monitored with the full facilities of intensive care. However, the faster the rewarming, the less time the medical attendants and the patient's body have to solve the complex metabolic, chemical and cardiac change as they occur (Mills, 1980, 1983a). There is therefore some advantage in rewarming at a moderate rate rather than fast. If the patient is allowed to rewarm slowly the body will probably sort out the biochemical abnormalities produced by hypothermia without the necessity for outside intervention (Golden in Marcus, 1979a; Maclean in Marcus, 1979a).

Once it has been decided to restore the body temperature to normal, there are several methods to choose from:

(1) Spontaneous rewarming, i.e. preventing further heat loss to the environment and allowing the body to rewarm without supplying any additional heat from an external source.
(2) Active rewarming, i.e. supplying additional heat which may be through two main routes:
    (a) surface heating;
    (b) central rewarming.
(3) Combinations of a number of different methods.

Central rewarming means that the heat is being supplied to the 'core' first, and rewarming proceeds from within out. This has many theoretical advantages in that the heart, which is the organ most at risk from hypothermia, is warmed first and there is no initial drop in temperature. The methods of central rewarming which have been used to date are:

(1) Extracorporeal blood warming:
    (a) Cardiopulmonary bypass
    (b) Haemodialysis
(2) Irrigation of body cavities:
    (a) Mediastinal irrigation
    (b) Pleural irrigation
    (c) Peritoneal dialysis
(3) Other methods:
    (a) Intragastric and intracolonic balloons
    (b) Intravenous infusion
    (c) Diathermy
(4) Airway warming

In deciding which method of rewarming should be used, it is important to consider the degree of access to the patient for monitoring or resuscitation allowed by the method, and also to consider the methods available in the hospital (Paton, 1983b). Mortality rates not warming rates should dictate the choice of therapy (Myers *et al.*, 1979). However, many patients will die despite being rewarmed successfully because they had a pre-existing underlying condition which may also have precipitated the hypothermia and in some series this was the most important factor for survival (Kurtz, 1982; Maclean and Emslie-Smith, 1977; Simpson, 1974).

In addition to the methods of physically increasing the body heat, there are a number of other measures which have been suggested or tried as adjuncts to rewarming and these must also be considered.

In the assessment of any method of treating accidental hypothermia there are three important factors which must be considered:

(1) Heat gain. This must be evaluated not only in terms of absolute quantities of heat gain, which will include both the heat added and any heat loss prevented, but also from the aspect of where the heat gain occurs.
(2) Other effects on the body. These may be beneficial or adverse, and should include consideration of cardiovascular, cerebral, respiratory and renal function.
(3) Where the method can be used (practical potential). Each method has to be evaluated as to its safety and utility through the whole medical sequence from discovery of the victim, through first aid treatment, transport, treatment at base or hospital, to ultimate recovery

14 SPONTANEOUS REWARMING

Technique

This involves insulating the patient from the environment to prevent further heat loss from the body surface and rewarming therefore occurs spontaneously through conservation of the metabolic heat produced by the patient.

Equipment

Blankets and sleeping bags are useful but any spare clothing may also be used. It is sometimes recommended that wet clothing should be removed when the victim is found (Holdcroft, 1981; Lilja, 1983) before adding dry clothing but, in the field situation, it is often better, and safer, to add layers on top of the wet clothing (Foray and Salon, 1985), especially a layer that is impervious to wind and water. The reasons for this are that the vigorous movement needed to remove the wet clothing may precipitate ventricular fibrillation, and, while it requires 30 kcal of body heat to warm 1 litre of water in the clothes from 4 °C to 34 °C (warm skin temperature), evaporation of 1 litre of water would remove 580 kcal of body heat (Kaufman, 1983). Wet clothing should therefore only be removed when the person is in warm shelter out of the wind, and carefully even then (Dubas, 1980).

It is important when applying the insulation to remember the head (Lilja, 1983) since large amounts of heat may be lost, e.g. with an air temperature of −4 °C, half the metabolic heat production of a resting normothermic man may be lost through the head (Froese and Burton, 1957). At −15 °C, 70 per cent of the total heat production can be lost through the head (Danzl, 1983). In a hypothermic victim the heat loss from the body surface is reduced by vasoconstriction but vasoconstriction does not occur over the head and therefore the proportion of heat lost through the head in hypothermia may be even greater. The importance of covering the head is frequently forgotten and is omitted in many rescue manuals.

Some means of providing shelter from the wind is essential (Holdcroft, 1981) in improving insulation, and this may take the form of a lifeboat cabin, hut, tent (possibly a special rescue one with no poles which is supported inside by six people round the edge (Jones in

Marcus, 1979a)), a large survival bag, or in an emergency a large sheet of material held in place (Frankland, 1983) or even just finding a place out of the wind in a snowhole or behind a large boulder.

Advantages

This method can obviously be applied anywhere, with whatever material is available. It is the method at present used as initial treatment by the rescue services (British Mountaineering Council, 1974; Golden, 1972; Mountain Rescue, 1968) and for field use has been the only practical treatment (Pugh, 1966).

Disadvantages and Hazards

In the field, where perfect insulation is difficult to achieve, the depressed metabolic heat production sometimes leads to the death of the sufferer before safety and warmth are reached — a distressing occurrence within the experience of many rescue teams (Freeman and Pugh, 1969). This may be due to continuing cooling of the core (Keatinge, 1969), to faulty carrying technique or movement (Dalgleish, 1969; Freeman and Pugh, 1969; Golden, 1973b) or, as discussed earlier, through changes in cardiovascular status. Rescue teams are advised that in many cases the ideal is not to evacuate a hypothermic casualty at once to habitation, but to make camp, insulate the casualty, and allow spontaneous rewarming with the possible additional heat from another person within the insulation (Freeman and Pugh, 1969; Mountain Rescue, 1968). However, the reduction in metabolic heat as a result of hypothermia may result in a prolonged camp for the rescue team with possible additional hazards from deteriorating weather conditions, and teams may opt to evacuate the casualty for his own and the team's safety (Zingg, 1967), and in practice many teams do choose this option. Even in hospital where there is every possibility of having perfect insulation the rate of rewarming varies greatly, with most series reporting rates of 0.14 to 0.5 °C/hour. Individuals have rewarmed faster, e.g. 1.1 °C/hour (Laufman, 1951), but it was suggested that this patient had an abnormally active metabolism. Laufman's case and many others suggest that even unconscious patients will revive once further cooling has been prevented (Pugh, 1967). Nevertheless, the lower the body temperature, the lower the metabolic rate, and the less heat production available for rewarming. In the literature are scattered reports, e.g. 'no change (of temperature) in 6 to 24 hours' (Maclean *et al.*, 1968), illustrating the fact that even in hospital the minimal heat loss may result in failure to rewarm. In some cases of subchronic and chronic hypothermia the rate of spontaneous rewarming may become too rapid, resulting in intercompartmental fluid shifts of body fluid. This may lead to cerebral and/or pulmonary oedema and, if severe, this may cause death. A study of the reports of patients treated (Atukorale, 1971; Duguid *et al.*, 1961; Laufman, 1951; Lovel, 1962; Maclean *et al.*, 1968; Prescott *et al.*, 1962; Sadikali and Owor, 1974; Sprunt *et al.*, 1970; Tolman and Cohen, 1970) shows that young people, people suffering from acute hypothermia, and those whose hypothermia was precipitated by drug overdose, had a very high survival rate if allowed to rewarm spontaneously, the only deaths being due to the severity of the drug overdose or severe underlying disease. However, in the elderly, with their high proportion of subchronic hypothermia, and in the similar subchronic hypothermia associated with malnutrition, there is a very high mortality rate and, while some of this may be due to underlying disease (BMJ, 1978b), there were far too many, 52 out of 96, who died while still hypothermic (Duguid *et al.*, 1961; Maclean *et al.*, 1968; Sadikali and Owor, 1974; Sprunt *et al.*, 1970). The only series where there were no deaths during rewarming elderly patients were those in which the patients were treated in an intensive care unit (Ledingham and Mone, 1980; Tolman and Cohen, 1970).

Conclusions

Insulation of the patient to prevent further heat loss and allow rewarming to occur spontaneously has the virtue of simplicity in that it requires no specialised equipment and can be used at any and all stages in the rescue and treatment of the hypothermic casualty. The dangers are (1) that perfect, total insulation is difficult to achieve and therefore the patient may not rewarm and may indeed continue to cool; (2) that death may occur due to cardiovascular problems; or (3) that a patient with subchronic hypothermia may rewarm too rapidly and die because of fluid shifts.

Space Blanket

One material which has had a tremendous amount of publicity, and has consequently been widely adopted, has been metallised plastic sheeting (MPS — the so-called space blanket) and there is a considerable body of opinion that lightweight blankets or exposure bags made of MPS would be of great value for protection from a cold, wet, windy environment and should therefore be widely provided. As a result, many civilian and mountain rescue organisations and private individuals have equipped themselves with this material, under the impression that this MPS provides all the insulation necessary.

As the name suggests, the substance was developed for use in space. However, the position of the space-walking astronaut is unique in that there is no convective or conductive heat exchange at the clothing surface and the only route of heat exchange is by radiation (Marcus *et al.*, 1977) with intense solar radiant heat on one side and on the other side a radiant temperature approaching absolute zero (Kerslake, 1969). In the more normal situation, the 'space blanket' layer can be applied on the outside or the inside of protective clothing. In still air the amount of heat lost by convection and radiation are about equal, which has led to the claim that metallised clothing will halve the rate of heat loss. In fact this is only true if the air movement is low and the clothing insulation is zero. The better the insulation of the clothing and the higher the wind the less benefit from metallising the clothing. On a cold night out of doors the sky may be effectively colder than the air (e.g. ground frost conditions) and a reflecting layer becomes theoretically more attractive, but the effect of air movement would remain and significant protection would only be given at low wind speeds. The addition of a metallised layer may also markedly reduce the permeability of clothing. This may result in condensation of water vapour in the clothing beneath, with consequent reduction of its insulating power. The reflecting layer might therefore be more effective on the inside where the air movement is lower. However, when clothing layers are close together, the conduction of heat between them through to air is much greater than the radiant heat transfer, and metallisation is of little value. It would therefore be best to use a loosely fitting blanket or sleeping bag, metallised on the inside. However, the air in the bag will be humidified by water loss from the skin and condensation will occur on the inner metallised surface thereby destroying its reflecting property. If sufficient circulation of air is allowed between the sleeping bag and the occupant, condensation can be prevented but the benefit of the reflecting layer will be reduced since heat will be lost to the ventilating air (Kerslake, 1969).

In a test carried out under laboratory and field conditions to evaluate MPS (Marcus *et al.*, 1977) it was found that heavyweight MPS was of some value as water and wind protection, but other materials such as polythene or ripstop nylon were equally effective and are cheaper and more robust. Sheets of any material were found to be unmanageable at windspeeds above 20 mph and it was only with extreme difficulty that they could be wrapped around an inert 'casualty'. Flapping soon produced gaps in the covers and the wind quickly carried them away. The exposure bags were easier to handle but, when made of lightweight MPS, quickly disintegrated at windspeeds over 20 mph. Even when correctly applied, the lightweight MPS was easily punctured by stones or twigs, and then tore. Bags of 4.12 mm polythene and of lightweight ripstop nylon withstood wind speeds of 40 mph even when holed intentionally. Reflection of the body's infra-red radiation by an MPS exposure bag is soon prevented by condensation on the aluminised surface and, at sub-zero temperatures, this condensation soon freezes. In this situation MPS offers no advantage over the cheaper alternatives. Finally MPS was found to be of no value even as a radar location aid in survival. This was despite the fact that the tests were made at sea, where there are few distracting radar echoes, the sea conditions were fairly calm during the test and the operators knew the positions of the dinghies in advance. When two casualty survival bags were tested under field conditions (Light and Norman, 1980) it was found that the presence of an MPS layer made no difference to the thermal properties of the bags, and in a further field trial, a simple heavy gauge polythene bag was found to give as much thermal protection as a survival bag manufactured from MPS and the casualty bag incorporating MPS (Light *et al.*, 1980).

In practical use after a marathon, the author's personal experience was that a large thick paper towelling sheet was more effective than a space blanket, even in wind and rain (Lloyd, 1983b). The MPS supplied is too thin and too small and is therefore difficult to hold wrapped round the body, tending, even with the slightest breeze, to flap about and look more like Batman's cape than thermal protection.

In hospital MPS has been recommended, on theoretical grounds, for use in the operating theatre, with any part of the body not needed for the operation being wrapped in MPS (Dyde and Lunn, 1970; Newton, 1976; Shanks, 1975a, b; Vale, 1973; White, 1980). However, in the neurosurgical operating theatre, using a heavy duty 'space blanket' with two layers of MPS separated by a fibre layer, there was no difference in the rate of cooling between those patients who were wrapped up completely in MPS except for the head, and those who were not (Radford and Thurlow, 1979). In most other types of surgery the needs of surgical access will reduce the area of the body which can be covered and therefore the possible benefit. Bourke *et al.* (1984), again in operations on the head and neck, found a significant benefit from the use of MPS as compared with operating drapes alone. However, that gain may have come from the careful wrapping of the MPS round the patients since this would have prevented evaporative and convective heat loss as well as radiant loss, and it would have been interesting to compare their results with similar patients wrapped in polythene alone. Even though convinced of the benefits of MPS, Bourke *et al.* (1984) only recommended its use if the operation was going to last more than two hours and if more than 60 per cent of the body surface can be covered. In the operating theatre, if the diathermy is faulty, and there is an almost inevitable break in the thin layer of plastic covering the metallised sheet, the MPS can conduct electricity and cause electrical burns or even electrocution (Chambers and Saha, 1979; Cundy, 1980; Hill, 1980).

There are in addition other practical disadvantages. MPS produces a continual crackling noise when in use, and this is aggravated by any movement. This noise is very distressing to a confused hypothermic patient, especially the elderly. At the other end of the age scale a 'silver swaddler' has been advocated to prevent the loss of heat in the new-born baby. Unfortunately, when the principle on which it works is not understood, it can do more harm than good, as was described by Hey (1972). He visited a large maternity hospital where babies requiring resuscitation were wrapped in a 'silver swaddler' before being placed under a servo-controlled radiant heat canopy. The staff could not understand why the babies still became cold since they failed to realise that most of the radiant heat canopy was being reflected off the baby by the 'silver swaddler'. As a final disadvantage MPS has been found to be highly flammable. Despite all this evidence the 'space blanket' is still recommended (Burton, 1981; West, 1980; White, 1980).

Conclusion

It would seem to be logical to abandon the 'space blankets' and replace them with polythene bags on the grounds of effectiveness, robustness, cheapness and safety. Certainly the army during the Falklands campaign in 1982 took polythene bags as primary anti-cold protection and not bags with MPS. The continued use of MPS sheets at the end of a marathon appears to be related more to a shiny advertising gimmick for TV purposes than to the thermal protective function.

15 ACTIVE SURFACE WARMING

Rapid

Despite moral objections, and ignoring the fact that the hypothermia was acute immersion induced, the Nazi experiments (Alexander, 1945) are regularly quoted as showing that rapid rewarming in a hot bath is the treatment of choice for hypothermia. This view was supported by experimental work (Burton and Edholm, 1955) again following immersion hypothermia, and the abysmal results achieved by the early workers treating hypothermia in hospital (Emslie-Smith, 1958; Duguid *et al.*, 1961), though in these hospital cases treatment was by moderate surface rewarming, the cause of hypothermia was other than cold water immersion, and many of the cases were elderly and therefore probably suffering from subchronic hypothermia. In addition the Nazi victims were thin, malnourished and often diseased, and many had lost the will to live — very dissimilar from the typical cases of acute hypothermia that the rescue services meet. These latter are mainly young people, reasonably fit though occasionally exhausted, with everything to live for and, certainly in temperate and colder countries, with a good layer of subcutaneous adipose tissue.

Technique

Despite the almost universal recommendation of the hot bath as a method of rewarming, the men of the rescue teams who have to treat the victims are nevertheless left in some doubt as to the details of this method of treatment. The standard advice is to maintain the temperature of the bath between 40 and 45 °C (Freeman and Pugh, 1969; Mountain Rescue, 1968; Keatinge, 1977; Paton, 1983b) though one author recommends a temperature as high as 50 °C (Davies, 1975b), and Rees (1958) started with a bath temperature of 37.5 °C. A three-year-old child was warmed from a core temperature of 17 °C using a water temperature of 37 to 38 °C (Anderson *et al.*, 1970). There is in addition conflicting advice as to whether the hot bath should only be used in the mild cases or also in the severe ones; whether the clothes should be removed or not; whether the body should be totally immersed or the limbs kept out; and whether the dangers inherent in the method are such as to require the presence of a doctor or not (Burton and Edholm, 1955; Dalgleish, 1969; Frankland, 1975, 1981; Freeman and Pugh, 1969; Golden, 1973a; Keatinge, 1969; Lathrop, 1972; Mountain Rescue, 1968; Zingg, 1967). Davies (1975a, 1979) gives a detailed description of the technique which he uses in every case of hypothermia brought off the hills, and reports many cases of successful resuscitation of patients who were pulseless and apnoeic on arrival.

Since a hot bath raises the body temperature by the physical transfer of heat through the body surface without relying on any contribution from intrinsic metabolism, rewarming should be more rapid if the clothes of the victim were removed before immersion in the bath, and certainly shorn sheep rewarmed in a bath faster than unshorn sheep (Lloyd *et al.*, 1976a). However, the vigorous movement of the victim necessary to remove the clothing may precipitate ventricular fibrillation (VF) (Freeman and Pugh, 1969; Golden, 1973a; Lloyd, 1973). For ease of handling the patient should be supported on a canvas sling with the head on a waterproof pillow (Paton, 1983).

Advantages

One of the advantages claimed for the hot bath is that by suppressing shivering, the oxygen demand and therefore the load on the heart is reduced (Golden in Marcus, 1979a). Immersion in hot water is also the fastest way of transferring heat to a patient and a hot bath is an unsophisticated piece of equipment which has a wide distribution outside hospital. Another advantage claimed for the hot bath is that the fast rewarming reduces the depth and duration of the dangerous after-drop (Burton and Edholm, 1955; Freeman and Pugh, 1969; Golden, 1973a; Keatinge, 1969). However, as discussed elsewhere, the occurrence of ventricular fibrillation precipitated by the after-drop is a theoretical danger which has probably been overestimated.

Disadvantages and Hazards

While immersion in a hot bath does reduce the depth of the after-drop as measured in the rectum, when the temperature is measured in the heart, the hot bath causes a definite after-drop which is not present when the patient rewarms spontaneously (Hayward *et al.*, 1984a), and, for survival, cardiac temperature is far more important than rectal temperature.

Less oxygen is carried by cold blood than by warm blood and

therefore if cold blood perfuses warm cells, there may be insufficient oxygen for the metabolic needs of the cells. In surface warming of hypothermia the surface cells are warm but the blood is coming from the still cold core and this may be a possible cause of the acidosis which is seen during surface warming (Paton, 1983b).

Though the hot bath has been used in semiconscious and unconscious patients, the problem of maintaining the airway of the unconscious subject must increase the hazards of the method and, in the event of cardiac arrest, the manoeuvres necessary for effective cardiorespiratory resuscitation cannot be performed (Belopavlovic and Buchtal, 1980; Paton, 1983b). Even if the person is removed from the bath before defibrillation is attempted, the charge may run over the wet skin to earth and not only will it therefore be ineffective but it may cause burns (Cooke in Marcus, 1979a; Paton, 1983b). Major injuries are also relative contraindications to the method (Freeman and Pugh, 1969) because of the associated difficulties in treatment (Barwood in Marcus, 1979a).

Some experts now feel that rapid rewarming in adults is unnecessary, and that the only real value of the hot bath is if a person is hypothermic through immersion and can be transferred to the hot bath within 20 to 30 minutes of rescue from the water (Keatinge, 1969; 1977) because this is a period during which the most dangerous changes occur (Hayward *et al.*, 1984a). During this period it may reduce the depth and duration of the after-drop (Keatinge, 1969), restore the hydrostatic squeeze (Golden, 1980), though its true value may lie in the effect on body fluid shifts. After 20 to 30 minutes the body temperature gradients will have stabilised and the primary after-drop will be completed. The hot bath could then be dangerous. The recommended time interval raises practical problems in that when a sufferer is first located, e.g. on a mountain or in a small boat at sea, evacuation to a hot bath cannot be achieved in the time because of distance (Andrew and Parker, 1978), though the availability of a helicopter might cause a reappraisal of time in any individual case. Even if habitation is reached in the time, there is no guarantee that hot water will be immediately available, nor in sufficient quantities to maintain the desired water temperature. (The cold body and clothes immediately and markedly lower the water temperature and more hot water must be run in. This topping up of the hot water has to be repeated frequently and to do this properly, around 40 gallons of water are necessary (Frankland, 1981). This volume is likely to exceed the capacity of the hot water system.) The potential use of this method is thus greatly reduced in practice because of logistical difficulties. For example, the use of a hot bath is not possible in a lifeboat at sea (Guild in Marcus, 1979a) and as an ex-commando Arctic Warfare Trials Officer wrote (Tuck, J., pesonal communication, 1975):

> The War Office recommended treatment of hypothermia was rapid rewarming in a hot bath with the arms and legs hanging out, but quite how you would find a bath in the medical centre of a commando unit, let alone in a forward position in the Arctic, was never established.

The hot bath is not recommended for the elderly.

Slow to Moderate

The techniques used, which vary in the rate of heat transfer (Harnett *et al.*, 1983a) though all are slower than the hot bath, have included hot-water bottles (Bristow *et al.*, 1977; Read *et al.*, 1961; Rees, 1958), hot-water-circulating blankets (Vaagenes and Holme, 1982) or sarong, hot packs (Vaagenes and Holme, 1982), heated cradles (Ledingham and Mone, 1980; Linton and Ledingham, 1966; Rees, 1958), a heat ceiling (Madsen, 1983), electric blankets (Emslie-Smith, 1958; Fell *et al.*, 1968; Fernandez *et al.*, 1970; Lash *et al.*, 1967; Siebke *et al.*, 1975) and a temperature-controlled cabinet (Forrester, 1958; Lee and Ames, 1965). A portable 'sarong' has been developed for field use (Paton, 1983b). This weighs 3.3 lb (1.5 kg) and the water is heated on a camp stove and circulated by a modified bilge pump. The Hibler technique used by the Bavarian Mountain Rescue is to fold a linen sheet 32 times and then pour one litre of very hot water into the folds. This hot wet pack is wrapped round the chest and the patient is then covered with blankets and aluminium foil. It is claimed that heating lasts about two hours. Hot packs applied to areas of high heat loss, e.g. the neck and groin (Neureuther, 1979), have been tried, and in the French Alps a heating bag is placed on the thorax and abdomen under the insulating layers (Foray and Salon, 1985). One method of warming sometimes used by mountain rescue teams is for a member of the rescue team to climb into a sleeping bag with the victim (Mountain Rescue, 1968). In the extreme survival situation, freshly voided urine, at about 36 °C, in a plastic bag may provide some worthwhile heat (Gavshon and Rice, 1984). The Norwegian Defence Research Establishment has developed a charcoal burner which is laid on the chest or abdomen and a battery-operated fan circulates warm air under the clothing and covers.

It has been suggested that immersing only the arm in hot water can produce safe rewarming (Lawson, 1976; Matthew, 1975; Pugh, 1966) and the Danish Navy treat mild hypothermia by immersing the hands and feet in hot water (Dressler, 1982; Vanggaard, 1985). While heat is certainly applied to the surface the effect is claimed to provide central rewarming since the heated blood is transported directly to the heart, and the large surface area to mass ratio ensures rapid heat uptake (Vanggaard, 1985).

In one series of experiments it was claimed that the heat supplied by a radiant heat cradle was the main source of heat benefit (Ledingham, 1979; 1981; 1983a; Ledingham and Mone, 1980) but it is impossible to calculate the amount of heat supplied to the patient. The one temperature chart shown (Ledingham, 1979; 1981; 1983a; Ledingham and Mone, 1980) was of a 48-year-old man suffering from barbiturate and alcohol overdose and the rate of rise of temperature was about 1 °C/hour.

Problems Associated With Surface Heating

Effectiveness of Heat Transfer

Though most patients do rewarm with surface heating, this is not always so. To be effective surface heating requires the presence of an adequate peripheral circulation and, when this is absent, heat transfer is ineffective (Ledingham and Mone, 1980). The peripheral circulation is obviously reduced when the cardiac output is too low to sustain an adequate blood pressure and Ledingham (1979) does state that, in this situation, surface warming using the heat cradle technique was less effective. Another factor is that, with the marked vasoconstriction present in severe hypothermia, the peripheral circulation may be effectively absent, as was illustrated by the fact that dogs cooled to a core temperature of 25 °C failed to rewarm under a heat cradle (Ledingham, 1983a). In another example hot-water bottles (Read *et al.*, 1961) failed to raise the rectal temperature of one patient in the eleven hours before she died. Even a hot bath (Jessen and Hagelsten, 1978) at 40 °C only raised the core temperature of one victim 0.6 °C in 2.25 hours because of the absence of circulation.

Superficial Burns

The local effect of any temperature on a body tissue depends on a balance between the total heat supplied and the heat removed. The heat supplied depends on the thermal capacity of the substance, the absolute temperature and whether or not a change in physical state occurs. Any variation in tolerance to heat is due to the rate at which heat is removed which in turn is governed by the variation in blood supply to the tissues. Even in the induction of hyperthermia it has been shown that for any particular degree of heat applied to the tissue the temperature within the tissue is directly dependent on the flow of blood through that tissue (Hornback, 1984). The body responds to cold by vasoconstriction, especially in the limbs and subcutaneous tissues, with a decrease in the ability to remove heat and a resulting increased susceptibility to thermal damage (Crino and Nagel, 1968; Danzl, 1983). Therefore it could be dangerous to assume that because normothermic people can tolerate any particular temperature, that that temperature is necessarily safe for hypothermic victims. For example volunteers coming out of the cold Puget Sound with marked vasconstriction in the skin, found that water temperatures above 26 °C caused pain, even though their core temperature was only 35 °C (Hayward and Steinman, 1975) and another mildly hypothermic victim found 26 °C water was painful (Low, 1982). Similarly in a young patient, where the surface warming with hot wet towels and hot-water bottles was only part of the total rewarming package, the patient suffered burns on the thighs (Bristow *et al.*, 1977) and burns have been caused to limbs, chest and groin by hot-water bottles which were only filled with 'hand warm' water (de Pay, 1982). Even a normothermic young man developed leg ulcers following burns from hot-water bottles which were not too hot to touch (Curley and Almeyda, 1979).

The patients that Davies (1975a, b) treated apparently tolerated a water temperature of 50 °C without discomfort or skin damage. The explanation may be that the reduction in vasoconstrictor tone which accompanies the initial stages of spontaneous rewarming may have been aggravated by the movement necessary in transporting a casualty from the mountain and therefore the heat from the water would be rapidly removed from the skin, preventing skin damage and producing a rapid rise in core temperature.

Cardiovascular Stability

Moderate surface warming is usually condemned (Weltz *et al.*, 1942;

Burton and Edholm, 1955) for the following reason: As the heat reaches the surface the peripheral vessels dilate and the blood flow increases. This, however, does not warm the core since the small amount of heat supplied is dissipated in the cold shell, and it is cold blood which reaches the core. This initial cold flow may lower the core temperature 4 to 6 °C and thus further embarrass an already cold and inefficient heart, resulting in cardiac failure or ventricular fibrillation. However, as discussed earlier there does not seem to be any convincing evidence for this mechanism and there are probably other causes. In the clinical cases treated with surface heating there are many reports of cardiovascular instability (Anderson *et al.*, 1970; Phillipson and Herbert, 1967), a drop in blood pressure (Coopwood and Kennedy, 1971; de Pay, 1982; Madsen, 1983; Rees, 1958), confusion (Coopwood and Kennedy, 1971), convulsions (Rees, 1958), ventricular fibrillation requiring external cardiac massage (de Pay, 1982; Linton and Ledingham, 1966; Madsen, 1983; Siebke *et al.*, 1975), or just general deterioration leading to death (Fell *et al.*, 1968). Even after a hot bath there has been post-treatment anuria (Vaagenes and Holme, 1982).

Shivering

The hot bath abolishes shivering which may be an advantage since this will reduce the oxygen demand and therefore the work on the heart (Golden in Marcus, 1979a). However, as discussed elsewhere, any measure which raises the skin temperature depresses shivering and, while the hot bath provides sufficient heat to warm the patient without shivering, with many methods of external warming the quantities of heat supplied may be very small and the abolition of shivering may then put the person severely at risk. This is probably one factor which explains why the worst mortality in cases of profound accidental hypothermia occurs when treatment is by exposure in a warm room (Lilja, 1983). Another factor is that if the treatment gives a sensation of warmth to the skin, the cold-induced vasoconstriction will be abolished, resulting in a drop in blood pressure, and if this is not accompanied by a significant heat input, the patient will probably die.

Survival

The first six hypothermic patients treated by Duguid *et al.* (1961) were given active surface heating with 100 per cent mortality before reaching normothermia. Using active rewarming Emslie-Smith

(1958) also had 100 per cent mortality. Duguid *et al.* (1961) then allowed their later cases to rewarm spontaneously with a marked improvement in survival. Roe (1963) surveyed the results from 23 papers from 1953 to 1963 and of 39 patients who were actively warmed by surface heat only 5 survived, whereas of 44 patients allowed to rewarm spontaneously, 22 survived. These results led to the decision that moderate surface rewarming should never be used, especially in the elderly. Unfortunately no account was taken of the ages of the patients (Roe, 1963) nor was it appreciated that the elderly are usually suffering from subchronic hypothermia with the fluid shift problems, and all the patients treated by Emslie-Smith (1958) and Duguid *et al.* (1961) were elderly. Fernandez *et al.* (1970) after treating three cases with hypothermic mattresses claimed, because all three survived, that rapid rewarming was safe whereas moderate rewarming was dangerous. Unfortunately the three cases were all under 60 and had taken drugs and alcohol and therefore would be acute (immersion type) rather than subchronic hypothermia. In another report of 15 cases of hypothermia associated with drug overdose (Lee and Ames, 1965) treated with moderate surface warming, all 15 survived. Similarly young patients treated with surface warming (Atukorale, 1971; Bristow *et al.*, 1977; Siebke *et al.*, 1975) had a very high survival rate though not without problems. It has been claimed (Dressler, 1982) that there have been no reports of deaths in a hot-water bath. On the other hand, active external rewarming in a whirlpool bath was found to have a much higher mortality rate than spontaneous rewarming or airway warming (Miller *et al.*, 1980) and Mills (1983a) felt that the deaths of two people treated by rewarming in a hot bath was due to the sudden return to the circulation of metabolic acids from frostbitten limbs. A death from cerebral infarction within two hours of rewarming in a hot bath was attributed to combined anoxia and hypotension from the treatment (Vaagenes and Holme, 1982). When another series of patients treated with moderate surface rewarming is analysed as to age, it becomes clear that the elderly have a high mortality whereas younger patients have a high survival rate (Coopwood and Kennedy, 1971). The hot bath was used for a semiconscious 86-year-old man with a rectal temperature of 27.8 °C after the slower methods of surface warming, blankets and hot-water bottles had failed to raise the temperature (Rees, 1958). The man rewarmed completely though requiring intensive care because of cardiovascular instability but unfortunately he suffered a pulmonary embolism nine weeks later and died. It must be remembered that the young victims of hypothermia have become hypothermic acutely (immersion or exhaustion types) whereas the majority of the elderly have subchronic hypothermia. In an animal experiment, many dogs died during rewarming in a hot bath after prolonged hypothermia (Fedor *et al.*, 1958). The reason the Nazi experiments (Alexander, 1945) had convinced people of the superiority of the hot bath as a method of rewarming is easily understood once it is realised that the victims were hypothermic through acute immersion and were immediately immersed in the hot bath. Similarly the high success rate achieved by Davies (1975a, b) was with young exhaustion type hypothermic patients. The evidence appears to suggest that the type of hypothermia is more important for survival than the type of rewarming. One author considers the hot bath to be obsolete because of its risks and complications (Laessing, 1982).

Conclusions

Surface heating requires equipment of varying degrees of sophistication but each method has the potential for being available in the pre-hospital as well as the hospital phase of treatment. There are, however, problems associated with surface heating which are potentially very hazardous and therefore surface heating probably cannot be recommended unless intensive monitoring can be applied as well.

16 EXTRACORPOREAL BLOOD WARMING

Cardiopulmonary Bypass

Technique

Over the past years cardiac bypass has become an almost routine procedure for open heart surgery. Total body cooling protects the tissues of the heart from the deleterious effects of anoxia during the period of cardiac standstill necessary for the surgical procedure. After the operation the patient is rewarmed before being taken off the bypass equipment. The body temperature is adjusted by cooling or warming the blood while it is passing through the external oxygenator. For rewarming, the simplest extracorporeal circuit (involving the least surgery) uses large bore cannulae to remove blood from the femoral veins. The blood is oxygenated, warmed and returned to the circulatory system via the femoral artery (Davies *et al.*, 1967; Fell *et al.*, 1968; Kugelberg *et al.*, 1967; Turina and Hossli, 1979; Wickstrom *et al.*, 1976). Occasionally thoracotomy with venting of the left side of the heart is also required (Fell *et al.*, 1968). A disposable oxygenator and heat exchanger (Roberts and Robinson, 1970) may be primed with only 70 ml of a solution containing no blood (Truscott *et al.*, 1973). Cardiopulmonary bypass has been used with (Althaus *et al.*, 1978; 1982) and without (Dorsey, 1983) the inclusion of an oxygenator.

Heat Gain

Unfortunately, since the technique involves a continuous flow of blood from the patient through the heat exchanger, it is impossible to calculate the actual heat supplied by the method.

Advantages

In hypothermia the greatest danger is that the heart should stop pumping blood either becasue of asystole or ventricular fibrillation. The main advantage of extracorporeal rewarming is that the heart is perfused almost directly by heated blood thus reducing cardiac irritability and, if cardiac standstill does occur, the circulation to the brain and other vital organs is maintained by the equipment until the cardiac function can be restored. As long as the heart is rewarmed before the other body tissues, shock due to depressed cardiac function is unlikely and, if hypovolaemic shock should occur due to peripheral vasodilatation, a warm heart can compensate far more successfully than a cold heart. Extracorporeal blood cooling is claimed to be faster than surface techniques for lowering body temperature (Bernhard, 1956) and the same claim could be expected for rewarming. There is no conceivable situation in which this method should not be successful. Hypothermia with intractable ventricular fibrillation or asystole is an obvious indication for extracorporeal warming (Braun, 1985; Foray and Salon, 1985; Muhlemann, 1979; Towne *et al.*, 1972), and the case in which a woman was rewarmed from 22 °C despite ventricular fibrillation and respiratory failure (Truscott *et al.*, 1973) is proof of its efficacy.

Disadvantages and Hazards

In the proper hands, the procedure can be reasonably safe but it is a complicated, highly invasive procedure that requires special training and equipment. The risks of extracorporeal rewarming are mainly those of the extracorporeal techniques themselves rather than through any effect on recovery from hypothermia. The bypass equipment may cause damage to red cells sufficient to result in a marked haemolysis. Arteriovenous cannulation involves the risk of severe damage to the vessel, the possibility that plaque material may be released into the circulation to produce emboli, the possibility of air leaking into the circuit and circulation, and the risk of ischaemia due to spasm of the vessel. Because of the need to heparinise the patient, bleeding, whether this is internal (e.g. ulcers or cerebrovascular accident) or external (e.g. trauma), is an obvious absolute contraindication to the use of extracorporeal blood warming as also are any other conditions which may be adversely affected by the use of anticoagulants.

One of the main claims made in advocating the use of this procedure as a method for treating accidental hypothermia, is that it produces almost ideal rewarming conditions (Harnett *et al.*, 1983b). This may be true in cardiac surgery under anaesthesia but the hypothermic victim is likely to have profound vasoconstriction and therefore though cardiopulmonary bypass will rewarm the circulated tissues there may be large volumes of the body in which there is no circulation and therefore no warming. As a result though the core temperature may have returned to normal, this gives no indication of the state of the total body heat, and on one occasion (Fell *et al.*, 1968) the core temperature dropped 4 °C after stopping warming and remained low for 13 hours with J waves on the ECG, indicating that only a small part of the total body mass had been rewarmed and in addition the BP became unrecordable and remained so for 18 hours. Finally the post-rewarming period has often been stormy, with oliguria (Davies *et al.*, 1967) or even anuria which sometimes requires peritoneal dialysis (Althaus *et al.*, 1982; Fell *et al.*, 1968; Kugelberg *et al.*, 1967), circulatory and respiratory problems (Davies *et al.*, 1967; Kugelberg, *et al.*, 1967) and abnormalities of the electrolytes. In one case (Fell *et al.*, 1968) there was some doubt for a considerable time as to the cerebral function of the patient. Intensive care had therefore to be provided.

There is the additional practical disadvantage that the complex equipment necessary for extracorporeal circulation is too expensive for small hospitals (Foray and Salon, 1985) and will therefore only be available in a small number of large hospitals which are usually a long way from the areas where hypothermia most commonly occurs (except urban cases). The equipment takes a considerable time to prepare and even if equipment is maintained in a ready state it may be in use for cardiac surgery, and therefore unavailable, when a hypothermic patient arrives.

Haemodialysis

Haemodialysis was used to treat barbiturate poisoning (Lee and Ames, 1965), and, with the dialysis set at 37 °C, patients who were hypothermic rewarmed at a rate of 0.5 °C. Lee and Ames (1965), however, also state that 'all patients with hypothermia were treated by rapid total body rewarming in specially heated cubicles' so the details of the heat exchange are obscure. In addition to the haemodialysis the patients also had artificial ventilation and forced alkaline diuresis. In another series of cases (Laessing, 1982) haemodialysis achieved a rewarming rate of 1 to 2 °C/hour, but in these cases the metabolism had not been depressed by drug overdosage. The general benefits and dangers are similar to those described for cardiopulmonary bypass.

Conclusions

Extracorporeal blood rewarming is a method that can and has been used successfully for the treatment of accidental hypothermia by properly trained personnel in hospital. It involves a surgical procedure, requiring a high level of technical and medical competence and has significant hazards and post-treatment problems. Consequently, extracorporeal bypass as a means of rewarming in accidental hypothermia should be considered only in a major hospital as a final life-saving measure for cases that do not respond to more conservative methods.

17 IRRIGATION OF BODY CAVITIES

Mediastinal Irrigation

Unfortunately there is a limited availability of pump-oxygenators and artificial kidneys and, even in hospitals which possess these items, they may be unavailable because they are already in use for a surgical procedure. If the equipment is free but not assembled there may be a considerable delay (Fernandez *et al.*, 1970) and to avoid this delay Linton and Ledingham (1966) performed thoracotomy and irrigated the mediastinum with physiological saline solution at 40 °C. (No figures are given from which heat gain due to the method could be calculated. Nevertheless, from the clinical course of the case the method is an efficient means of transferring heat to the heart.) Intensive care was continued because of problems with both cardiovascular and respiratory status and the patient was also treated with forced diuresis to eliminate the barbiturate. Rewarming was successful, and the method has been used on other occasions (Althaus *et al.*, 1982; Coughlin, 1973; Foray, 1983; Foray and Cahen, 1981; Ledingham and Mone, 1980). The method has not always resulted in survival of the patient with three cases having died (Foray, 1983). Defibrillation is also more difficult during rewarming with pericardial irrigation than during cardiopulmonary bypass (Althaus *et al.*, 1982).

This method has most of the limiting problems associated with cardiopulmonary bypass requiring a high level of surgical competence and sophisticated facilities and, being an open method, there is an increased risk of infection (Paton, 1983b). It should, however, be a procedure which can be available in a greater number of hospitals than the two extracorporeal systems, but, like them, should probably be reserved for final life-saving emergencies.

Peritoneal Dialysis

Technique

Peritoneal dialysis is used in the treatment of renal failure and drug overdosage with the toxic substances diffusing from the body into the dialysate which is replaced regularly to maintain a large blood/fluid gradient and diffusion rate. The technique involves inserting a large needle through the abdominal wall into the peritoneal cavity and a suitable liquid is passed through this needle directly into the cavity and allowed to bathe the surfaces of the organs and tissues in the abdomen before being drained and replaced by fresh fluid. When peritoneal dialysis is used for rewarming, the technique should be the standard procedure except that the fluid should be warmed to a higher temperature (40.5 °C to 42.5 °C is probably satisfactory (Doolittle, 1977)). The heated fluid is left in the peritoneal cavity until most of its surplus heat has been given up to the tissues and it is then removed and replaced by a fresh, warm supply. The heat is transferred to the contents of the peritoneal cavity, which includes the liver, kidneys and the intestinal mesentery with its extensive vascular network. The inferior vena cava with blood from the lower limbs is heated directly and also returns heated blood from the other organs straight to the heart. Conductive heat transfer through the diaphragm provides some additional heat to the heart and lungs. The rate of heat input can be increased by changing the dialysate more frequently, the time interval being determined by measuring the temperature of the fluid being removed and the core temperature of the victim. One approach (Harnett *et al.*, 1983b) would be to begin with a short exchange interval and increase it until the removed dialysate is found to have lost much of its heat in relation to the core temperature. Jessen and Hagelsten (1978) describe the use of a two-catheter dialysis system with suction at the outflow to achieve high throughput rates (12 l/hour). It might be possible to simplify the technique for rewarming by developing equipment to allow the continuous heating and circulation of the dialysate through a closed-loop system. This would also reduce the volume of fluid needed to accomplish rewarming, but would eliminate the possibility of electrolyte adjustments or removal of drugs.

Heat Gain

There are several reports of cases of accidental hypothermia which have been successfully treated with peritoneal dialysis (Bristow, 1978, 1981; Grossheim, 1973; Jessen and Hagelsten, 1978; Jessen *et al.*, 1974; Johnson, 1977; Klarskov and Amter, 1976; Lash *et al.*, 1967; Pickering *et al.*, 1977; Reuler and Parker, 1978; Schissler *et al.*, 1981; Soung *et al.*, 1977; Stine, 1977), and it is interesting to examine the actual heat exchange and rewarming rates achieved. The first case reported (Lash *et al.*, 1967) described peritoneal dialysis as providing 'rapid' rewarming, though the rectal temperature only rose from 21 °C to 21.1 °C over two hours, and the rapid rise of temperature (4 °C in two hours) did not start until the dialysis was supplemented by surface warming with possible additional contributions from warmed intravenous fluids and a humidifier attached to the ventilator. The next 8 °C came at 1 °C/hour. It is often difficult to be sure of the actual quantities of heat supplied since, though the temperature of the fluid is known before being infused, it is not reported when the fluid comes out, and it is always assumed that the temperature will be that of the patient's core. However, some rough calculations can be made. In the above case, with the core temperature at 21 °C, 2 litres of fluid at 37 °C were instilled and left for one hour. The procedure was then repeated. The heat gained therefore was 64 kcal over the two hours that the temperature rose 1 °C. In a case in Winnipeg (Pickering *et al.*, 1977), where the temperature rose from 26 °C to 32 °C in 1.5 hours, 2 litres of fluid at 38 °C was run into the patient at 26 °C, and, on the assumption that 15 minutes were enough to give complete equilibration, the total heat supplied would be 24 kcal. The third treatment would give 12 kcal, with the second, therefore, about 18 kcal (a total of 54 kcal in 1.5 hours). In a 70 kg man, 56 kcal is required to raise the body temperature by 1 °C (mean specific heat of body tissues being 0.8 kcal per kilogram (Burton and Edholm, 1955)) and, if the 'core' is 50 per cent of the total body mass, 28 kcal is required to raise the 'core' temperature by 1 °C. The two cases discussed above were both young women and were therefore unlikely to weight 70 kg but in both the core temperature should have risen about 2 °C (actual 0.1 and 6 °C). There must therefore have been other factors, heat loss or gain, in both equations. In one other case (Jessen and Hagelsten, 1978), after immersion in a hot bath at 40 °C for 2.25 hours had only raised the core temperature from 23.4 to 24 °C, peritoneal dialysis raised the core temperature 6.2 °C in 2.3 hours. This is the exact result expected from a calculation of the heat supplied by the peritoneal dialysis. The body was therefore rewarming as if it was an inanimate object, which may have been the case since this patient did not survive. Similar calculations can be made for the other cases treated though, since heat was usually available from other sources in addition to the peritoneal dialysis, it is hard to attribute all the temperature rise to the peritoneal dialysis. Nevertheless these cases confirm that peritoneal dialysis is an efficient method of heat transfer.

Advantages

With peritoneal dialysis the temperature gradients throughout the body are more normal than those found during surface rewarming (Patton and Doolittle, 1972) and in addition to being an effective means of transferring heat to a victim, peritoneal dialysis has a definite beneficial effect on many organs. Cardiac function is improved as measured by heart rate, ECG configuration, arterial pressure, cardiac output, peripheral resistance and left ventricular work (Patton and Doolittle, 1972) and with peritoneal dialysis any cardiac irregularity tends to revert spontaneously to sinus rhythm (Klarskov and Amter, 1976). Direct warming within the peritoneal cavity also offers the advantage of revitalising the liver, thus allowing it to resume its functions of detoxification and conversion of lactic acid to glucose (Harnett *et al.*, 1983b) and the method has been shown to accelerate return of post-hypothermic renal function to normal (Patton, 1976), thus reducing the risk of post-rewarming anuria sometimes encountered after other methods of rewarming (Basycharov *et al.*, 1978; McKean *et al.*, 1970), e.g. surface heating (Darim and Reza, 1970; Vaagenes and Holme, 1982) and cardio-pulmonary bypass (Althaus *et al.*, 1982; Davies *et al.*, 1967; Fell *et al.*, 1968). Peritoneal dialysis also stimulates other vital functions (Jessen and Hagelsten, 1978) and therefore in cases of hypothermia with drug overdose, peritoneal dialysis could have a double benefit.

As a technique peritoneal dialysis is simple. It does not require highly trained personnel, or expensive complicated equipment, and can be set up in a few minutes (Lash *et al.*, 1967; Lightman, 1978; Mattocks and El-Bassiouni, 1971). It also has the advantages of not requiring access to blood and is no strain on the cardiovascular system (Lightman, 1978).

Disadvantages and Dangers

There are some problems and complications inherent in the technique (Jones, 1971):

(1) Recent abdominal surgery (Lightman, 1978) or massive trauma of the peritoneal cavity (Harnett *et al.*, 1983b) are major contraindications, though the initial insertion of the catheter can be used as a diagnostic test of intraperitoneal bleeding.

(2) There is the danger of inducing hypovolaemia through faulty technique (Lightman, 1978; Soung *et al.*, 1977) and this risk would increase with the high flow rates recommended by Harnett

et al. (1979) and Jessen and Hagelsten (1978). Too vigorous dialysis may also cause electrolytic imbalance (Holdcroft, 1981).

(3) The pressure of fluid in the peritoneal cavity predisposes to basal collapse and consolidation in the lungs and therefore any respiratory insufficiency is a relative contraindication (Lightman, 1978). A high flow rate might be expected to aggravate the problem.

(4) Infection is related to the length of dialysis, the efficiency of the aseptic procedures used during the introduction of the catheter and the administration of the dialysis fluid, and the use of closed drainage techniques. Infection can also pass down the catheter track from the skin. Though infection is very rare if the dialysis is continued for less than 72 hours (Leigh, 1974) — longer than is required for the treatment of accidental hypothermia — the procedure nevertheless requires to be done with full aseptic and sterile precautions (Lightman, 1978).

(5) Perforation of bowel or major blood vessel may be a tragic complication of peritoneal dialysis, but if care is taken to avoid old operation scars and patients with a history of peritonitis, this complication is fortunately very rare (Lightman, 1978). It should be remembered that the hypothermic patient may be unable to give a history.

There have been four deaths in patients rewarmed with peritoneal dialysis even under total physiological control though these were attributable to severe hypothermia and extensive frostbite rather that to the method of rewarming (Mills, 1983a).

Conclusions

Peritoneal dialysis is an efficient method of rewarming the core, and it also has beneficial effects on many organ systems. It is, however, an invasive technique with dangers and complications and one would not expect to see it used as a first aid measure. The major problem is the difficulty in carrying out a sterile procedure in the field as well as the necessity for a certain amount of diagnosis by non-medical personnel to determine the indications and contraindications in any individual case. The procedure does have the advantage that the equipment required for its application is minimal and should be readily available at any hospital.

Pleural Irrigation

Intra-pleural rewarming has been suggested (Blades and Pierpoint, 1954) though it has only been used in experiments with dogs and in one clinical case. The method requires an open thorax, and saline warmed to 45 °C is allowed to flow over the lungs and pleura and the excess siphoned off. In the clinical case hypothermia had previously been induced by the use of cold saline applied by the same technique. It should be possible to carry out pleural irrigation through catheters as with peritoneal dialysis though there must be an increased risk of pulmonary collapse and other pulmonary complications. If any of the underlying organs were to be damaged during insertion of the catheters the result is likely to be more dangerous than in the peritoneal cavity. This method appears to have no advantages over either of the other two irrigation techniques and probably has no place in the range of practical treatments for accidental hypothermia.

18 OTHER METHODS OF CENTRAL REWARMING

Rewarming Via the Gastrointestinal Tract

The possible approaches are warm drinks, gastric lavage, warm enemas and intragastric and intracolonic balloons.

Techniques

It is recommended that victims of hypothermia be given warm fluids by mouth (Lilja, 1983) but there is a limit to the quantity that can be given and the patient must be conscious.

Intragastric balloons are normally used for cooling the gastric mucosa to control bleeding due to ulceration (Barnard, 1956). It has also been used to induce hypothermia (Moss, 1966), but only recently has the technique been used to try to rewarm hypothermic patients (Pickering *et al.*, 1977). A double lumen tube transports fluid to and from the balloon with a provision for negative pressure removal of water from the balloon to keep its size constant in the stomach (Khalil, 1958). In addition Ledingham (1983a) has now described a technique using a modified Sengstaken tube through which Ringer's lactate solution is circulated at 41 °C.

Intracolonic balloons have been used for controlling the body temperature of animals (Cooper and Ross, 1960), but have not so far been used in man.

Enemas and gastric lavage have also been described (Bristow *et al.*, 1977) but require larger amounts of fluid than the closed-loop balloon systems and the fluid must be safe.

In any of the techniques using fluid the temperature of the liquid should probably be restricted to 40.5 to 42.5 °C as recommended for peritoneal dialysis (Doolittle, 1977; Khalil, 1958).

Heat Gain

In one case (Pickering *et al.*, 1977), where surface rewarming by circulating-water blanket and warm intravenous saline were used in addition to gastric lavage, the core temperature initially fell 1 °C over two hours. In another case (Bristow *et al.*, 1977) gastric lavage was supplemented by hot enemas plus hot wet towels and hot-water bottles, and a rise of 2.8 °C was achieved over 1 hour 25 minutes. In both cases the heat being supplied through other routes makes it impossible to calculate the quantity of heat supplied by gastric lavage. Rewarming using the modified Sengstaken tube with the double balloon (Ledingham, 1983a) is obviously an effective method of rewarming (though heat transfer calculations are impossible) since greyhounds rewarmed from 25 °C at a rate of 2.5 to 3 °C using this method, whereas similar greyhounds under a heat cage showed no rise of temperature in four hours. In a clinical case (Ledingham, 1983a), after the heat cage had produced a temperature rise of only 1.5 °C in twelve hours, the Sengstaken tube rewarmed the patient at 1.0 to 1.3 °C per hour.

Advantages

The intragastric and intracolonic routes both supply heat to the core through structures (stomach and large intestine) which are located in the peritoneal cavity and could therefore be expected to have effects similar to peritoneal irrigation, e.g. stimulation of the metabolic processes of the liver (Khalil and MacKeith, 1954), without penetrating the skin. If the balloon systems are used the rate of exchange of the rewarming medium is completely under external control and if a closed-loop circulation was developed, it might theoretically allow the circulation of a fluid with high specific heat but which was not biocompatible but there would be dangers if the balloon ruptured. The intragastric approach has the advantage that the heat is being supplied closer to the heart than through the colonic route and the modified Sengstaken tube could be expected to have some additional direct warming effect on the heart from its oesophageal component.

Disadvantages and Dangers

The actual surface area for heat exchange is small (Paton, 1983b) and trauma or surgical intervention involving the gastrointestinal tract would be a major contraindication to using intragastric or intracolonic balloons or lavage for core rewarming.

Gastrointestinal warming should be without serious risk. However, at temperatures below 28 °C the heart is very sensitive to mechanical irritation and the stimulation associated with the insertion of an intragastric balloon could trigger ventricular fibrillation (Hegnaur *et al.*, 1951). However, though endotracheal intubation has a similarly dangerous reputation, in several series of patients in which this technique was regularly used no case was reported in which ventricular fibrillation occurred during intubation (Ledingham and Mone, 1980; Lloyd, 1973; Miller *et al.*, 1980). Similarly in a series of animal experiments no arrhythmias were reported despite a Sengstaken tube being inserted at a core temperature of 25 °C (Ledingham, 1983a). As a note of caution, however, Schissler *et al.* (1981) reported a case where they had no doubt that intubation precipitated ventricular fibrillation and O'Keefe (1977) found two cases in a review of 62 patients where fibrillation followed some sort of manipulation. In another case the passage of an endotracheal tube provoked the onset of ventricular fibrillation (Osborne *et al.*, 1984). A more realistic danger associated with the passage of an intragastric balloon is the possibility of damage to the teeth, especially if there is trismus (Evans *et al.*, 1971), and the hypothermic victim's teeth may be so tightly clenched as to make passage of the tube impossible (Laufman, 1951). Even the insertion of a Guedel airway may be impossible because of muscle spasm (Frankland, 1983).

With gastric lavage fluid may pass into the duodenum and intestine and the patient may therefore receive large volumes of fluid (Paton, 1983b). There is also the possibility of regurgitation (de Villota *et al.*, 1973; Paton, 1983b) or vomiting resulting in inhalation/aspiration of gastric contents. This danger is obviously much greater with gastric lavage than with the use of a balloon system, but a balloon system is less efficient with regard to heat transfer (Paton, 1983b) and regurgitation can still occur up the outside of a balloon tube. If external cardiac massage is needed it cannot be done with gastric lavage because of the danger of emptying the full stomach resulting in pulmonary aspiration (Paton, 1983b).

At the lower end of the gastrointestinal tract, the membranes of the colon are thin, and traumatic injury is possible, particularly with elderly patients. In addition for core rewarming deep colonic penetration is desirable but this may be difficult to achieve and maintain against the peristaltic movements of the gut which tend to eject the balloon.

Conclusions

Intracolonic, and more particularly intragastric, balloons offer some promise as a core rewarming therapy without the requirement for the sterile precautions necessary for the peritoneal dialysis. It should be possible to carry out intragastric balloon rewarming at any hospital, though before it could be recommended for use in the field further experimental work is needed both with respect to the clinical benefits to be obtained and as regards equipment which must provide fluid at a safe temperature.

Intravenous Infusion

It is very easy to calculate the heat given to a patient by intravenous infusion (IV) but the danger of fluid overload and possible pulmonary oedema will limit the use of this method of heat transfer in pure hypothermia. However, if fluids are being given, they should be warmed (Paton, 1983), though this might be difficult in the field or during evacuation (Danzl, 1983), and even in hospital many blood/ IV fluid warmers are unsatisfactory in use (Russel, 1974).

Diathermy

Techniques

There are three systems which are used for therapeutic purposes (Lehmann, 1971) and all act by transmitting energy through superficial tissues to deeper ones where the energy is converted into heat. The three types were considered by Harnett *et al.* (1983b) and the following technical information is taken from that paper.

Ultrasonic Diathermy. With ultrasonic diathermy, high-frequency acoustic vibrations (0.8 to 1.0 MHz) are propagated at intensities of 1 to 4 watts/cm^2 in the form of longitudinal compression waves and the heating results from tissue particle movement as a result of the wave propagation. Wave intensity diminishes exponentially with depth but reflection can occur at the interface between different tissues and especially at bone and surgical implants. Fat and bone absorb much more of the energy than does muscle but because most of the conversion to heat occurs in the tissue proteins (Carstenson *et al.*, 1953; Piersol *et al.*, 1952) the main generation of heat occurs in the muscles with relatively little in the subcutaneous fat. Ultrasonic waves will not propagate through air, so physical contact with the transducer is required and therefore ultrasonic diathermy should be applied with a heavy oil as a mediator between the transducer and the patient's skin.

Short-wave Diathermy. In short-wave diathermy the patient is part of a circuit through which a high-frequency current (13.56 to 40.68 MHz) is passed, using either a capacitance or an induction device. Heating is produced at a depth which is between that produced by superficial heating agents and that produced by low-frequency microwave or ultrasound, and appears to be an efficient agent to heat musculature up to a depth of 1 to 3 cm (Lehmann, 1971). Surgical patients have been rewarmed by using a standard diathermy unit, with the induction coil wrapped around the pelvis (Swan *et al.*, 1955) and rewarming was as rapid as immersion in water at 45 °C. However, occasionally, for no apparent reason, the method appeared to be inefficient. Bigelow *et al.* (1952) found that the short-wave treatment on a frequency of 13.56 megacycles was most effective for heating the deep tissues of large animals, and if the diathermy coils were spaced half an inch from the body, adequate heat could be generated without burning the subcutaneous tissues. All the dogs and monkeys resuscitated by this technique from 21 °C to normal body temperatures survived with no burns, no signs of vascular collapse and no post-rewarming change in behaviour or intelligence. This finding was repeated with rhesus monkeys (Olsen and David, 1984). Whole-body animal rewarming led to the recovery of the animal 'with puzzling rapidity' (Holzloehner *et al.*, 1942) and these results stimulated the human experiments at Dachau. However, 'short wave' diathermy of the heart had no demonstrable beneficial effect when used at Dachau (Alexander, 1945) though no technical details are provided and the equipment available at the time did not permit whole-body treatment of the human subjects.

Microwave Diathermy. Microwave diathermy has also been used (Leese and Schuette, 1980; Westenskow and Wong, 1980; Westenskow *et al.*, 1979), and with this method the energy is in the form of electromagnetic radiation (915 to 2,450 MHz) and heat is created by the resistance of the tissues to the radiation. The longer wavelength (915 MHz) usually used for industrial, scientific and medical purposes transfers more power to deep tissues than does 2,450 MHz (Guy *et al.*, 1974). With 2,450 MHz the absorption is so great in the muscle layer that the depth of penetration is only 1.7 cm and the fat/muscle interface produces a 'hot spot' in the fat layer one quarter wavelength from the muscle surface. It is also difficult to predict the proper therapeutic level for individual patients since the thickness of subcutaneous fat varies widely and this affects the amount of power reaching the deep tissues (Guy *et al.*, 1974). On the other hand, with

915 MHz there is minimal fat heating and the heating pattern is reasonably uniform. With 915 MHz microwaves 50 per cent of the energy available at the muscle surface is available at a 3 cm depth while it is available to only a 1 cm depth with 2,450 MHz (Lehmann, 1971).

Heat Gain

Apart from the clinical evidence of the effect of short-wave diathermy the heat gain from the other methods would have to be calculated in each case. However, in one experimental series the rewarming rate using diathermy was much faster than using airway warming (White *et al.*, 1984).

Advantages

The ability to heat tissues below the subcutaneous fat layer is the primary advantage for diathermy rewarming, especially using ultrasound and low-frequency microwaves. If cardiac arrest occurs the coils can be positioned over the pelvis and this would allow external cardiac massage to be used to support the circulation until the patient had rewarmed sufficiently for spontaneous defibrillation to occur or till the cardiac temperature was high enough for electrical defibrillation to be effective.

Disadvantages and Hazards

Short-wave and microwave diathermy are liable to cause superficial burns as a result of the use of excessive energy, moisture on the patient's skin, or improper positioning or movement of the applicator during treatment and it can result in severe, deep and slow-healing burns (Paton, 1983b). For short-wave diathermy the induction coil applicator reduces the risk and with modern ultrasound equipment the energy output is automatically reduced if there is transducer movement. A more difficult problem is the determination of proper treatment dosage. Verbal feedback from the patient is generally used in physical medicine to determine control settings on a diathermy unit. A semiconscious or unconscious hypothermia victim would be unable to provide information about the heating effect of the treatment and even if the patient was conscious, because of the loss of skin sensation due to the cold, the danger of extensive burns exists even though constant supervision is provided by a physician (Alexander, 1945). Swan *et al.* (1955) regularly used the technique on surgical patients applying the therapy intermittently, two minutes on and one minute off. Nevertheless it is undoubtedly true that diathermy can 'cook' the tissues, and this is most likely to occur where there is no circulation to transport the heat generated to other parts of the body. Under these circumstances even a heart in asystole may be burned (Umach and Unterdorfer, 1979a).

The complete lists of contraindications are given by Lehmann (1971) and include:

(1) any question of haemorrhage;
(2) areas of sensory loss;
(3) moist dressings or adhesive tape;
(4) regions of unsuspected malignancy;
(5) presence of phlebitis;
(6) tuberculosis;
(7) haemorrhagic diathesis;
(8) areas of occlusive arterial disease;
(9) areas containing metallic implants;
(10) patients with pacemakers;
(11) during pregnancy or menstruation; and
(12) spinal area after laminectomy.

The region of the eyes must be avoided because of the danger of damage caused by cavitation of the fluid. In addition fluid accumulation in the body cavities, including the joints, may cause problems since selective heating of these may occur. Areas of oedematous tissue should also be avoided, which is a problem since oedema may be a consequence of hypothermia. For short-wave and microwave diathermy, wet clothing should be removed and the patient should be thoroughly dried so that hot spots and burns do not develop on the body surface. This must increase the risk of ventricular fibrillation because of the movement necessary. To prevent burns, terry cloth is usually used with short-wave diathermy to absorb any residual moisture or perspiration and to help space the induction heating coils at least 1 cm from the skin. Short-wave therapy by induction coil heating is recommended rather than capacitance heating with large plates. Since metallic implants or pacemakers are contraindications for short-wave and microwave diathermy, any patient to be rewarmed by these methods should be thoroughly checked for scars on the thorax or joints which might suggest implants in or near the regions to be heated. Also, due to the danger of strong locally induced heating, all metallic objects such as rings or bracelets should be removed prior to treatment.

There are also worries that microwave radiation may have some possibly hazardous non-thermal effects (Hornback, 1984).

Conclusions

Diathermy requires sophisticated and therefore expensive equipment but it is commonly operated by technicians. The equipment may be made reasonably portable but requires a supply of electric power. Diathermy has an undoubted potential for delivering significant amounts of heat. However, the practical scope for the use of this type of therapy must be severely limited in the emergency situation by the difficulty of identifying all the features which are contraindications to the use of diathermy, especially if the patient is not fully conscious, by the problems of finding dosimetry guidelines which are effective yet safe in the absence of reliable feedback from the patient and finally by the difficulty in ensuring that a person is completely dry before treatment.

19 AIRWAY WARMING

This is a relatively new method of treatment, having first been suggested as being of potential benefit in 1971 (Lloyd, 1971). Since that time there have been divergent views as to its value, ranging from marked enthusiasm to outright hostility, and because of this, the following examination of the method is more detailed than was applied to the more established methods.

Technique

As will become evident from the calculations below, airway warming works mainly by preventing the heat and moisture loss which normally occurs through respiration. The equipment for airway warming therefore has to fulfil this requirement. This can be done in a number of ways, and the range of possible equipment has been reviewed (Lloyd, 1986). The currently available practical equipment is as follows:

(1) A condenser humidifier traps the heat and moisture during expiration and returns both to the next inspiration. There are a number of designs with different levels of efficiency and any type could be incorporated in a breathing system. Two versions have been suggested for practical use (Lloyd and Croxton, 1981; Soininen and Linden, 1982). One design (Lloyd and Croxton, 1981) only weighs 85 g (3 oz) complete (Figure 19.1) and should be used tucked under the outer clothing for the greatest thermal benefit (Figure 19.2).

(2) Heat and moisture can be provided by a conventional electrically powered humidifier (Lloyd, 1973). One version has been developed which is powered by a portable generator and is used in crevasse and mountain rescue in the French Alps (Foray and Cahen, 1981). This weighs 6 kg without the generator (Legrand, 1984).

(3) Another device has been developed (Hayward, 1979) which heats water over a gas burner and the steam is injected into a breathing circuit with the inspired air temperature being

Figure 19.1: Respiratory Insulator — Exploded View

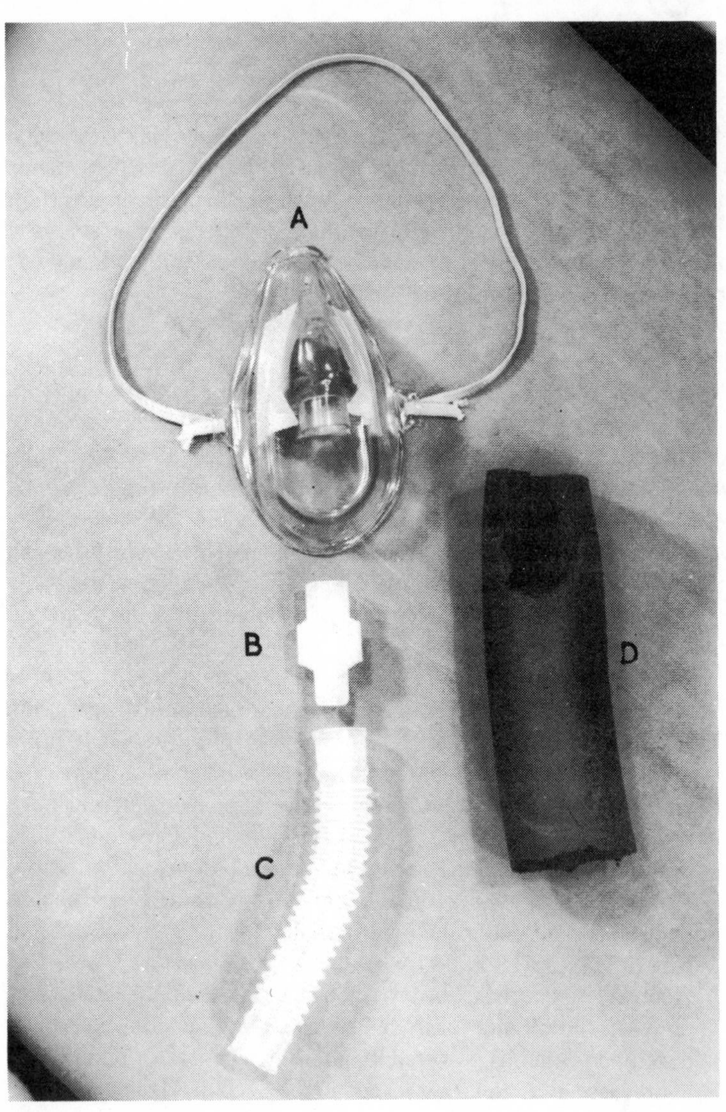

A Mask
B Portex condenser humidifier
C Tubing
D Neoprene insulating tubing

Figure 19.2: Respiratory Insulator in Use

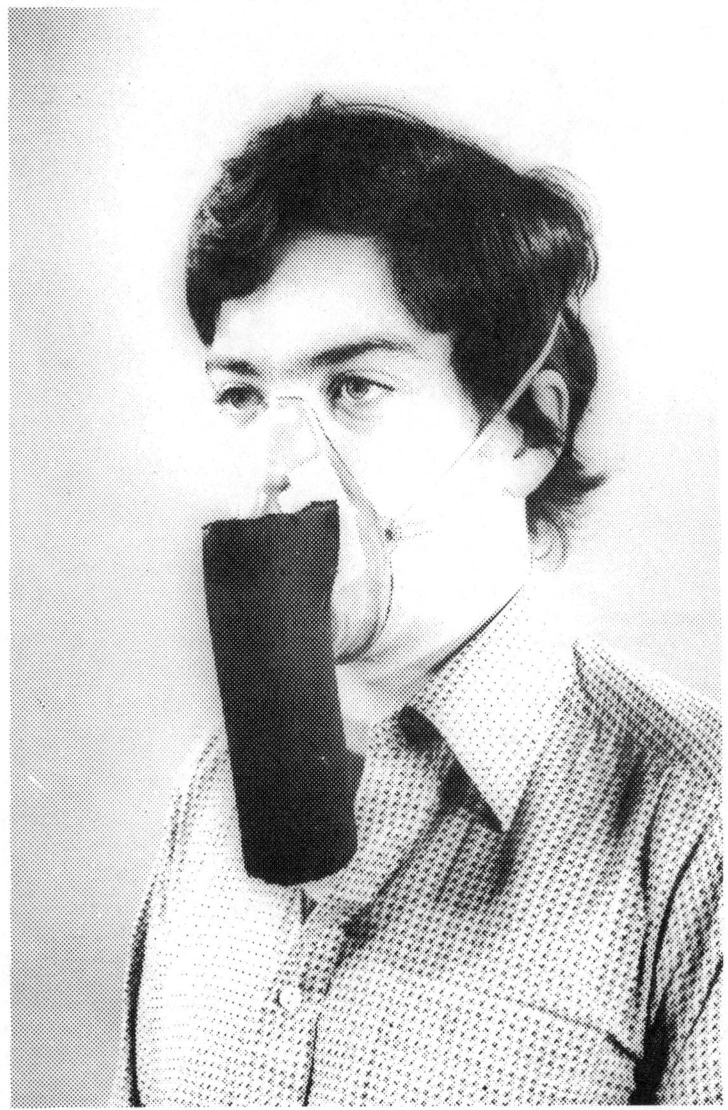

Note: end of tubing should be under the clothing and the insulation should cover the condenser humidifier and mask.

Figure 19.3: Lightweight Portable Airway Warming Equipment — Exploded View

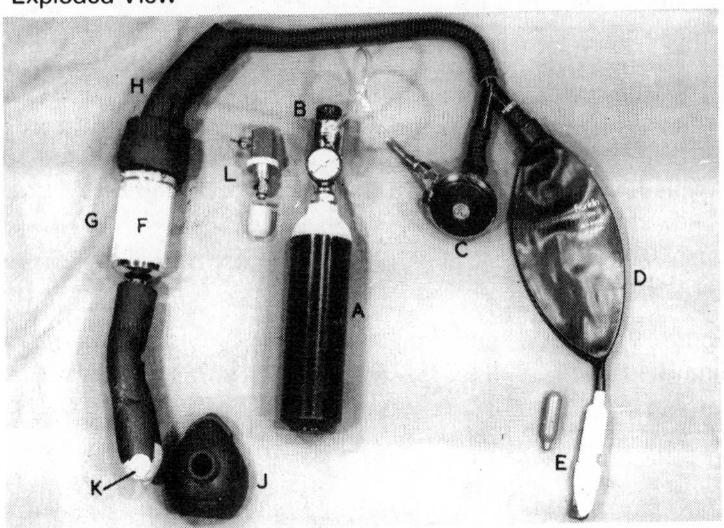

A Oxygen cylinder
B First stage reducing valve and gauge
C Demand reducing valve with manual override to allow reservoir bag D to be filled if ventilation requires to be assisted
D 2-litre reservoir bag
E Corkette (sparklet corkmaster) — with the distal portion of the needle removed and inserted into the tail of the reservoir bag, spare sparklet alongside
F Soda lime
G Paediatric Waters canister
H Insulation — neoprene foam tubing
J Face mask
K Thermometer registering mean air temperature at mask inflow
L Adaptor for refilling small oxygen cylinder from a large cylinder

Instructions for use

Empty one sparklet cylinder into system by using corkette (E). Open the valve (B) on the oxygen cylinder (A). Apply the face mask (J) to the patient. If desired the reservoir bag (D) can be partially inflated by depressing the centre of the demand valve (C). Thereafter the system will work on demand. The thermometer (K) should be observed. This will rise steadily into the working temperature range and when the temperature again drops to 35 °C, place a new sparklet cylinder in the corkette (E) and by depressing the lever allow CO_2 to flow for three seconds. This may be repeated whenever the thermometer temperature drops to 35 °C until the second sparklet is empty. Where possible the Waters canister (G) should be vertical rather than horizontal to reduce the risk of the gases channelling along the side of the canister. The gauge on the oxygen cylinder should be checked regularly to ensure that it is not empty.

After use the oxygen cylinder should be refilled from a large cylinder using the adaptor (L). The soda lime (F) should be replaced in the Waters canister (G), ensuring by tapping and shaking that the canister is completely full and that no channelling of gases can occur along the side when the canister is not vertical.

controlled by adjusting the proportion of admixture with the cold ambient air. There is a thermometer in the face mask. This weighs a minimum of 3.36 kg without the gas cylinder.

(4) The first equipment described (Lloyd *et al.*, 1972) utilised the reaction between carbon dioxide and soda lime to produce heat and moisture and the victim breathes through the hot, moist soda lime. The original closed-circuit prototype weighed about 3 kg plus the weight of the oxygen cylinder (5 kg). However, further development has produced a version (Figures 19.3 and 19.4) weighing only 3 kg including the oxygen (Lloyd and Croxton, 1981).

Figure 19.4: Lightweight Portable Airway Warming Equipment in Simulated Use

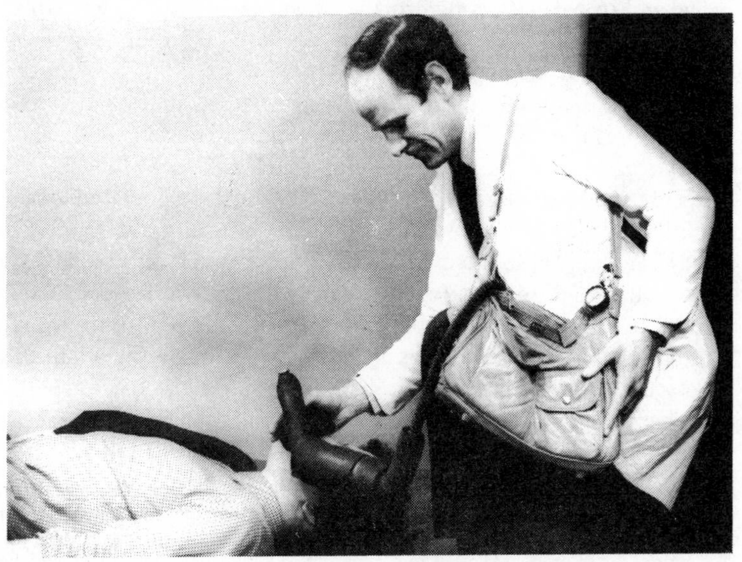

(5) A number of versions of equipment using the carbon dioxide/soda lime reaction but with an open, non-return breathing circuit. The most sophisticated version (Guild, 1978) weighs 4 to 5 kg but is not commercially available. The designs commercially available are the 'Reviva' (Bell, P.M., personal communication, 1976) which weighs 5.3 kg, and the 'Little Dragon' (Mitchell, M., personal communication, 1976) which weighs about 3 kg. Both these models have been used in the field in mountain rescue and cave rescue.

The choice of design depends on the particular circumstances of any rescue service.

Heat Gain

Theoretical Calculations

Because of the very low thermal conductivity of air, ventilation with warm dry air will provide negligible heat gain and, being dry, may cause a net heat loss from the body. Moritz *et al.* (1945) calculated that if 500 ml of dry air at 142 °C is inhaled and then exhaled at 38 °C, 13 cal of heat is given up. If, however, 500 ml of equal parts of steam and air are inhaled at 125 °C and exhaled at 38 °C, 175 cal would be given up by condensation of the water vapour and only 12 cal and 26 cal in the cooling of the gas and condensed water, a total of 213 cal compared with 13 cal from the hotter drier air. It must be emphasised that the experiments of Moritz *et al.* (1945) were very artificially designed to try to produce burns of the lungs and all the temperatures used would cause severe burning to the skin of the face or laryngeal spasm and oedema before the lungs could be affected. The only significant quantity of heat available to be liberated is that from the condensation of water vapour, i.e. 540 cal/g at 100 °C and somewhat more at lower temperatures (Hudson and Robinson, 1973).

The quantities of heat lost through respiration were calculated (Lloyd *et al.*, 1972) using the formulae provided by Burton and Edholm (1955) but several assumptions were made including the false one that the respiratory minute volume is the same at hypothermic temperatures as at normothermia. An average man at rest has a total lung ventilation of about 8 l/min (480 1/hour). If a person inspires air at 20 °C and exhales at 37 °C, heat is lost in raising the temperature of the air by 17 °C and in saturating the inspired air with water vapour. The specific heat of air at normal atmospheric pressure is 0.24 cal/g/°C. 480 litres of air will have a mass of 576 g (density of air = 0.012 g/ml) and to raise this mass of air by 17 °C will require $576 \times 0.24 \times 17 = 2{,}350$ cal (2.35 kcal). The loss of heat through saturating the inspired air with water vapour, i.e. the heat loss by evaporation, is considerably greater, about 9 to 11 kcal/hour, so altogether the heat loss by warming the inspired air is 11 to 13 kcal/hour, which is negligible when compared with the heat production of a normal resting man (70 to 100 kcal/hour). If, however, a hypothermic situation is envisaged the calculation changes. At a core temperature of 30 °C the heat production has been reduced by 50 per cent (Bigelow *et al.*, 1950) to 35 to 50 kcal/hour. In the situation where hypothermia occurs the air temperature will be much lower, e.g. 0 °C, and drier, so that the calculation of the heat loss now reads (core temperature 30 °C) 576 × 0.24 × 30 = 4,147 cal/hour = 4.1 kcal/hour + 13 to 15 kcal/hour as evaporative loss from the lower temperature, a total of 17 to 20 kcal/hour. This heat loss is about 30 to 50 per cent of the heat production of the hypothermic person compared to 10 to 15 per cent in the normothermic example. If a third example is taken of the same hypothermic patient breathing air saturated with water vapour at a temperature of 45 °C, the heat gained will be 576 × 0.24 × 15 = 2.1 kcal/hour and no heat will be lost in evaporation from the respiratory tract. Hudson and Robinson (1973) calculated that if a hypothermic patient was ventilated for 1 hour at 8 l/min with air saturated with water vapour, and if all this water vapour were to condense, the quantity of heat released would be about 13 kcal. However, because only a part of the inspired water vapour condenses in the body a more realistic figure was likely to be 2.1 kcal (Hudson and Robinson, 1973). There will therefore be a heat gain of 2 to 13 kcal/hour from the condensation of the water vapour and a possible further 2 kcal/hour through the cooling of the condensed water. Therefore instead of a heat loss of 17 to 20 kcal/hour there will be a gain of 2.1 kcal/hour plus 2 to 13 + 2 kcal/hour, a difference in the equation of at least 21 and possibly 35 kcal/hour. If the temperature of the inspired gas is raised to 60 °C the heat gained for the hypothetical victim would be 576 × 0.24 × 30 = 4.2 kcal/hour. However, the higher the temperature the greater the danger of burning the tissues of the body, especially the face and larynx, and therefore the increase of 2.1 kcal/hour is so negligible that there is no advantage in raising the temperature of the inspired gas above about 40 to 45 °C. The assumption that the temperature of the exhaled air is at core temperature whereas it is on average 4 °C cooler (Hudson and Robinson, 1973) affects the calculations very little, amounting in fact to about 0.5 kcal/hour difference in the heating only. Similar figures for respiratory heat loss and gain were calculated by Shanks and Marsh (1973). To summarise, if the hypothetical victim at 30 °C is breathing direct to the environment he will have 15 to 33 kcal/hour with which to rewarm providing there is no continuing loss of heat from the body surface. If, however, airway warming is used he will have from 56 to 85 kcal/hour with which to rewarm, a worthwhile gain but only if the far greater heat loss from the body surface has been stopped by insulation.

Guild (1978) using the Institute of Heating and Ventilation Engineers psychrometric charts and airway temperatures based on figures given by Cole (1953a, b; 1954a, b), Walker *et al.* (1961) and Webb (1951) and his own studies, produced a table which showed the heat gains and losses under a variety of conditions of body and air temperatures and ventilation rates. Unfortunately there was a minor error in one of the calculations which had the effect of diminishing the apparent benefit of airway warming. Table 19.1 gives the correct figures and also an indication of the potential benefit of the use of airway warming in terms of anticipated rise in core temperature. The other problem is that 30 °C is the lowest temperature considered in the calculations and in the operational requirements (Guild, 1978) when in fact considerably lower temperatures are possible in the field.

Hudson and Robinson (1973) criticised the concept of airway warming by means of calculations but unfortunately they used 1.0 kcal/kg/°C as the specific heat of the body and not 0.8 kcal/kg/°C (Burton and Edholm, 1955). They also only calculated the heat input and its effect on the total body temperature and ignored the prevention of the normal respiratory heat and moisture loss and the fact that any heat benefit would be concentrated in a small core. In fact it was noticed that in spontaneous rewarming and airway warming (AW) the skin temperature was very slow to rise (Hayward *et al.*, 1984a). In an experiment with sheep (Lloyd *et al.*, 1976a), the temperature of the aortic blood was always lower than the temperature of the blood in the pulmonary artery and the introduction of airway warming was the only factor which raised the temperature of the aortic blood above that of the pulmonary artery (Figure 12.1). This is added support for the idea that the heat gain from airway warming is concentrated in the core.

The vital core of the body consists of the brain, heart, kidneys and hepato-portal system and this comprises 8 per cent of the body mass in contrast to the muscles and skin which make up 52 per cent of the body mass and other tissues, presumably including bone and cartilage, make up the remaining 40 per cent (Aschoff and Wever, 1958; Carlson and Hsieh, 1965). However, in the basal non-shivering state the muscles and skin only produce 25 per cent of the metabolic heat whereas the 8 per cent core produces 56 per cent of the heat (Aschoff and Wever, 1958; Carlson and Hsieh, 1965). In the hypothermic situation the position is worsened because not only is the

Table 19.1: Calculated Respiratory Heat Losses at Various Ambient and Core Temperatures, and Ventilation Rates, with the Potential Benefits of Airway Warming

								Rise in Core Temp. from Available Heat	
Body Temp. °C	*Ventilation l/min*	*Basal Metabolic Rate kcal/hour*	*Heat Loss kcal/hour*	*Heat Left for Rewarming kcal/hour*	*Heat Gain with Airway Warming kcal/hour*	*Heat Available for Rewarming kcal/hour*	*% Improvement*	*Without Airway Warming °C/hour*	*With Airway Warming °C/hour*
37	5	72	– 8.0	64				1.8	
37	10	90	–16.0	74				2.1	
30	3	35	– 3.2	32.8	+ 6.2	39	19	0.9	1.1
30	10	35	–10.6	24.4	+20.5	55.6	128	0.7	1.6

Environmental temperature of air = 0 °C
Airway warming air temperature = 45 °C with 100% relative humidity
Source: Adapted from Guild (1978)

total heat production reduced but the proportions produced by the different tissues will also be altered. The heat generated by a tissue is dependent on the absolute temperature and therefore lowering the temperature reduces the maximum heat-generating ability of that tissue. Since the main muscle masses and skin will lie in the cold shell of the body their temperature will be much lower than normal and they will therefore be producing even less than the 25 per cent of heat produced at normothermia. The temperature of the organs making up the 8 per cent of the core will be much nearer normothermia than the superficial tissues and these organs will therefore be producing more than the normothermic 56 per cent of the total heat being produced. As there will be heat produced from the respiratory muscles a possible estimate is that in the hypothermic person 10 per cent of the body mass will be producing 80 per cent of the body heat. Therefore if any net heat gain can be concentrated in this 10 per cent of the body instead of the whole 70 kg man or even in the 50 per cent suggested as being the maximum core, only 5.6 kcal would be required to raise the temperature by 1 °C. The net heat gain from airway warming of 19 to 15 kcal/hour could therefore produce a rise in temperature of the 10 per cent core of between 3 and 6 °C/hour. The concentration of the heat gain in the active 10 per cent could have an additional spin-off benefit to the patient since every degree rise of temperature increases the metabolic heat production of the tissues. (The Q_{10} factor for metabolism is 3 which means that if the body temperature rises by 10 °C heat production is trebled (Maclean and Emslie-Smith, 1977).) It is therefore theoretically enticing to try and concentrate the available heat in this metabolically most active part of the body. This theoretical concept is reinforced by the observation that in patients who had become hypothermic while under anaesthesia, the intercostal muscle temperatures rose after the initiation of spontaneous ventilation but there was no rise of temperature in the deltoid, biceps or forearm muscles until voluntary movement started (Lunn, 1969).

The main thermal value of airway warming therefore lies in the prevention of the loss of respiratory heat and of respiratory moisture heat, with only a small benefit from the additional heat supplied. Therefore increasing the tidal volume without increasing the minute volume would result in negligible thermal benefit. On the other hand, if the minute volume is increased using saturated gases, the increased condensation of the water vapour might increase the rate of rewarming but would also increase the risk of precipitating ventricular fibrillation through the rapid alteration of the acid base status. On theoretical grounds the aim of airway warming as a practical measure must be to regard it as a means of insulating the respiratory heat loss and this can be done by providing a warm humid atmosphere for the victim to breathe and while the gas temperature should be above the core temperature of the victim, 40 to 45 °C should be the maximum.

Rate of Rewarming

Airway warming is similar to spontaneous rewarming in that the main thermal input comes from the body's own metabolic heat production. This makes it difficult to compare the rates of rewarming reported in case reports of individual patients which have been rewarmed by airway warming. However, one study reported 37 cases of which 19 were treated with airway warming and 18 were allowed to rewarm spontaneously (Lloyd, 1986). The rates at which the patients rewarmed are shown in Table 19.2 for the airway-warmed group and Table 19.3 for the spontaneously rewarmed group.

In many of the cases treated by airway warming there was a period before airway warming could be introduced and the rate of change of temperature during this period was recorded. Similarly it was not always possible to continue with airway warming until normothermia was reached and the rate of change of temperature during this period was also recorded. In the cases treated with airway warming, the rate of rewarming with airway warming was faster than the rate before treatment was started and, when airway warming was stopped before rewarming was completed, the subsequent rate of rewarming was always less than the rate during airway warming. The mean rate of rewarming during airway warming was 0.76 °C/hour compared with −0.25 °C/hour, for the 13 patients from whom readings were obtained in the period before treatment started, and with 0.24 °C/hour for the 12 with readings from the post-airway-warming period. Three of the airway warming group started to cool after airway warming stopped, because of the neurological damage which had precipitated the hypothermia, but the mean rewarming rate for the rest, post airway warming, was 0.39 °C/hour which is very similar to the mean for the spontaneous rewarming group which was 0.34 °C/hour. This confirms the findings of the animal experiments (Lloyd *et al.*, 1976a) that airway warming accelerates rewarming and, as would be expected since the method increases the heat available to the core, there was no initial drop of temperature as a result of the treatment. In fact any after-drop had probably been completed before the treatment started.

Table 19.2: Rates of Rewarming in Patients as Influenced by Airway Warming

			Pre-treatment Change			*Temp. at Start of Treatment*	*Change with Airway Warming*			*Temp. at End of Treatment*	*Change After Treatment*		
Case	*Sex*	*Age*	*Temp. °C*	*Time Hours*	*Rate °C/hour*	*°C*	*Temp. °C*	*Time Hours*	*Rate °C/hour*	*°C*	*Temp. °C*	*Time Hours*	*Rate °C/hour*
A 2	M	55	—	4	—	27	3	3	1.00	30	7	9	0.78
A 3	F	22	—	4	—	34	1.5	2.75	0.55	35.5	–0.75	5	–0.15
						34.75	3	4.25	0.71	37.75	—	2	—
A 7	F	23	–1	1	–1	29	7.5	13	0.58	36.5	1	11	0.09
A 8	F	39	–3.5	3	–1.2	30	6	12	0.50	36	2.5	8	0.30
A14	M	50				33	1	2	0.50	34	4	15	0.27
A17	M	56	—	1.5	—	28.5	7.7	4.5	1.70	36.2	1.5	3	0.50
A18	F	39	–0.5	0.5	–1	30.5	2.5	4	0.63	33	4.5	8.5	0.53
A 1	F	61	–2	10	–0.20	34.8	1.8	2	0.90	36.6			
A11	F	75	–6	24	–0.25	31	6	30	0.20	37			
A13	M	38	–5	24	–0.21	32	4.5	12	0.38	36.5	–2.5	12	–0.21
A 5	F	75				28	3.3	5.5	0.60	31.3			
A 6	F	80	—	2	—	25.5	1.8	3	0.60	27.3			
A15	M	84				23	4	6	0.67	27			
A16	F	81				28	7	5	1.40	35			
A 4	F	57	—	7	—	28	0.6	1.5	0.40	28.6			
A19	F	60				28	7	7.25	0.97	35	–3.5	9	–0.39
A12	F	70	3	6	0.5	33	2	2.5	0.80	35	2	5	0.4
A 9	F	75				32.5	1.5	1.5	1.00	34	3	4.5	0.67
A10	F	86	0.3	2	0.15	24.6	11.2	11	1.02	35.8	1.75	19	0.09

Note: Case A3 was treated twice with airway warming with an interval during which no airway warming was given. This was because the author was called away after the first period and because of the drug overdose there was no further temperature rise until airway warming was restarted (Lloyd, 1986).

Table 19.3: Rates of Spontaneous Rewarming in Patients

Case	*Sex*	*Age*	*Temp. (°C) at Start*	*Temperature Rise*		
				Temp °C	*Time Hours*	*Rate °C/hour*
S 3	M	30	30.8	7	10	0.7
S 6	F	24	28.7	9.3	14	0.66
S 7	F	56	29.4	8	11.5	0.73
S 1	F	76	33.5	0.3	0.5	0.6
S15	F	79	25	5	10	0.5
				6	8	0.75
S 2	F	76	29.6	6	27	0.22
S 4	F	69	31	6.5	16	0.41
S 5	F	82	33.5	1.9	10	0.19
				0.6	23	0.03
S 8	M	83	33.2	4	29	0.14
S 9	M	69	33	3	9	0.3
S10	F	67	28	9	20	0.45
S11	F	77	25	11.4	43	0.27
S12	F	90	26.5	8.5	17	0.5
S13	F	75	33.75	3	11	0.27
S14	F	85	28	9	24	0.38
S16	M	old	31.8	3	21.5	0.14
S17	F	86	34.5	0.7	8	0.09
				3.3	14	0.24
S18	F	86	27.5	9.5	27	0.35

Note: In Cases S15, S5 and S17 the temperature charts showed periods with distinctly differing rates of rewarming (Lloyd, 1986) and so the periods are shown separately.

Comparison With Other Methods

The hot bath is undoubtedly a faster method of providing heat to a hypothermic victim than airway warming (Harnett *et al.*, 1980; Hayward *et al.*, 1984a; Lloyd *et al.*, 1976a; Marcus, 1978), though discomfort may force a lower initial water temperature and may therefore slow the rate of rewarming to one similar to airway warming (Collis *et al.*, 1977; Hayward and Steinman, 1975). A similar claim has been made for hot-water-circulating systems (Marcus, 1978), though this has been disputed (Harnett *et al.*, 1980) and in comparison with other methods of supplying heat which are available for field use, airway warming performed as well as any other method (Harnett *et al.*, 1980).

Some experiments have found in animals (Auld *et al.*, 1979) and man (Marcus, 1978) that if the subject is shivering, airway warming does not increase the rate of rewarming to a statistically significant degree, but the same criticism applies to the use of heating pads in shivering subjects (Collis *et al.*, 1977). However, other studies in man have found that rewarming with airway warming was faster than with shivering alone (Conn, 1979b; Hayward *et al.*, 1984a). If shivering is absent, airway warming accelerates rewarming (Lloyd *et al.*, 1976a; Pavlin *et al.*, 1976; Wessel *et al.*, 1966) and, under certain circumstances, the introduction of airway warming can change the situation from one in which the subject is continuing to cool into one in which the subject is rewarming, even if slowly (Brock *et al.*, 1977; Lloyd *et al.*, 1976a; Pavlin *et al.*, 1976; Shanks, 1974b). In the one study which claimed that there was no benefit from airway warming (Auld *et al.*, 1979) there is one flaw in that the group in which airway warming was used without shivering, the shivering had been abolished by muscle relaxants. In addition to abolishing shivering heat production, the heat produced by the activity of the respiratory muscles and general muscle tonus is also abolished by the muscle relaxant and heat production is also decreased by the use of mechanical ventilation (Mikat *et al.*, 1984).

One patient was rewarmed from 25 °C to 31 °C in four hours using airway warming plus gastric lavage. This achievement was more impressive since ventricular fibrillation had occurred at 25 °C and defibrillation was unsuccessful. Active resuscitative measures were needed till defibrillation was successful at 31 °C (Osborne *et al.*, 1984).

Other Effects

Mortality

Mortality is an important consideration for any method of treatment, but it must be remembered that, for many patients especially in the urban scene, the factor which precipitated the hypothermia is likely to prove fatal in the longer term. However, it should be possible to hope that none will die hypothermic before the diagnosis is made. In the study which compared patients treated with airway warming with another group allowed to rewarm spontaneously mentioned above (Lloyd, 1986), the airway warming group is likely to contain a higher proportion of problem cases than the spontaneously rewarmed group, because any difficulty with rewarming, e.g. failure to rewarm, continued cooling after admission to hospital or becoming hypothermic in hospital, would be referred for additional treatment. It is useful to divide the patients into groups depending on whether the onset of hypothermia was relatively short or prolonged. the mortality of the patients rewarmed by the two methods is shown in Table 19.4.

In the airway warming group all the younger patients, A2 to A18,

Table 19.4: Survival of Patients in Various Categories

	Case Number	*Sex*	*Age*	*Temperature on Admission*	*Airway Warming Method*	*Outcome*	*Death during Rewarming*	*Pre-existing Condition Causing Death*
I	A 1	F	61	34.8	IPPV	D		X
	A11	F	75	31	SV	D		X
	A13	M	38	32	IPPV	D		X
II	A 4	F	57	28	SV	D	X	
	A 5	F	75	28	SV	D	X	X
	A 6	F	80	25.5	SV	D	X	X
	A 9	F	75	32.5	IPPV			
	A10	F	86	24.6	IPPV	D		X
	A12	F	70	33	SV	D		X
	A15	F	84	23	SV	D	X	
	A16	F	81	28	SV	D	X	X
	A19	F	60	28	SV	D		X
III	A 2	M	55	27	IPPV/SV			
	A 3	F	22	34	IPPV/SV			
	A 7	F	23	29	SV			
	A 8	F	39	30	IPPV/SV			
	A14	M	50	33	IPPV/SV			
	A17	M	56	28.5	SV			
	A18	F	39	30.5	IPPV/SV			
II	S 1	F	76	33.5		D	X	
	S 2	F	76	29.6				
	S 4	F	69	31		D		
	S 5	F	82	33.5				
	S 8	M	83	33.2		D		
	S 9	M	69	33				
	S10	F	67	28		D		
	S11	F	77	25				
	S12	F	90	26.5				
	S13	F	75	33.5		D		X
	S14	F	85	28		D		
	S15	F	79	25		D	X	
	S16	M	?	31.8		D	X	
	S17	F	86	34.5				
	S18	F	86	27.5		D		
III	S 3	M	30	30.8		D		X
	S 6	F	24	28.7				
	S 7	F	56	29.4				

I Those that became hypothermic in hospital
II Slow-onset hypothermia including elderly and malnutrition
III Others, mainly young and/or drug overdose

D Death
IPPV Intermittent positive pressure ventilation
SV Spontaneous ventilation

rewarmed without problems, but they had hypothermia of relatively short onset mainly following drug overdose, except A17 who had a head injury. The similar group who rewarmed spontaneously, S3 to S7, also had no rewarming problems. Case S3, though young, was a diabetic with known complications which put him in a high-risk group (Gale and Tattersal, 1978; Tolman and Cohen, 1970) and though he rewarmed successfully, he died later. The three patients — A1, A11, A13 — all became hypothermic in hospital as a result of neurological damage and this explains the long pre-treatment times (Table 19.2). Though they rewarmed without problems, they all eventually died, and Hunter (1971) considers that all who, having been normothermic, develop hypothermia in hospital will die because the hypothermia has been caused by cerebral damage and the patients therefore have a poor prognosis.

The other main subdivision is those who have had a prolonged onset of hypothermia, which includes most of the elderly who may have a low total body heat even before the final precipitating incident. Malnutrition is another contributing factor to this group. In this study (Lloyd, 1986) all the elderly patients were considered to have slow onset hypothermia. Of the patients treated with airway warming, in addition to the elderly patients, A4 was known not to have been seen for at least two days and malnutrition was a previously known problem with A19. Of this group of nine, five died during rewarming and in all there were signs of possible cerebral and/or pulmonary oedema (Lloyd, 1986). Of the four that rewarmed successfully, A19 was relatively young, A12 had a very mild degree of hypothermia which had been precipitated by the cerebro-vascular accident (CVA) which later killed her, and A9 and A10 were rewarmed using intermittent positive pressure ventilation (IPPV). A10 later developed a fatal CVA some days after rewarming successfully. The death of A19 can also be understood since, though she rewarmed without any problems, she was unable thereafter to maintain her temperature (Table 19.2), even though she was in an environment with minimal cold stress. This is a common feature of hypothermia associated with malnutrition (Brooke, 1972a, b and c; Howitt, 1971; Lawless and Lawless, 1972; Sadikali and Owor, 1974). Since she had been rewarmed to normothermia before again becoming hypothermic, this places her in the category of having become hypothermic from normothermia while in hospital, and therefore in the group in which death is considered to be inevitable (Hunter, 1971).

Of the 15 slow-onset elderly group who rewarmed spontaneously, three died during rewarming (Table 19.4). S15 was rewarming successfully at 0.5 °C/hour but died when the rate of rewarming accelerated to more than 0.5 °C/hour and S1 warmed at 0.6 °C/hour during the half-hour before she died (Table 19.3). S16 was a vagrant male who was admitted unconscious. He never regained consciousness, and his cardiovascular status gradually deteriorated during the attempted rewarming. Six patients survived and were discharged or transferred to other hospitals. The other six died because of some problem which developed after they had successfully rewarmed.

Bloch (1965; 1967a, b) found that, if patients had been hypothermic over a period of days, too rapid rewarming (even if spontaneous) produced cerebral and/or pulmonary oedema because the reversal of the intercompartmental fluid shifts occurred too rapidly for the vascular compartment. It has been suggested that the maximum safe rewarming rate is 0.55 °C/hour (Bloch, 1965; Maclean and Emslie-Smith, 1977). All the airway-warmed patients rewarmed at more than 0.55 °C/hour, except the 57 year old, A4, and the cause of her hypothermia, and not being seen for two days, was unknown. IPPV counteracts cerebral and pulmonary oedema and this is the probable reason that A9 and A10 rewarmed safely, A10 from 24.6 °C. In the spontaneously rewarmed group, all those who rewarmed successfully did so at a rate less than 0.5 °C/hour. Since airway warming accelerates rewarming, it should not be used for the elderly unless there are facilities for using IPPV, and this means intensive care.

Miller *et al.* (1980) found that airway warming was a safe method of treatment with the only deaths being due to pre-existing medical conditions. Some of the deaths in the cases treated by surface heating and spontaneous rewarming did not have underlying disease. This is despite airway warming with intubation being chosen for the more severely hypothermic.

In Oregon airway warming is the only method of treatment now used for hypothermia cases down to a core temperature of 29 °C and in 60 cases treated there have been no deaths or complications (Oksenholt, E.J., personal communication, 1982).

Cardiovascular Effects

With airway warming the heat flow through the airways (Wessel *et al.*, 1966) and the other structures of the mediastinum could warm the heart from the pericardium inwards and the return of warm blood from the lungs would heat the endocardium and the myocardium via the coronary perfusion and this could minimise the possiblity of ventricular fibrillation (Lloyd and Mitchell, 1974) and potentiate increased cardiac output (Rose *et al.*, 1957; Sabiston *et al.*, 1955).

In a study with an unanaesthetised human subject (Hayward *et al.*, 1984a), within the 10 to 20 minutes needed to raise the water temperature to 42 °C, the hot bath caused a 35 per cent increase in cardiac output on top of the 64 per cent increase produced during cooling, and the heart rate had a 55 per cent increase to add to the 25 per cent increase from cooling. Despite these marked increases, there was a marked fall in blood pressure probably as the result of the fall in peripheral resistance. With spontaneous rewarming and airway warming the cardiac output returned to pre-immersion values within 30 minutes of starting treatment and, since the peripheral resistance remained steady, there was no catastrophic fall in blood pressure, though the blood pressure remained higher with airway warming than with spontaneous rewarming. In this study the subject had not been cooled to a level which would cause cardiac depression.

In animal experiments with anaesthetised sheep (Lloyd *et al.*, 1976b) cardiac depression had occurred during cooling and there was no shivering. The effects of airway warming were compared with spontaneous rewarming and immersion in a hot bath (Figure 7.4). The changes in spontaneous rewarming and immersion were discussed earlier in Chapter 7. The cardiac output rose with each method as the temperature rose but, by contrast with the other two methods, with airway warming there was no drop in peripheral resistance and in fact it rose later as rewarming progressed. The only measurement which showed an early rise with airway warming was the blood pressure. It is interesting that in Germany, since active external rewarming was abandoned in favour of airway warming, there have been no problems with rewarming collapse (de Pay, 1982).

In the clinical cases treated in Edinburgh (Lloyd, 1986) (Tables 19.2 and 19.3) the effects of airway warming on pulse and blood pressure (BP) were noted and compared with the effects of spontaneous rewarming. In two patients (A3, A14) no pulses were palpable when heating started and in others (A4, A6, A17, S11) the BP was unrecordable on admission because the peripheral pulses were absent. Four of these cases make interesting comparisons. A3 and A4 were both young girls suffering from drug overdose. A3 was the worse clinically, but her BP became recordable after two hours of treatment with airway warming whereas with case A4 airway warming was introduced late into the management and the BP had only become recordable after seven hours using other treatment.

Cases A6 and S11 were both elderly women and, whereas airway warming restored the BP of A6 within three hours and at a core temperature of 27.5 °C, in case S11 the BP was not recordable for 22 hours and then only when the core temperature reached 33 °C. Case A17 had the BP restored within half an hour of starting airway warming after it had been absent during the previous one and a half hours, and in case A14 the BP was restored within two hours. In cases A9, A12, A18, A19, S1 and S16 the BP which had been present on admission became unrecordable but in all the patients treated with airway warming the BP improved rapidly, e.g. within one hour in case A18, whereas with S1 and S16 the improvement was slower. Shanks and Marsh (1973) described the rewarming of a 50-year-old man, whose pulse had become impalpable at a nasopharyngeal temperature of 26 °C, who had his BP restored after 40 minutes of airway warming.

Cardiac Rhythm

In animals rewarmed with airway warming in addition to hot-water blankets, ventricular ectopics occurred which were not seen when the blankets were used without airway warming (Roberts *et al.*, 1983). In an experiment rewarming similar dogs from a similar low temperature using either diathermy or airway warming, there were no arrhythmias and the heart remained in sinus rhythm throughout rewarming (White *et al.*, 1984). This latter observation agrees with the experiments on sheep (Lloyd *et al.*, 1976b) in which no arrhythmias were noted during airway warming. The results of Roberts *et al.* (1983) may be due to the particular combination of rewarming methods which is unlikely to be used in the field. It should be noted, however, that even in this study there were no instances of ventricular fibrillation (Roberts *et al.*, 1983).

In the clinical cases (Lloyd, 1986) (Tables 19.2 and 19.3), cardiac arrhythmias attributable to hypothermia (J waves and ventricular and supraventricular extrasystoles) disappeared rapidly on commencing airway warming and normal sinus rhythm was established often at very low temperatures, e.g. by 27 °C in case A10. In another study (Miller *et al.*, 1980) three patients developed ventricular fibrillation during spontaneous rewarming and one during active surface rewarming but none when airway warming was used either via a mask or via an endotracheal tube, and in another case, rewarming using airway warming and peritoneal dialysis converted a pulse of 35/min with huge J waves and ST depression at 26 °C, to a rate of 70/min with normal complexes at 29.5 °C (Rankin and Rae, 1984).

If the ventilation is being assisted, hyperventilation should be avoided since a sudden drop in carbon dioxide tension in the blood may precipitate ventricular fibrillation (Brown and Miller, 1952).

Effects on the Central Nervous System

During treatment with airway warming, warming of the brain may occur by direct conduction from the nasopharynx and by circulation of warmed arterial blood (Hayward and Steinman, 1975). The early rise in jugular venous temperature following the introduction of airway warming in cooled sheep (Lloyd *et al.*, 1976a) gives measurable support to this theory. The more rapid rewarming of the brain would reverse the cold-induced depression of the respiratory centres and might stimulate the conscious level of the severely hypothermic patient. In the study mentioned above (Lloyd, 1986) several patients (A2, A3, A7, A8 and A18) whose respiratory drive had been depressed by drug overdose returned to normal before the core temperature had risen 1 °C and Shanks and Marsh (1973) described a similar effect. In a further four patients (A3, A7, A14 and A18) the pupils, which had been dilated and non-reactive, returned to normal size and reactivity very rapidly, in the cases A3 and A7 before any rise in core temperature could be recorded. This contrasts with case S11 where the pupillary response did not return for several hours. This apparent selective improvement in cerebral function with airway warming occurred with or without an endotracheal tube.

Oxygen Uptake

In animal experiments, when one lung was ventilated with dry gas and th other with humid, the oxygen uptake through the 'dry' lung fell from 56 per cent to 30 per cent whereas the oxygen uptake through the 'humid' lung rose from 44 per cent to 70 per cent (Fonkalsrud, 1975).

Effect on Shivering and Oxygen Consumption

In the rescue situation the inhibition of shivering may be beneficial in that it will reduce the oxygen requirement and reduce the blood flow requirements of the limbs, thus reducing the cardiac load (Golden in Marcus, 1979a) and the rate of heat loss, and therefore making more efficient use of the available energy resources. These effects might occasionally be critical, e.g. if there are respiratory difficulties either from pre-existing problems or a chest injury the extra oxygen consumption caused by shivering might be sufficient to precipitate hypoxia. The decrease in metabolic demand through the abolition of shivering may be of equal value if there is a lack of metabolic substrate as occurs in exhaustion hypothermia. Surface heat inhibits shivering (Collis *et al.*, 1977; Golden in Marcus, 1979a) but it also inhibits endogenous heat production (Adolph, 1950) and the reduction in oxygen consumption associated with warming of the skin will be accompanied by a net reduction in the metabolic heat available for rewarming. Airway warming also causes an immediate decrease in the amplitude of shivering of a hypothermic subject, possibly through receptors in the nose or through hypothalamic warming by heat transferred via bone (Pozos and Wittmers, 1983). It also causes a decrease in goosepimples and blushing on the backs of some subjects. This is unrelated to a rise in core temperature since the onset is very rapid, and conversely when a subject breathes cold air there is an equally rapid immediate increase in the amplitude of the shivering (Pozos and Wittmers, 1983).

Shivering increases not only the metabolic heat production but also ventilation minute volumes (Auld, 1977; Morrison *et al.*, 1979) and therefore increases the absolute quantities of heat which can be conserved by airway warming. At the start of rewarming there is a high minute volume but, unless this is maintained artificially by the inhalation of carbon dioxide, the ventilation rates fall as rewarming progresses (Conn, 1979b; Morrison *et al.*, 1979). The oxygen consumption decreases to basal levels as the subjects rewarm. However, the total oxygen consumed during the rewarming period is least with hyperventilation airway warming, more with unforced airway warming and greatest with spontaneous rewarming with shivering (Conn, 1979b). The oxygen requirement of the victim, both in immediate and total consumption, is reduced by airway warming and this decrease in oxygen consumption might be of vital importance in a victim who has other problems, such as chronic chest disease or injuries, and could also make a difference when exhaustion is superimposed on, or predisposing to, the hypothermia since in this situation the metabolic substrate available for heat production is severely reduced.

When the heat balance is considered there were some interesting observations (Conn, 1979b). Obviously with shivering there is a net respiratory heat loss, whereas with unforced and hyperventilation airway warming there is a net heat gain. However, as can be seen in Table 19.5, airway warming decreases the metabolic heat rate, with the result that the total heat available is almost identical whether the

Table 19.5: The Effects of Airway Warming on Available Heat and Oxygen Consumption During Rewarming

	Shivering	*Airway Warming*	*Hyperventilation*
Respiratory heat kcal/hour	−9.7	20.2	40.4
Metabolic heat kcal/hour	217.8	182.2	146.6
Total heat kcal/hour	208.1	203.1	187.0
Mean VO_2 1/min	0.76	0.64	0.51
Percentage heat available to core	10.7%	14.7%	24.9%

Source: After Conn (1979b)

rewarming is by shivering alone or with airway warming. With hyperventilation airway warming, the total heat available for rewarming is actually reduced and is less than in the other two groups (Conn, 1979b). Despite this the rate of core rewarming is faster with hyperventilation airway warming than unforced airway warming (Conn, 1979b; Morrison *et al.*, 1979), and the rewarming is faster with unforced airway warming than with shivering (Conn, 1979b).

Therefore though airway warming does inhibit shivering, the net heat available for rewarming is not reduced (Conn, 1979b) and calculations showed that with shivering only 10.7 per cent of the total heat was available to the core whereas with airway warming there was 14.7 per cent and with hyperventilation airway warming 14.9 per cent (Conn, 1979b).

The observation that, in the experimental treatment of hypothermia, the use of airway warming using air produced an improvement in blood gases (Roberts *et al.*, 1983) could be due either to improved oxygen uptake or reduced requirement.

Hazards and Complications

Thermal Effects

One of the fears voiced about airway warming is that it might cause tracheobronchial burning (Soulski *et al.*, 1983) but provided the larynx is bypassed the trachea can tolerate dry heat up to 350 °C (Moritz *et al.*, 1945) and a review of many experimental reports (Lloyd and MacRae, 1971) shows that steam at 94 to 104 °C is required to produce consistent thermal damage. However, 47 °C on the face can become unpleasant within a very short time in some subjects (Guild, 1976). This variation in tolerance to heat is due to the differing blood supply to the different tissues. Since the whole of the cardiac output from the right side of the heart and some of the output from the left side passes through the respiratory system there is an adequate blood supply to make respiratory burning unlikely. Nevertheless Klein and Graves (1974) have reported respiratory burning which they call 'hot pot' tracheitis. On the other hand dogs exposed in a sauna at 65 °C for twelve minutes daily for six weeks showed only minor changes in the respiratory tract and even 85 °C for ten minutes daily for 60 days produced only minor reversible changes and only the trachea and main bronchi were affected (Heino, 1980a, b).

There were no respiratory problems during or after the use of airway warming in those patients who survived and, when post-mortem was carried out there was no evidence of damage to the larynx or trachea in the sheep (Lloyd *et al.*, 1976a) or in the human cases (Lloyd, 1986) except in A10. In this case the patient had been treated with airway warming by intermittent positive pressure ventilation (IPPV) with the inspiratory tube lagged which would result in the temperature of the gases in the trachea being almost the 80 °C set at the humidifier, and this produced some laryngeal oedema and mild tracheal scalding. The rate of rewarming with this very high temperature was not significantly greater than the rate of rewarming achieved with the lower temperatures normally used and confirms the calculations of heat exchange considered earlier. With further knowledge the temperatures used in A10 are now considered to be dangerously high, with 45 °C being the maximum recommended temperature.

Humidification

Questions have been raised regarding the possibility of 'drowning' a patient by the delivery of large quantities of water-saturated gas over an extended period (Soulski *et al.*, 1983). It should not be forgotten that inhalation of warmed, humidified gas is a natural physiological process since in the quietly breathing individual the nose and mouth serve to warm and humidify the inspired air as it passes to the trachea. The normal respiratory tract can transfer vast volumes of fluid into the vascular system. Toung *et al.* (1970) found that an ultrasonic nebuliser could deliver to the trachea of an intubated animal, suspended mist in the range of 160 to 190 mg/litre which can amount to eight litres of water in mist form in 24 hours. Despite this there was no change in pulmonary mechanics with either acute or chronic exposure (Modell *et al.*, 1967) nor was there any loss of pulmonary surfactant as a result of water deposition (Shakoor *et al.*, 1968; Toung *et al.*, 1970). Modell (1976) did find that saline was more likely to produce a picture similar to bronchopneumonia than was distilled water and the water from humidifying (not nebulising) equipment can only deliver distilled water.

As mentioned earlier, fluid in the respiratory system is a not uncommon finding in hypothermia, and the effects of the inhalation of water vapour may depend on the nature of this excess fluid. If the congestion is due to pulmonary oedema, the condensation of additional water may compound the problem. The ability to absorb fluids is dependent on a favourable balance between osmotic and hydrostatic pressures and upon the normal functioning of blood vessel membranes. The existence of pulmonary oedema is prima facie evidence of the failure of one or more of these elements to preserve the fluid contents of the vasculature. Therefore there might be some reason to doubt the reliability of the fluid transfer mechanisms to contend with condensing inhalation vapour in addition to pulmonary oedema existing in a victim of hypothermia.

The preceding situation contrasts with that of an alternative source of pulmonary congestion which occurs as the result of the accumulation of mucus and other secretions. This is the result of impairment of ciliary function through cooling and/or drying and airway warming by providing warmed humidified air should liquefy the tracheobronchial secretions, reactivate ciliary activity (Danzl, 1983; Soulski *et al.*, 1983) and clear pulmonary opacities as was seen in Case A9 (Lloyd, 1986). This aspect is illustrated in Figures 6.2 and 6.3.

There is a suggestion that use of a humidifier may produce infection (Soulski *et al.*, 1983) but this is less likely with a humidifier than a nebuliser and there has been no evidence of infection in clinical cases treated.

Contraindications

Harnett *et al.* (1983b) suggest that traumatic injury to the face would be one possible contraindication to airway warming in that other first aid measures might take precedence. However, the most important first aid measure would be control of the airway either by tracheostomy or with an endotracheal tube and in either case airway warming could easily be instituted.

A more important contraindication is chronic or subchronic hypothermia because the acceleration of rewarming produced by airway warming will increase the reversal of fluid shifts and the risk of cerebral and/or pulmonary oedema. In these cases airway warming should not be used unless there is possibility of using intermittent positive pressure ventilation, either from the start as prevention or as soon as there is any evidence of oedema.

Practical Potential of the Method

The equipment designs described earlier are all intended to be used in the field as immediate care measures and the original prototype carbon dioxide/soda lime equipment (Lloyd *et al.*, 1972) was carried on the successful Everest expedition (Figure 19.5) (Bonnington, 1977) and tested and found to provide inhaled heat and moisture at 20,000 feet (Lloyd, 1977, 1979b). If any method of treatment is intended for use in the field it is essential to assess its effect in practice, but because of the sheer practical difficulties of the environment in which rescue teams work it is obviously impossible for the case reports to provide much in the way of detailed measurements. However, clinical case reports can be very informative and some are given below:

Case 1 (Lloyd and Frankland, 1974), 1st May, 1974. An inexperienced potholer had got himself trapped in a narrow rift and lay there without a wet suit partially in water, for about five hours. The position underground was such that he could not be carried out and it took a couple of hours for him to crawl out with help. When he reached the surface he was shivering vigorously, slightly ataxic, ketotic and felt very cold indeed although his cerebration was not impaired. He had a mouth temperature of 33.5 °C. He was put in a heated Landrover ambulance, wrapped in blankets and given airway warming with oxygen for 20 minutes. During this time his condition improved, the shivering stopped, he felt much better and his mouth temperature was 37 °C. He stated that he felt the benefit from the airway warming (Frankland, J., personal communication, 1974).

Case 2 (Schroder, L., personal communication, 1977), 29th August, 1975. Nine members of a hiking group, ranging in ages from 12 to 41 years, became engulfed in an unseasonal rainstorm lasting two days. Because the group carried no rain gear and had inadequate

Figure 19.5: Airway Warming Equipment on Mount Everest 1975 with the Khumbu Ice-fall in the Background

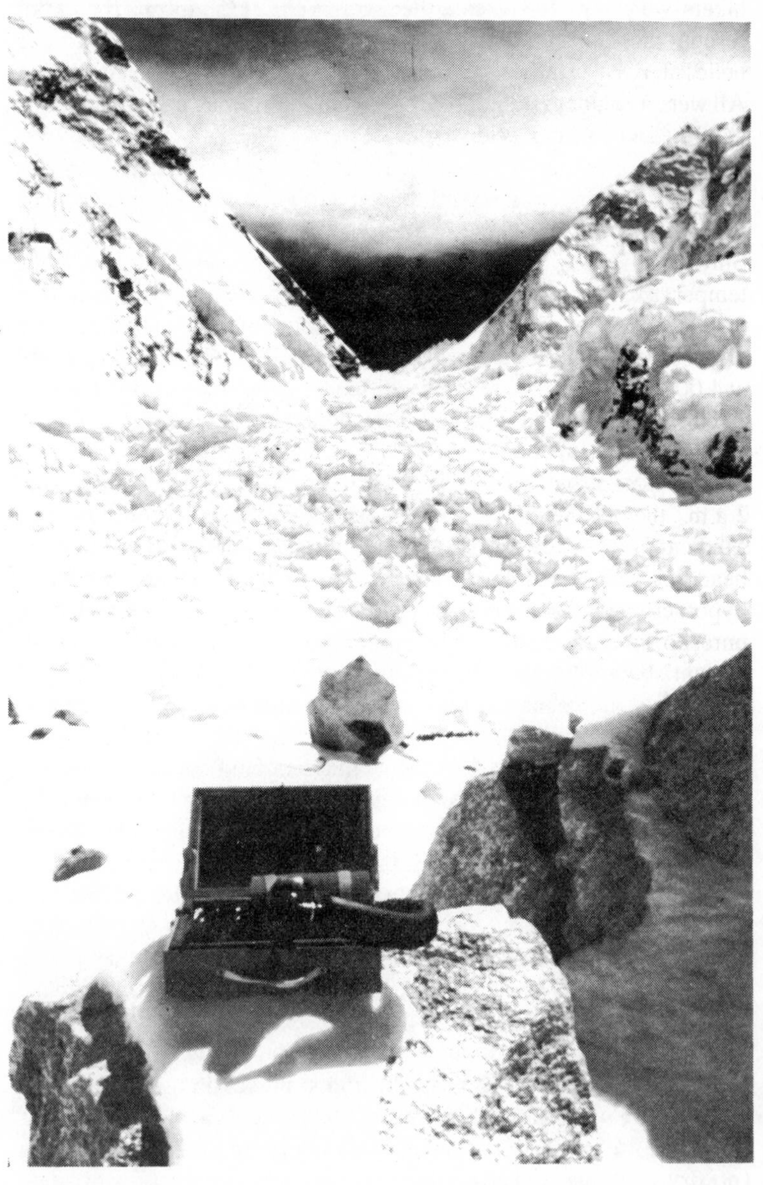

shelter, they were completely wet with no extra dry clothes. Within ten miles of the trailhead it became evident to some that several of the weaker members were becoming hypothermic. Two of the stronger hikers were sent for help while the remainder rested and ate. The rescue team with airway warming equipment arrived by Navy helicopter just as the bulk of the hiking party was leaving the trailhead. All were weak but satisfactory with the exception of the youngest who exhibited symptoms of advanced hypothermia. His behaviour was erratic, skin colour was pale and his oral temperature was below 33.5 °C. The patient was wrapped in a dry blanket and given airway warming in the back of a truck. Warm liquids were also given. Shivering became evident but subsided within a few minutes. Oral temperature was normal within one hour of treatment.

Case 3 (Schroder, L., personal communication, 1977), 15th October 1975. A man, 29 years of age, after shooting a mountain goat at 4,000 feet, fell approximately 75 feet. The time of the accident was 1 p.m. and rain and snow had been falling throughout the day. The victim was placed on his kill by his companions and covered with two thin sleeping bags. The victim was reached by rescue personnel at 2 a.m. the following day. An examination by three Emergency Medical Technicians disclosed severe bruising of the lower extremity, head lacerations and an apparent head injury as well as acute hypothermia. The patient was semi-conscious and, on the report, unresponsive to customary examination and questioning. Intermittent shivering was noted. Airway warming was applied at 3 a.m. (when the equipment arrived) and the patient began to respond after 30 minutes of manual intermittent positive pressure ventilation at an operating temperature of 57 °C. After one hour he was shivering violently and showing a very belligerent resistance to treatment. By approximately 4.30 a.m. shivering was intermittent and he was more willing to accept therapy. He was evacuated by helicopter at 7.30 a.m. The temperature on arrival at hospital was 35.5 °C.

Case 4 (Schroder, L., personal communication, 1977), October 1975. A 39-year-old man, a member of the rescue group aiding Case 3 above, was found to be unresponsive to his companions when they wakened at dawn, having bivouacked a short distance from the main rescue party. The subject was highly predisposed to hypothermia having had no sleep in 20 hours, being thoroughly wet and exposed to wind under only a light cover. When the subject's condition was noticed he was immediately given additional covering (no dry covering was available) and when Case 3 was evacuated airway warming was applied. The core temperature was estimated to be between 32.5 and 35.5 °C. Shivering was violent and uncontrollable though this diminished after 20 minutes of airway warming at 49 °C. Hot soup was also given. He was able to move unaided after one hour of treatment.

Case 5 (Bell, P.M., personal communication, 1977) 28th December, 1976. A girl who had been walking in the fells in the Lake District lost her way and when she was found, she was lightly unconscious and very cold with signs similar to light anaesthesia. Airway warming was used during the evacuation and she regained consciousness after some time. On arrival at hospital (Palmer, H.M., personal communication, 1977) her temperature was 35 °C and she was fully conscious. Her recovery thereafter was uneventful though there was amnesia for a part of the time, during which she had appeared to be fully conscious.

Case 6 (Bell, P.M., personal communication, 1977). An experienced climber was out in very bad conditions of low temperature and freezing mist with snow and ice on high ground. His first problem was that when he came to take a bearing, his hand co-ordination was so poor that he could not even get his hands into his pocket to extract the compass, let alone use it. He continued to walk but was confused about his position. Luckily a passer-by appreciated the situation and, after making contact with someone on the hill to call for help, protected him from the elements. When found by the rescue team he was cold and shivering but conscious and able to say who he was and who his companions were. With airway warming for half an hour his condition showed a marked improvement and he was then transported down to a rendezvous with a helicopter. He made a complete recovery but had total amnesia from the time when he tried to use the compass and the next thing he could remember was the helicopter engine noise.

In Oregon airway warming is taught to ambulance crews and pararescue personnel, with the result that in some cases the treatment in the ambulance has almost resolved the hypothermia on the way to the hospital and in 60 cases treated this way there have been no deaths or complications (Oksenholt, E.J., personal communication, 1982). In experiments in the French Alps at 3,800 metres in a temperature of −8 °C with a windspeed of 15 to 20 kph, the rectal temperature only fell 1.3 °C in 1.5 hours because of the use of airway warming (Foray and Cahen, 1981) and airway warming in addition to surface insulation is recommended as the initial measure for hypothermia victims in the field if suitable equipment is available (Danzl, 1983; Foray and Salon, 1985; Lilja, 1983). In the field situation it has been noticed that airway warming produced a feeling of well-being with a rise in morale (Foray and Cahen, 1981; Foray and Salon, 1985).

Conclusion

Airway warming, in conjunction with surface insulation, appears to provide a worthwhile increase in the rewarming rate and it has additional benefits on the vital functions of the body. It is recommended as part of the immediate first aid treatment not only for mountain hypothermia but also in some other areas (Banssillon, 1985), and it may help to prevent some of the deaths which occur following the rescue of a hypothermic victim in the field. The method, which is one of the few which can be used as soon as a hypothermic victim is found (Foray and Salon, 1985; Lloyd, 1979b), can be continued to and in hospital, even while the wet clothing is being removed (Foray and Salon, 1985). It appears to be at least as safe as other methods except for patients with subchronic hypothermia, e.g. the elderly and those with malnutrition. While all cases of accidental hypothermia should be rewarmed in an intensive care unit (Braun, 1985; Emslie-Smith, 1982, Ledingham and Mone, 1980; Mills, 1983a), this is especially true of elderly patients. In elderly patients, airway warming should not be used without intensive care facilities because the accelerated rate of rewarming may precipitate cerebral and/or pulmonary oedema.

20 OTHER TREATMENT

Combinations of Methods of Rewarming

There are many case reports where a variety of methods of supplying heat to the patient have been used concurrently, e.g. surface warming by circulating-water blanket plus warm intravenous fluids plus gastric lavage plus peritoneal dialysis (Pickering *et al.*, 1977; Sekar *et al.*, 1980). In fact at first sight the possibilities for combinations are only limited by the equipment available at any particular hospital. However, there are limitations, e.g. the hot bath cannot be used with pericardial irrigation. Diathermy should not be applied in the area while either intragastric or intracolonic balloons are being used or while the peritoneal cavity is being irrigated. This is particularly the case for ultrasonic and low-frequency microwave diathermy due to the penetration depths they can achieve and their undesirable effects on accumulations of water. Airway warming, on the other hand, appears to have the potential for use irrespective of any other method of rewarming which may be contemplated (Foray and Cahen, 1981). Airway warming has been used in combination with peritoneal dialysis (Foray and Salon, 1985; Rankin and Rae, 1984) and it has also been used in combination with gastric lavage and warmed intravenous infusion during four hours of cardiac massage. The patient warmed 6 °C during the time, and defibrillation was then successful (Osborne *et al.*, 1984).

Other Measures

General

While a number of measures can be used in hospital, e.g. low molecular weight dextran (Foray and Salon, 1985), there is much less that can be done in the field. It is most important that all hypothermic casualties should be handled gently to avoid the risk of precipitating ventricular fibrillation (Danzl, 1983; Merrifield in Marcus, 1979a). This may not always be possible in the emergency, and rough handling is almost inevitable during helicopter rescue and transport (Golde in Marcus, 1979a) and during rescue and transport in a lifeboat (Guild in Marcus, 1979a). In the emergency it is more important to get the person out of the water even if the only means is by a rope looped round the victim's neck (Frankland, 1983). Rubbing of the limbs, recommended by Barron de Larry after Napoleon's retreat from Moscow, is now universally condemned in the management of hypothermia since it may damage the skin and its only other possible effect might be to suppress shivering either by giving a sensation of warmth or by increasing the blood flow to the skin (Danzl, 1983), thus aggravating the cooling of the core or impairing vasomotor tone.

Exercise

It used to be suggested that, in cases of hypothermia, exercise was better than inaction (Lloyd, 1964), and there was an attitude in hill climbing circles that sufferers should be forced to continue walking to maintain heat production rather than take shelter. It is still suggested that, since exercise increases heat production, when someone is mildly hypothermic exercise is a reasonable measure to increase body temperature rather than allowing further heat loss (Kaufman, 1983). Unfortunately in most cases hypothermia only develops as the person is becoming exhausted and therefore will have great difficulty in increasing his heat production. The other problem is that unless the person is close to safety, he is liable to become totally exhausted and he will then be unable to make proper shelter and the rate of heat loss is greatly increased. It is not known how many people have died because of the attitude of continuing to exercise, but cases are regularly reported in the newspapers (*Scotsman*, 1981). It is now considered that exercise is dangerous (Frankland, 1975, 1981; Freeman and Pugh, 1969; Harnett *et al.*, 1983a) and that, not only should the hypothermic victim be prevented from exercising (Dubas, 1980), but parties should take shelter early in severe risk situations. The basis for this advice is that maximum heat loss occurs when a person is exhausted (Witherspoon *et al.*, 1971) and therefore exhaustion is to be avoided if possible. In addition, by taking shelter early, the environmental heat loss is markedly reduced and energy is conserved to maintain heat production without being suppressed by exercise. There are now many reports in newspapers of people who have taken this advice and not only have they survived weather conditions which were so severe that the rescue services had expected a fatal outcome, but when the weather eased they were able to walk out of the hills apparently undistressed. In the rescue situation, forcing a person to get up and exercise may cause a secondary after-drop of cardiac temperature (Hong and Nadel, 1979) or death through a sudden loss of vasomotor tone.

Drugs

General. Most drugs are either ineffective in the hypothermic patient or are dangerous to use because of the increased cardiac irritability (Maclean and Emslie-Smith, 1977).

Glucose. Despite the fact that hypoglycaemia was an important factor in one series of hypothermia cases admitted to hospital (Fitzgerald and Jessop, 1982), high blood glucose levels are sometimes found in non-diabetic cases of hypothermia (Jones in Marcus, 1979a) but this may be due to an inability of the cold muscles to utilise glucose, and as metabolism recovers with rewarming, the blood glucose level may drop precipitously. Hypothermia may be the first and occasionally the only sign of hypoglycaemia in both conscious and comatose patients (Hanson *et al.*, 1984) and in non-hypothermic hypoglycaemia the clinical signs may closely mimic those of hypothermia (MacInnes, 1979), hypoglycaemia may precipitate hypothermia and if gluconeogenesis is impaired by alcohol glucose reverses the hypothermia (BMJ, 1979). In addition if there is hypoglycaemia in the central nervous system this may impair the function of centres controlling peripheral heat production (Mager and Francesconi, 1983), and in cases of exhaustion hypothermia glucose may be necessary to restart rewarming. All these facts suggest that glucose should be given to young people in the rescue situation (MacInnes, 1979).

Corticosteroids. There is a great deal of controversy regarding the use of steroids in hypothermia. This started when Duguid *et al.* (1961) gave steroids to their patients following the observation that hypothermia depressed the output of corticosteroids (Bernhard, 1956; Hume *et al.*, 1956). This observation was made in patients whose response had been altered by anaesthesia and whose hypothermia was rapidly induced whereas Duguid's patients were elderly with probably subchronic hypothermia. The effect of steroids was not dramatic nor was any benefit noted in the other type of subchronic hypothermia associated with malnutrition (Sadikali and Owor, 1974), though Prescott *et al.* (1962) felt from clinical observation that the use of steroids eased the control of blood pressure

Client: 1608   SCHWEIZER VERLAGSHAU No.: 9304030098
03/04/93   ZUERICH   Ref.: CDE TEL. 2.4.93

Code art.: **C022308**   Ref.ligne: CDE TEL. 2.4.93/CK   cdmq
Qte cdee.: 1   Qte a fact.: 1 Remise: 0,00   C

Remise en fact.: CCR 9304020164   No.fact: 301035408

Editeur: CROOM CROOM HELM LTD Coll.:
Auteur : LLOYD E.   No.Coll.:
Titre: HYPOTHERMIA AND COLD STRESS Tome: 0   Fac.:
ISBN : 0-7099-1665-5
Ref.fourn.:   Prix: 0,00

Litige N - Verif Serv. D - Urgence 0 - Entre   12111

Fr. 158.90   252   Representant :
Auto. Retour :
Transporteur :
Echeance : 03

in subchronic hypothermia. Despite this non-evidence steroids were recommended as routine treatment in hypothermia (Duguid *et al.*, 1961; Hockaday, 1969). When cortisol levels were measured in hospital in eleven cases (Tolman and Cohen, 1970) the levels were high but ten out of the eleven were diabetic or alcoholic and in another series, cortisol levels were high in eight out of eleven cases and low in none (Miller *et al.*, 1980). Similarly in 34 elderly patients only four had low cortisol levels (Sprunt *et al.*, 1970) and during recovery the levels in most patients fell, though some remained up for several days. The position as far as elderly patients is concerned can be summarised by saying that cortisol levels are raised in most patients with accidental hypothermia, and cortisol utilisation, which is poor during hypothermia, is related more to plasma cortisol levels than to the severity of the hypothermia. Utilisation, however, improves during rewarming and cortisol levels rise and remain high for several days after rewarming. Hypotension was associated with high cortisol levels rather than with low levels and in fact patients with low cortisol levels survived better than those with high levels (Maclean and Emslie-Smith, 1977).

In the experimental situation, immersion in water at 25.5 °C did not result in any increase in cortisol production (Weihl *et al.*, 1981) but the immersions were short and the temperature of the water was above the 20 °C necessary to cause hypothermia. In other experiments with healthy young males it was found that cold stress caused an increase in cortisol production (Jansky, 1979; Wilkerson *et al.*, 1974; Wilson *et al.*, 1970), possibly 50 per cent above normal (Mager and Francesconi, 1983). Even in water at 23.9 °C, with prolonged exposure, some subjects developed significant adrenocortical stress and subsequent adrenocortical insufficiency (Beckman and Reeves, 1966).

In the outdoor situation MacInnes *et al.* (1971) found that a hard day on the hills in bad weather caused a rise in cortisol production. However, when investigating five climbers who had collapsed with exhaustion, though three had raised cortisol levels two had unexpectedly low levels.

There are other pieces of information which complicate the already murky picture. Some very ill patients have very low cortisol levels which do not respond to the administration of ACTH (Greig *et al.*, 1971; McKee and Finlay, 1983), which suggests adrenal exhaustion. In addition even in normothermic patients on a long-term steroid treatment exposed to the stress of surgery, arterial hypotension and low plasma cortisol levels are not invariably linked (Kehlet and Binder, 1973; Kehlet *et al.*, 1974; Oyama, 1969). This does not, however, contraindicate the routine giving of corticosteroid in the treatment of any hypotensive episode not due to blood loss, and the blood pressure rises whatever the plasma cortisol level (Lloyd, 1981c).

It is possible to hypothesise a sequence of events which explains the conflicting evidence. Cold stress causes a rise in cortisol production but, if the cold stress is very severe, hypothermia will develop before the adrenal cortex is exhausted, and therefore not only will plasma cortisol levels be raised but there will be no problem during resuscitation. If the cold stress is very mild there may be no rise in cortisol production. Nevertheless the cold stress may be sufficient to cause gradual loss of body heat, especially in the elderly or those with malnutrition, and the person may drift into hypothermia or have a final superimposed short acute episode. In these cases the plasma cortisol level would be low or normal and, since there is no adrenal cortical exhaustion, the cortex can respond to the stresses of rewarming with increased cortisol production. There is, however, an intermediate group where the environmental stresses, including cold, are sufficient to cause a rise in cortisol production. If the stresses are sufficiently prolonged, the adrenal cortex may become exhausted and the plasma cortisol levels will then drop, i.e. a functional adrenal insufficiency (Felicetta and Green, 1979). The level found in any one case will therefore depend on precisely how far this drop has gone, i.e. the levels may be high, normal or low, and in these cases supplementary steroids will be necessary and may be life saving if the condition is extreme.

There is one other possible scenario. It is known that patients with adrenal failure have high circulating levels of β-endorphin which can be reduced by the administration of steroids (Holaday and Loh, 1981). It is also known that many of the features of shock – haemorrhagic, septic and spinal — can be reversed by a β-endorphin antagonist (Holaday and Loh, 1981). The two items together, plus the fact that β-endorphins are released under stress (Vidal *et al.*, 1983), suggest that, though steroids can reverse the severe hypotension in hypothermia, the symptomatology may be due to β-endorphin excess precipitated by prolonged stress and the raised cortisol levels may be secondary to raised β-endorphin levels.

Some people recommend steroids in mountain hypothermia on clinical empirical experience (Jones in Marcus, 1979a) and in addition steroids have been given as a last resort to climbers who have collapsed and are apparently moribund (MacInnes, 1971) and at least some have been successfully revived.

Hypothermia often occurs in conjunction with other conditions and steroids may be necessary in these circumstances. Near-drowning is often an associated problem and, though steroids had no beneficial effect in a carefully controlled study of near-drowning in dogs (Calderwood *et al.*, 1975), it has been suggested that the danger of cerebral oedema — a frequent complication of drowning — may itself be regarded as an indication for the early administration of steroids (Golden, 1980) though recent evidence suggests that in fresh-water drowning, steroids have no effect on the pulmonary lesion and do not prevent the rise in intracranial pressure (Conn and Barker, 1984). In hypothermia associated with drug overdose, steroids are contra-indicated because they may impair or delay metabolism of the drugs (Matthew, 1975).

Oxygen

This is again a controversial subject. Oxygen supplied to the myocardium is decreased in hypothermia through a combination of a decreased coronary vascular flow (Hegnauer *et al.*, 1950) and decreased oxygen dissociation (Callaghan *et al.*, 1961) and therefore the possibility of ventricular fibrillation from a limitation of myocardial energetics is enhanced (Hicks *et al.*, 1956). The administration of oxygen might be expected to reduce this risk (Collis *et al.*, 1977) and it may also be expected to counter the tendency towards anoxic pulmonary oedema. However, the use of 100 per cent oxygen may not be desirable (Negovskii, 1962). Pure 100 per cent oxygen can certainly cause pulmonary toxicity (Kafer, 1971; Morgan, 1968) but Heino *et al.* (1981) found that while 100 per cent oxygen caused some pulmonary damage after 24 hours, there was none after twelve hours. Nevertheless tracheitis was noted on bronchoscopy after only six hours of 100 per cent oxygen (Hedley-White *et al.*, 1976). There are also other possible problems. Pure oxygen may cause marked depression of ciliary activity in normothermic patients resulting in an impairment of mucus flow (Hedley-White *et al.*, 1976). This may contribute to the production of pulmonary oedema. Surfactant activity may also be impaired (SMJ, 1972) and certainly prolonged oxygen therapy has been blamed for a condition similar to adult respiratory distress syndrome found in deaths following secondary drowning (Glauser and Smith, 1975;

Nash *et al.*, 1967).

Pure oxygen was used to resuscitate 20 dogs after being clinically dead for five minutes (Romanova, 1956). Oxygen therapy was continued after the resuscitation of some of the dogs. Fifteen died within the first five days and five were sacrificed 14 to 90 days after resuscitation. In the 15 animals dying within the first five days, characteristic findings included abundant small haemorrhages in all parts of the brain, swollen vascular endothelium and separation and homogenisation of the walls of some vessels. These changes were not seen to such a pronounced extent in animals not receiving oxygen, even after longer periods of clinical death. Haemorrhages and changes in vascular walls were also found in the heart, lungs and liver. Circumscribed changes in the brain, including structural changes, death of nerve cells and scar formation, were found in animals dying in a moderately prolonged period of time only when oxygen therapy was given. It has been suggested that the oxygen concentration during resuscitation should not exceed 30 to 40 per cent (Romanova, 1956) or 50 per cent (Dembo, 1957). In fact 3 to 4 per cent oxygen is sufficient in the resuscitation from acute anoxia with the exception of carbon monoxide poisoning (Swann, 1950; 1951).

Oxygen therapy was examined in the Dachau experiments because the clinical picture of dyspnoea with the formation of foam at the mouth was reminiscent of early oedema of the lungs (Alexander, 1945). However, oxygen inhalation had no effect upon either respiration or heart function, and Holzloehner *et al.* (1942) felt that the markedly bright colour of the arterial blood (observed in other human experiments) made it unlikely that additional oxygen would have any beneficial effect.

Cyanosis and dyspnoea are absent in hypothermia (Ledingham and Norman, 1964; McNicol and Smith, 1964) and it has been suggested that the respiratory response to carbon dioxide is suppressed in hypothermia with spontaneous respiration being maintained by hypoxia (Grosse-Brockhoff, 1950). This is rarely the case (Merrifield in Marcus, 1979a) and in their case report Linton and Ledingham (1966) found that in fact the patient maintained a normal carbon dioxide level but was unable to maintain oxygenation without ventilatory assistance. The importance of hypoxia in hypothermia is now emphasised (Freeman and Pugh, 1969; Gregory and Patton, 1972; Jessen and Hagelsten, 1972; Ledingham, 1979; Ledingham and Mone, 1972, 1978, 1980; Linton and Ledingham, 1966; Patton, 1974) and in hospital oxygen is given routinely

(Tolman and Cohen, 1970) or the blood gases are monitored and oxygen given to correct any hypoxia. Oxygen should therefore be given if available to hypothermic patients (Dubas, 1980; Golden in Marcus, 1979a; Holdcroft, 1981; Lilja, 1983; Merrifield in Marcus, 1979a).

There is one possible additional danger of oxygen being given in the field illustrated by a case report (Legrand, 1984). A victim was rescued alive from an avalanche and since the respirations were feeble, mouth-to-mouth respiration was started. All was going well until a doctor arrived with an oxygen cylinder and insisted on taking over the ventilation of the patient, who died within a few seconds of this being started. Relevant points are that the air was cold and the cylinder had in addition been lying on the snow for some minutes while the respiratory circuit was being assembled. The patient was then suddenly changed from warm, humid mouth-to-mouth ventilation to ventilation (?hyperventilation) with very cold, dry oxygen. This would increase the respiratory heat loss with the additional possibility of bronchospasm but whatever the cause, death was immediate.

Intensive Care

When case reports are studied, especially those in which the victims have survived, it becomes obvious that survival had more to do with the fact that intensive care was available to control variables such as blood gas and acid-base status, cardiovascular instability or renal impairment, than with the method of rewarming (Mills, 1980; 1983a). The controversy between the conservative and aggressive management of hypothermia (Emslie-Smith, 1981; Emslie-Smith *et al.*, 1981; Ledingham, 1981b; Ledingham and Mone, 1982) does not appear to be about the rate of rewarming since some of the patients managed conservatively warm faster than some of those treated aggressively. There was, however, general agreement that the old traditional management of hypothermia, i.e. putting the patient in a quiet corner and awaiting developments, is no longer acceptable and hypothermic patients should be managed with intensive care monitoring. Intensive care should also prevent deaths occurring while the victim is still hypothermic (Ledingham and Mone, 1980). All the evidence in fact suggests that all cases of hypothermia admitted to hospital should be managed with full intensive care support (BMJ, 1978b; Braun, 1985; Dubas, 1980; Mills, 1980; 1983a; Paton, 1983b), and any hospital where this does not happen should admit that the standard of care provided is less than the optimal possible. As long as intensive care monitoring is provided, the method of rewarming is probably irrelevant and the method best suited to the hospital should be used (Mills, 1980; 1983a; Paton; 1983b). Intensive care is also advisable since some patients require temporary pacing of the heart following recovery from hypothermia (Faller and Rauscher, 1978) and intensive care also allows the use of low-dose heparin used to try to prevent the syndrome of diffuse intravascular coagulation which sometimes accompanies hypothermia (Foray and Salon, 1985; Laessing, 1982).

The microvascular sludging which occurs in hypothermia (Schmid-Schonbein and Neumann, 1985), and the thrombogenic changes which accompany cold exposure (Keatinge *et al.*, 1984), may be important factors in the aetiology of some of the problems associated with hypothermia, e.g. pancreatitis, and this is a justification for using low molecular weight dextran in the treatment of accidental hypothermia (Foray and Salon, 1985).

21 RESUSCITATION

In hypothermia signs of life may be severely depressed and are easily missed in the rescue situation and it was suggested (Zingg, 1967) that, in the disaster situation, since there was no adequate treatment, the problem could be ignored. However, at that time the only treatment considered adequate was immersion in a hot bath. There is nevertheless no point in the rescue teams investing in sophisticated equipment for diagnosing signs of life since even definite evidence of total cessation of cardiorespiratory activity does not preclude the chance of recovery. Information from induced hypothermia is not always valid for the accidental situation. For example it has been shown that after 40 minutes' cardiac arrest at 20 °C, irreversible brain damage is almost inevitable (Treasure, 1984) whereas a patient at a core temperature of 29 °C survived 45 minutes of severe but not complete brain ischaemia (Belopavlovic and Buchtal, 1980). In induced hypothermia the moment of circulatory cessation is known exactly whereas in the clinical accidental hypothermia situation there is a long period of steadily dropping blood pressure and slowing pulse during which time, because of the hypothermia, there is adequate circulation for the brain. In fact cardiac activity may persist for 10 to 15 minutes after respiratory arrest (Harries, 1982). Even the fact that the victim has been known to be submerged for a prolonged period cannot be taken as an indicator for not attempting resuscitation, especially if the water is cold and the victim is young, because cases have been successfully revived after periods of up to 40 minutes' known submersion in very cold water (see pages 298 to 302). This duration is again probably due to the fact that the cerebral circulation has certainly been maintained for the greater part of the time submerged. For example a six-year-old was submerged for a known 25 minutes in 4 °C liquid and, though his core temperature was only 31.8 °C when rescued, he survived (Theilade, 1977). One woman during induced hypothermia had a known period of cardiac arrest for one hour at a core temperature of 9 °C with complete mental and physical recovery (Niazi and Lewis, 1958) and six monkeys had periods of cardiac arrest of between 42 minutes and two hours at core temperatures of 4 to 9 °C and all recovered. The general consensus is that death in hypothermia can only be defined as failure to revive on rewarming. It has been claimed that this has resulted in extended effort and the use of costly resources such as cardiopulmonary bypass equipment which could be more efficiently used elsewhere (Lawrence, 1984). To try to avoid this, a hypothermia survival index (HSI) has been proposed to predict the outcome of hypothermia. This index uses (1) the presence or absence of cardiac function; (2) the duration of circulatory arrest; (3) core temperature; (4) medical and traumatic disorders; (5) serum potassium; and (6) hypothermia related abnormalities; and the index has successfully predicted the outcome in 49 out of 52 cases (Lawrence, 1984). Unfortunately this index is of no value for the rescue teams since none of the factors can be measured in the field except possibly for the core temperature and core temperature is no indicator of potential recovery, with clinical cases having recovered from as low as an estimated 16 °C (Laufman, 1951) and recovery being recorded fairly frequently from below 22 °C (Althaus *et al.*, 1982; Kugelberg *et al.*, 1967). Recent results have also shown that successful rewarming and resuscitation can be achieved without involving complex equipment such as cardiopulmonary bypass devices. (Frankland, 1983; Legrand, 1984; Osborne *et al.*, 1984; Pickering *et al.*, 1977; Sekar *et al.*, 1980).

If the body is frozen solid so that it is impossible to alter the person's position or if the mouth and nose are blocked with ice it is probably reasonable to diagnose death (Stewart, 1981). Similarly if the eyes are frozen or if the rectal temperature is equal to or lower than the ambient air temperature the person has probably been dead for some time and attempts at revival are unlikely to be successful and merely increase the hazards for the rescuers. It is also true that the statement about not accepting death in a cold body is easier to make in the warmth and comfort of a laboratory or hospital than in a storm at sea or on a windy and snow-swept mountainside. One successful resuscitation on a cold, gale-swept seafront (Frankland, 1983) shows what is possible.

The indications for the use of external cardiac massage (ECM) are still an area for argument (Banssillon, 1985). For example it has been stated that ECM should not be used in cases of hypothermia because of the danger of precipitating ventricular fibrillation (VF) in a heart which may still be in normal rhythm even though there may be no clinical evidence of activity (BMJ, 1977b; *Lancet*, 1972b). Even for a body in the water it was recommended that ECM should be used if it was a case of drowning but not if hypothermia was the cause of apparent death (Golden and Rivers, 1975) though it is now recognised that hypothermia may precede drowning (the two may be present together) and the management should be similar (Golden, 1980). Similarly it is frequently stated that endotracheal intubation (ETI) or insertion of an oesophageal temperature probe or intragastric balloon carry a very high risk of precipitating VF in the hypothermic heart (BMJ, 1977b; Coniam, 1979; Fell and Dendy, 1968; Holdcroft, 1981; Keatinge, 1969; *Lancet*, 1972b) though no evidence was presented. In fact one editorial (BMJ, 1977b) cited two articles as supportive evidence despite the fact that one of the articles (Lloyd and Mitchell, 1974) did not mention ECM, ETI or any other instrumentation and the other (Lloyd, 1973) specifically stated that ETI was carried out under continuous electrocardiographic monitoring without any evidence of cardiac arrhythmias even at a core temperature as low as 24.3 °C. Many authors from practical experience dismiss the dangers of VF resulting from ETI or other instrumentation (Johnson, 1977; Ledingham and Mone, 1980; Linton and Ledingham, 1966; Shanks, 1975d; Shanks and Marsh, 1973; Tolman and Cohen, 1970). As a cautionary point, however, it has been claimed that intubation precipitated VF in one case (Schissler *et al.*, 1981) and that in two other cases VF followed therapeutic manipulation (O'Keefe, 1977). In another case the passage of an endotracheal tube provoked the onset of VF (Osborne *et al.*, 1984). ETI should probably not be undertaken unless ventilation is inadequate or the protective reflexes are absent, and even then it should always be done as in anaesthesia, after some pre-oxygenation of the patient either from an oxygen source or from expired air resuscitation (EAR) (Dubas, 1980). When this has been done there have been no problems with rhythm (Lloyd, 1973; Miller *et al.*, 1980).

It was also stated (*Lancet*, 1972b) that there was no evidence that ECM and EAR would prolong survival in hypothermic cardiac arrest despite the fact that Freeman and Pugh (1969) recommended ECM and EAR to keep patients alive while rewarming was proceeding. The practical experience with many clinical cases confirms the fact that ECM and ventilation either by EAR or ETI and assisted ventilation can keep patients alive for periods of up to four hours (Bristow *et al.*, 1977; de Villota *et al.*, 1973; Evans *et al.*, 1971; Fell *et al.*, 1968; Kugler-Podelleck *et al.*, 1965; Kvittingen and Naess, 1963; Lash *et al.*, 1967; Legrand, 1984; Linton and Ledingham 1966; Osborne *et al.*, 1984; Paton, 1983b; Theilade, 1977; Wind, 1975). There are even cases reported where ECM and EAR with or without ETI have been used during helicopter evacuation lasting up to 2.5 hours and the patients have then been successfully rewarmed in hospital and survived (Althaus *et al.*, 1982; Muhlemann, 1979), and one patient was kept alive by ECM and EAR over a period of four hours during transport in a snow vehicle, ambulance and helicopter (Steinman, A.M., personal communication, 1984). One victim has been successfully resuscitated on the seafront using ECM and EAR after he had been hauled out of cold water, very cold and with no signs of life (Frankland, 1983).

There is now doubt about the mechanism by which ECM works (Harries, 1984). The traditional explanation that the heart was compressed between the sternum and the spine with the heart valves producing the circulation (Jude *et al.*, 1961; Kouwenhoven *et al.*, 1960) cannot now be accepted uncritically. Even though transducers have shown that the heart is squashed (Meier *et al.*, cited in Harries, 1984), in hypothermia the heart is hard and difficult to compress even on direct manual compression through a thoracotomy (Althaus *et al.*, 1982), and echocardiography shows that the valves in fact move very little during normal cardiopulmonary resuscitation (CPR) (Werner *et al.*, 1981). Recent work has shown that if the heart is compressed at between 90 and 150 compressions/minute, the valves do in fact work (Meier *et al.*, cited in Harries, 1984) but this rate is far in excess of what is used successfully in practice and would be impossible for rescuers to maintain for any length of time. The fact that one patient during prolonged VF kept himself conscious by repeated coughing (Criley *et al.*, 1976) led to the development of the thoracic pump theory of ECM. In this, compression of the chest squeezes the vascular bed in the lungs, and because there is a valve in the superior vena cava at the thoracic inlet, cephalic regurgitation of the blood is prevented (Fisher *et al.*, 1982). The diaphragm provides a similar though less efficient valve effect on the inferior vena cava (Fisher *et al.*, 1982). Clinical experience has shown that the duration of the compression is more important than the rate, with the ideal rate being about 40 to 60/min (Taylor *et al.*, 1977) and this fits the thoracic pump theory because the chest is a large capacity organ which will fill slowly. Increasing the intrathoracic pressure improves the forward flow and this can be achieved by abdominal compression to prevent inferior vena caval regurgitation (Harris *et al.*, 1967; Koehler *et al.*, 1983) and by ventilating the lungs at the same time as the chest is compressed (Rudikoff *et al.*, 1980). This 'new CPR' can only be done with ETI and there is an additional problem in that increasing the pressure results in decreased coronary perfusion, because coronary perfusion occurs during the diastolic pause. The coronary perfusion can be improved by the infusion of 10 ml 1:10,000 adrenaline down the endotracheal tube (Michael *et al.*, 1984). The practical recommendations, based on this knowledge, are that if there is no endotracheal tube, ventilation should alternate with ECM as is traditionally taught, but if ETI has been done, ventilation should be synchronous with ECM with the use of adrenaline (Harries, 1984). These last two manoeuvres are not really practical for the situations where ECM might be considered for a hypothermic victim.

The thoracic pump mechanism could be effective in hypothermia even though the cold heart may be rigid. In animal experiments with hypothermic dogs (Maningas, 1985) it was found that ECM could produce only 50 per cent of the coronary and cerebral blood flow produced by ECM in normothermic dogs. This was the result of the changes in the compressibility of the heart and the compliance of the chest wall. However, because of the reduced oxygen requirements of the tissues in hypothermia, the reduced circulation may be sufficient to maintain viability. However, these findings do discount the suggestion that ECM should be done more slowly in hypothermia, and in hypothermia ECM should be done at the same rate as in normothermia (Merrifield in Marcus, 1979a).

Some resuscitative measures recommended following animal experiments are impractical in the field, e.g. (Hillman, 1971):

(1) 'Abdominal pumping or jack-knifing the body instead of ECM'. The abdominal pumping would have an effect through the thoracic pump mechanism of ECM but it may cause trauma to the liver (Harris *et al.*, 1967) and in practical terms it would be liable to empty the dilated stomach with the danger of inhalation of the gastric contents. Jack-knifing is impossible because the victim's bodies are too rigid (Danzl, 1983).
(2) 'Intracarotid centripetal infusion'. Even if rescue teams had the appropriate cannulae and infusion fluids it would probably be impossible to identify a pulseless carotid artery.
(3) 'Ventilation with 95 per cent oxygen plus 5 per cent carbon dioxide'. This would involve extra weight and expense, both important considerations for rescue teams.

It is sometimes said that defibrillation of a cold heart is unlikely till the cardiac temperature is over 30 °C (Drew *et al.*, 1959; Freeman and Pugh, 1969; Lougheed, 1961; Paton, 1983b). However, if there has been direct core rewarming, defibrillation has been achieved at 28 °C (Bristow *et al.*, 1977; Linton and Ledingham, 1966), sinus rhythm has been restored at 27 °C (Lloyd, 1972b) and 22.5 °C (Kugelberg *et al.*, 1967) and a heart in asystole has started spontaneously at 24 °C (Kvittingen and Naess, 1963).

Rewarming an apparently dead body in the field is difficult since most of the methods of providing active rewarming are not available or require too much expertise. Surface warming is technically possible but the absence of circulation through the skin will mean that the technique is ineffective and there will be the risk of causing severe skin damage. The most efficient means of surface heating is immersion in a hot bath but even in the resuscitation of rats (Andjus and Smith, 1955) immersion in a hot bath was not used until the heart beat and respiration had been restored. In one human case where it was tried (Jessen and Hagelsten, 1978) the bath failed to produce any rewarming though peritoneal dialysis subsequently did. Cardiopulmonary bypass is recommended as being the only hope of resuscitation in a patient in cardiac arrest with a core temperature below 25 °C (Foray and Salon, 1985), though the fact that one patient was resuscitated from VF at 25 °C by means of airway warming and gastric lavage (Osborne *et al.*, 1984) suggests that the absence of cardiopulmonary bypass in a hospital does not preclude a successful outcome.

The rescue teams are therefore faced with conflicting evidence and advice as to what they should do if the victim is apparently dead. ECM can certainly cause VF in a hypothermic heart but on the other hand ECM and EAR have kept people alive till they reached hospital. A severely hypothermic person is in a 'metabolic ice-box' (Mills, 1980) and his chance of survival is likely to be reduced by anything which disturbs the equilibrium, whether this disturbance is due to continued cooling or active rewarming measures (Mills, 1980; 1983a). One or two breaths of EAR are unlikely to cause any harm and might be beneficial but ECM is more problematical. A cold person, who has had a slow undetectable sinus rhythm converted to VF by ECM, is in a worse state than before but it is impossible to distinguish clinically between slow undetectable sinus rhythm and asystole or VF. It is important for the rescuers to check the pulse and heart beat over a long period because the heart rate may be as slow as 6/min (Steinman, A.M., personal communication, 1984) and if a pulse or heartbeat is detected, however slow, ECM is contra-indicated. Two hypothermia victims had a detectable pulse when found but the pulse then disappeared during the rescue, cardiac arrest was assumed and ECM and EAR commenced and continued until hospital was reached and the patients rewarmed (Steinman, A.M., personal communication, 1984).

When a person has been resuscitated after prolonged cardiac arrest in hypothermia, there is the danger of a late onset of acute pulmonary oedema (Kvittingen and Naess, 1963; Osborne *et al.*, 1984; Siebke *et al.*, 1975, Wind, 1975) even when the victim has not been in water (Althaus *et al.*, 1982). This phenomenon has many similarities with secondary drowning and may be due to the loss of surfactant from anoxic damage to the pneumocytes lining the alveoli (Pearn, 1980), though it may also be related to the cold-induced pulmonary oedema discussed earlier. Cerebral oedema may also occur in the first few hours after rewarming from hypothermia (Pausescu *et al.*, 1969).

Conclusion

If a person is found apparently dead from hypothermia ECM should not be started unless there is sufficient manpower and skill to rewarm the person where he is found, or to maintain ECM continuously until the victim reaches hospital. Therefore a victim in a small boat at sea or in an isolated cabin in the wilds or on a mountain where the only possible evacuation involves prolonged transport over difficult terrain on foot is probably safer left in his 'metabolic ice-box' without ECM. If ventilation of the patient is being performed it should probably be by EAR or with the use of airway warming equipment if available. Once resuscitation is complete, the patient should be transferred to hospital in case of the late onset of cerebral or pulmonary oedema or secondary drowning.

PART 4: THE SIGNIFICANCE OF HYPOTHERMIA AND COLD STRESS IN PARTICULAR SITUATIONS AND APPROPRIATE PREVENTIVE AND THERAPEUTIC MEASURES

INTRODUCTION

Accidental hypothermia can occur in a wide variety of situations. Cases have been reported during caving (Lloyd, 1964) and during skiing (Foray and Cahen, 1981), hill walking or mountain climbing (Foray and Cahen, 1981; Foray *et al.*, 1977; Pugh, 1964; 1966) though the incidence is probably greater in mountain casualties than is reported in details of accidents and injuries (Freeman and Pugh, 1969). At sea men on fishing trawlers are at risk (Pugh, 1968; Richardson, 1981) nor are passengers on a pleasure cruise guaranteed immunity (Keatinge, 1965) and the introduction of oil exploration in the North Sea has increased the population at risk on drilling and production platforms, diver support and supply vessels and in the ferry helicopters if they were to crash (Cumming, 1975; Leese, 1981; Roythorne, 1981). Divers are also at risk anywhere (Bennett and Elliott, 1969; Rawlins, 1981) and the deeper dives with oxyhelium breathing mixtures increase the risks (Rawlins, 1981).

Hypothermia may also occur in indoor situations in towns among the elderly (Fox *et al.*, 1973d), the very young (Frederiksen, 1977) and those who have medical disorders or malnutrition, or following drug overdose (Cohen, 1968; Duguid *et al.*, 1961; Emslie-Smith, 1958; Howitt, 1971). Hypothermia can also occur during summer months (Rees, 1958), in operating theatres (Newman, 1971; Searle, 1971; Vale and Lunn, 1969), and with so many possible factors contributing to hypothermia — indoor and outdoor environment, nutrition, clothing, general health, age, etc. — it is hardly surprising that hypothermia has been reported from most parts of the world, including areas normally considered warm, e.g. Ceylon (Atukorale, 1971), Australia (Budd *et al.*, 1971), South Africa (Duckworth and Cooper, 1964; Thomas and Gerber, 1965), Tunisia (Ferchiou, 1972) and subtropical Texas (Coopwood and Kennedy, 1971; Tolman and Cohen, 1970), though in these reports, altitude or night frosts have been at least partial explanations. More surprising is the possibility of hypothermia in the balmy seas off Madiera (Keatinge, 1965), and even at low altitudes in the Sahara, night frosts and desert winds expose the traveller to the risks of hypothermia and frostbite (Barber, 1978). Finally when Sadikali and Owor (1974) wrote that 'Hypothermia is not uncommon' they forced the inevitable conclusion that nowhere in the world can be guaranteed to be entirely free from the risk of hypothermia because they were reporting on 24 cases of accidental hypothermia which had occurred in two years in tropical Kampala where the environmental temperature never dropped below 16 °C.

Accurate total figures for hypothermia cases are not easy to obtain because the possibility of hypothermia is often not considered and the diagnosis missed. The environments in which hypothermia occurs can be subdivided into the following groups:

- Hospital hypothermia
  - Anaesthesia
  - Burns
  - Drug overdose
- Urban hypothermia
  - Neonatal and infant hypothermia
  - The elderly
  - Down and outs
- Hypothermia outdoors
  - In the mountains
  - Caving
  - Water (immersion) hypothermia
  - Cold at work
  - Sport in the cold
- Diving

In each situation the predisposing causes are different and in each there may be a number of other factors which can interact with hypothermia to cause death. Finally preventive and therapeutic measures appropriate for one situation may be useless or dangerous in another and therefore each must be considered separately.

22 HOSPITAL HYPOTHERMIA

Hypothermia in Anaesthesia

In 1880 von Kappeler reported a lowering of body temperature in 20 surgical cases, but the problem of heat loss during anaesthesia was only really considered after about 1950. One possible reason for this is that prior to the introduction of curare, muscle relaxation was produced by deep anaesthesia but there would probably always be some residual muscle tone present resulting in metabolic heat production. This heat production would, of course, be abolished by curare. Also in pre-curare times cyclopropane was a popular anaesthetic agent and, as this was used with a Waters to-and-fro circuit, the carbon dioxide produced by the patient would react with the soda lime to produce heat and moisture and the gas delivered to the patient would therefore be warmed and humidified (Adriani and Rovenstine, 1941). With the general use of muscle relaxants, mechanical ventilators came into use along with other anaesthetic circuits and higher gas flows.

Precipitating Factors

Anaesthetic agents interfere with the fine control of thermoregulation by removing the influence of the extra-hypothalamic temperature sensors on the responsiveness to changes in hypothalamic temperatures, while leaving the central sensor system and the coarse control of thermoregulation relatively intact (Bligh, 1973). Anaesthesia also reduces metabolic rate (Burton and Edholm, 1955; Keatinge, 1969; Mackenzie, 1973; Wylie and Churchill-Davidson, 1966) though not by as much as sleep (Mikat *et al.*, 1984). Anaesthesia also depresses thermostatic reflexes (Hemingway, 1941) though the body can increase its thermoregulatory effort even under anaesthesia (Mikat *et al.*, 1984). Muscle paralysis abolishes muscle tone and muscle heat production and eliminates shivering (Hall, 1978; Holdcroft, 1981; Mackenzie, 1973; Mikat *et al.*, 1984; Newman, 1971) but the mere introduction of mechanical ventilation will decrease heat production (Mikat *et al.*, 1984). Finally anaesthesia increases heat loss by dilating the peripheral vasculature directly and by overcoming the vasoconstrictor response to cold (Wylie and Churchill-Davidson,

1966) but possibly the most important factors are the degree of vasodilation produced by extradural and spinal analgesia and by inhalation agents such as halothane (Hall, 1978). The importance of epidural anaesthesia as a cause of increased heat loss (Holdcroft *et al.*, 1979; Jenkins *et al.*, 1983) was shown by a case described by Searle (1971) where the core temperature cooled to 31.2 °C, though when the same patient had a similar operation three years later and was treated the same way, i.e. with heated infusion and a water mattress, but was under a general anaesthetic without the epidural used in the first operation, hypothermia did not develop (Wedley, 1974). Regional blockade, especially epidural, not only cause an increased incidence of hypothermia but the duration of hypothermia is longer and the rewarming rate is only half as fast as in cases of hypothermia occurring under general anaesthesia (Holdcroft, 1981; Vaughan *et al.*, 1981).

The induction of anaesthesia causes a redistribution of body heat (Ellis and Zwana, 1977; Holdcroft *et al.*, 1979; Vale, 1973) which is seen as a fall in core temperature in the first 15 to 30 minutes following induction, accompanied by a rise in skin temperature and therefore a narrowing in the core/shell temperature gradient. It is therefore important not to consider just the core temperature but also the total body heat as computed from core and skin temperatures. This drop in temperature is also seen in children (Calvert, 1962), in neonates (Calvert, 1962; Hercus, 1960) and in dogs and cats (Waterman, 1975). At the end of anaesthesia increased heat production occurs as anaesthesia becomes light, but the changes in muscle temperature follow rather than precede the general rise in body temperature. The intercostal muscle temperatures rise after the initiation of spontaneous ventilation, but there is no rise in the deltoid, biceps or forearm muscles until voluntary movement starts (Lunn, 1969). The temperature rise is therefore mainly due to non-muscular elements.

The problem of hypothermia during anaesthesia has been widely considered (Calvert, 1962; Clark *et al.*, 1954; Hall, 1978; Holdcroft, 1981; Lunn, 1969; Morris, 1971a, b; Morris and Wilkie, 1970; Roe *et al.*, 1966b; Vale, 1973; Vaughan *et al.*, 1981) and the individual factors in heat loss studied such as theatre environment, anaesthetic technique, duration of surgery, infusion of cold fluids and age — the very old and the very young. It has been calculated that a 2 to 3 kg neonate is losing about 8 to 9 kcal/hour in an ambient temperature of 24 to 25 °C (Day and Hardy, 1942; Roe *et al.*, 1966a). Hey *et al.*

(1970) felt that on an operating table mattress the conductive losses for a baby are small unless cold irrigating fluid is allowed to wash under the infant, though Calvert (1962) felt that radiation and heat conduction to the mattress were major sources of heat loss in children.

Reasons for Maintaining Normothermia

It is important to try to consider the reasons for maintaining body temperature at normal levels during anaesthesia in addition to the aesthetic reason of avoiding the sight of a miserable cold clammy post-operative patient whose circulation is unstable as he rewarms (Cundy, 1972; Newman, 1971):

(1) As the core temperature drops the risk of ventricular fibrillation rises (Newman, 1971).

(2) If the patient is cold the action of drugs (Weihe, 1973) and anaesthetic agents (Calvert, 1962) are impaired as is also neuromuscular conduction (Thornton *et al.*, 1976) and any residual depolarising muscle blockade is augmented (Rashad and Benson, 1967). In addition, if the patient is cold during the operation, the action of the non-depolarising muscle relaxants (NDMR), such as tubocurarine, is antagonised (Feldman, 1971) and therefore the anaesthetist may have to give additional doses of muscle relaxants to achieve adequate surgical muscle relaxation (Choi *et al.*, 1985). Since the metabolism and excretion of these drugs is also impaired by hypothermia (Choi *et al.*, 1985), at the end of the operation the serum level of NDMR is likely to be elevated through either or both of the two mechanisms. There is the added complication that, even if the neuromuscular blockade is adequately reversed at the low body temperature, recurarisation may occur on rewarming (Choi *et al.*, 1985), though this phenomenon has not been demonstrated in the experimental animal (Choi *et al.*, 1985). The net result of these observations is that if a patient becomes hypothermic during an operation there is a greatly increased chance of residual paralysis at the end of the operation.

(3) Cold will cause discomfort to the patient which may result in restlessness and the patient requiring more narcotic sedation.

(4) Preventing the heat loss may reduce the metabolic response to injury as has been shown in fracture patients (Cuthbertson *et al.*, 1968), in the treatment of severely burned patients (Barr *et al.*, 1968) and in paediatric surgery (Silverman and Sinclair, 1966). The idea of preventing cold stress in patients has received experimental support

(Caldwell, 1962; Campbell and Cuthbertson, 1966; 1967).

(5) For the neonate, on top of the six-hour pre-operative fast, hypothermia will cause a delay, sometimes very long, in restarting feeding following operation with all the additional metabolic problems (Calvert, 1962; Rickham, 1957). There is the added complication that hypoglycaemia is relatively common in the peri-operative period in children, especially small children (Payne and Ireland, 1984) and this increases the risk of and dangers from hypothermia.

(6) The heat loss which occurs during anaesthesia is regained after operation by a combination of shivering and vasoconstriction. Shivering increases the metabolic and circulatory demands (Rodriguez *et al.*, 1983), which may overwhelm patients with impaired cardio-pulmonary reserves and the elderly (Vaughan *et al.*, 1981) and vasoconstriction may have the following additional undesirable side effects:

(a) In a patient with arterial disease, anastomotic channels, which are barely able to provide a collateral circulation when fully dilated, may fail to maintain tissue perfusion when vasoconstriction occurs due to exposure to cold (Lunn, 1969).
(b) Sluggish circulation may jeopardise the success of vascular graft procedures.
(c) Blood volume, as indicated by a satisfactory venous pressure, may be adequate at the end of an operation during which peripheral vasoconstriction occurred but when rewarming takes place some hours later after the patient has returned to bed, the peripheral circulation opens up again, the central venous pressure falls sometimes rapidly and a state of hypovolaemia develops (Lunn, 1969). This may cause a fall in blood pressure or a marked drop in urine output (Dyde and Lunn, 1970).
(d) The relatively high incidence of deep vein thrombosis and of pulmonary embolism in countries where operations are performed under cold ambient conditions is in marked contrast with the virtual absence of these complications in warm subtropical regions. Long periods of reduced blood flow, together with local pressure on the calf muscles, would be expected to favour intravascular thrombosis (Lunn, 1969).
(e) Vasoconstriction may cause hyperpyrexia in the post-operative period as the patient's heart production increases (Vale, 1973; Vale and Lunn, 1969) and if the vasoconstriction is not

overcome, this increase in heat production may lead to a dangerous hyperpyrexia because of the Q_{10} effect (Vale, 1973) and hyperpyrexia increases mortality (Wedley, 1978).

(7) The necessity for an increase in heat production means that the oxygen consumption will increase in the post-operative period (Horvath *et al.*, 1956; Rodriguez *et al.*, 1983), with figures of 109 to 178 per cent (Vale, 1973) and 135 to 468 per cent with shivering (Bay *et al.*, 1968) being quoted. Even a drop in temperature of as little as 0.3 °C may cause a rise in oxygen consumption of 25 to 100 per cent (Roe *et al.*, 1966a). It is known that shivering itself can increase oxygen consumption by 400 per cent (Burton and Edholm, 1955). These enormous increases in oxygen consumption impose a further burden on a cardiovascular system which may already be depressed after prolonged anaesthesia (Hall, 1978). This depression will include factors such as increased pulmonary shunting (Vale, 1973) due to ventilation perfusion imbalance following the general anaesthetic (Nunn and Payne, 1962), residual paresis following muscle relaxants (Vale, 1973) aggravated if the patient is hypothermic, and inefficient grunting respiration due to pain (Vale, 1973). As the patient is recovering from the anaesthetic there is an increased risk of laryngeal spasm and bronchial obstruction from mucous plugs (Goldberg and Roe, 1966) and the elderly are at greater post-operative risk because they are more likely to have pre-existing pulmonary and cardiovascular disease (Goldberg and Roe, 1966; Newman, 1971). If oxygen is not delivered to the muscles to maintain aerobic metabolism, then anaerobic pathways are activated with the production of lactate and a metabolic acidosis.

Thus the patient who is maintained in normothermia, i.e. whose average skin temperature is above the critical level of 33 °C (Benzinger *et al.*, 1963), is unlikely to shiver, to increase his demand for oxygen, to increase the catabolic breakdown of his tissues or to suffer from inadequate tissue perfusion and he may in fact benefit from the advantages of peripheral vasodilatation (Bloch *et al.*, 1966; Irving, 1968).

Reducing Heat Loss

A number of methods of trying to reduce heat loss have been suggested:

(1) Evaporative heat losses can be reduced by avoiding the use of volatile solutions for skin preparation (Rashad and Benson, 1967).

(2) Any intravenous fluids given should be warmed (Boyan and Howland, 1963; Lunn, 1969; Mackenzie, 1973; Newman, 1971; Newton, 1975; Shanks, 1975 a, b).

(3) The environmental temperature of the theatre may be raised and the recommended figures have ranged from 21 to 26.8 °C (Calvert, 1962; Hall, 1978; Holdcroft *et al.*, 1979; Mackenzie, 1973; Morris, 1971b) with a relative humidity of 50 to 55 per cent (Mackenzie, 1973). However, an environmental temperature of over 22 °C is not tolerable for work (Calvert, 1962; Dyde and Lunn, 1970; Wyon *et al.*, 1968) and 18 to 21 °C is the temperature preferred by surgeons (Mackenzie, 1973; Morris, 1971b). Mackenzie (1973) found that provided the theatre temperature was over 21 °C there was no problem with the temperature of the patients, and between 19 and 21 °C heated water blankets would prevent cooling.

(4) The parts of the body not needed for the operation can have surface insulation by means of a heat-reflecting blanket — 'space blanket' (Dyde and Lunn, 1970; Newton, 1976; Shanks, 1975 a, b; Vale, 1973) but this recommendation was made on theoretical considerations alone. However, when a heavy-duty 'space blanket', with two layers of metallised plastic sheeting (MPS) separated by a fibre layer, was tested in neurosurgical patients it was found to give no protection against a drop in core temperature (Radford and Thurlow, 1979) though a similar study found a significant improvement from the use of MPS (Bourke *et al.*, 1984). The difference may have been due to the care with which the MPS was wrapped round the patient thus affecting convective and evaporative loss and no comparison has been made between the effects of MPS and polythene sheeting. Even those favourably impressed by MPS only recommend it when the operation is going to last more than two hours and when more than 60 per cent of the body surface can be covered (Bourke *et al.*, 1984). When using MPS there is the additional risk of electrocution if the diathermy is faulty (Chambers and Saha, 1979; Cundy, 1980; Hill, 1980) and its use will also be restricted because of the needs of surgical access (Mackenzie, 1973). When these facts are added to the general ineffectiveness of the 'space blanket' concept there would seem to be very little place for MPS in theatre. Despite this MPS is still being recommended for use in theatre (White, 1980). MPS may produce a dangerously high temperature if used on a restless patient (Dyde and Lunn, 1970) but the same problem would be likely to occur if simple polythene is used instead of MPS.

(5) For the neonate Shaw *et al.* (1970) suggested the use of a fibre-

optic 'hotpipe' system.

(6) Vale (1973) demonstrated a large decrease in heat loss during anaesthesia by the use of a heat-retaining mattress filled with methylcellulose gel. Warm-water blankets are recommended to prevent hypothermia (Evans *et al.*, 1973) and are used during small animal surgery (Waterman, 1975). Other investigators have achieved variable results using warming blankets, either electrical or water circulating, or heat-retaining mattresses (Calvert, 1972; Cundy, 1972; Goudsouzian *et al.*, 1973; Lewis and Mackenzie, 1972; Lunn, 1969; Mackenzie, 1973; Morris and Kumar, 1972; Newman, 1971). For neurosurgical procedures, where the body can be totally covered, a water-circulating piped suit has been used (Goldblatt and Miller, 1972). It has been pointed out, however, that water-circulating mattresses and electric blankets may cause skin burns (Andersen *et al.*, 1977) unless careful attention is directed towards ensuring good contact with the surface of the patient (Vale, 1971; 1973). Even so-called 'safe' warming blankets may generate a thermal burn in under-perfused tissues (Crino and Nagel, 1968) or may be ineffective in a cool room (Morris and Kumar, 1972). On the other hand, some heated water beds used to maintain thermoneutrality have a maximum thermostat setting of 26 °C and will therefore be acting as a cold stress on the patient (Brydon, 1977a). There is also a danger of producing hyperthermia especially in children if the thermostat is intentionally or accidentally set too high (Smith, 1983).

(7) Humidification of the inspired gases is now widely recommended as a measure to assist the control of body temperature during anaesthesia (Chalon *et al.*, 1979a, b; Newton, 1976; 1980; Ramanathan *et al.*, 1976; Rashad and Benson, 1967; Shanks, 1975a, b; 1977; Stone *et al.*, 1981; Tausk *et al.*, 1976; Vale, 1971), though it has been claimed to be ineffective (Lunn, 1967; 1969; Raffe and Martin, 1983) and further doubt has been expressed on the value of humidification of the inspired gases either as a means of controlling temperature or to protect the mucosa (BJA, 1976). Nevertheless in an experiment with rabbits, those ventilated with dry gases showed a fall in temperature, a 2 per cent loss of weight and had damage to the respiratory epithelium. None of these deleterious effects were noted in animals ventilated with humidified gas (Marfatia *et al.*, 1975). In another study one lung was ventilated with dry gas while the other was ventilated with humidifed gas (Fonkalsrud, 1975). In the 'dry' lung the oxygen uptake dropped from a pre-experiment 56 per cent to 30 per cent whereas in the 'wet' lung it rose from 44 per cent to 70 per

cent. In the 'dry' lung cilial activity was impaired, slowing clearance of debris, and there was an increase in surface tension, possibly through a depression of surfactant activity (Fonkalsrud, 1975).

Inhalation of dry gas at room temperature is a cause of heat loss which is increased by controlled ventilation with high gas flows and large minute volumes, but as compensation the vasoconstriction which occurs in hypocarbia may reduce radiant heat loss from the skin (Vale, 1973). Dogs ventilated with cold, dry gas cooled, whereas they remained normothermic when ventilated with warm, humidified gas (Brock *et al.*, 1977). Hyperventilation with cold, dry gas caused vasoconstriction even when hypocarbia was eliminated as a cause. Vale (1973) calculated that, since one litre of inspired gas required approximately 15 cal to raise its temperature from room temperature to 37 °C and to saturate it with water vapour, this contributed a loss of about 12 kcal/hour which could be halved by the use of a vapour condenser. Weeks (1975b) calculated that 22 ± 8 mg of water were needed per litre of ventilation. In actual experiments dogs ventilated with dry gas lost 15.7 kcal/hour whereas dogs ventilated with a humid gas lost 1.5 kcal/hour (Shanks, 1974a) and when the experiments were repeated in humans a dry gas caused a loss of 12.4 kcal/hour as compared with a 1.5 kcal/hour with a more humid gas (Shanks, 1974b). Similarly patients who inspired dry gas cooled at 1.5 °C/hour whereas if they inspired humidifed gas there was no heat loss and in fact two patients who were cool before the start of the operation rewarmed during the procedure (Newton, 1975). The combination of surface insulation, warmed intravenous fluids and humidification of the inspired gases can increase the body heat in operations involving the body cavity including vascular procedures (Shanks, 1975b). Vivori and Bush (1977) claimed that humidification and heating of the anaesthetic gases was not required in children and that other methods were sufficient, but this opinion is disputed by other authors (Berry *et al.*, 1973; Campbell *et al.*, 1975; Garg, 1973; Haller, 1975; Mackuanying and Chalon, 1974; Rashad and Benson, 1967; Wallace *et al.*, 1978) and one states that as in adults the introduction of airway warming can raise the temperature of a child who is cooling (Hendren, 1975).

The effect of different anaesthetic circuits on heat and moisture loss during anaesthesia has been extensively studied (Aldrete and Cubillos, 1981; Chalon *et al.*, 1973; Clarke *et al.*, 1958; Dery, 1971; 1973a; Dery *et al.*, 1967a, b; Newton, 1976; Ramanathan *et al.*, 1975; 1976; Shanks, 1973; Shanks and Sara, 1973a, b, c; 1974;

Weeks, 1975a) but, while some were better than others, none was as effective as adding a humidifier to the circuit. There are a variety of means of providing additional humidification (Benveniste and Pedersen, 1977; Berry *et al.*, 1973; Campbell *et al.*, 1975; Chalon *et al.*, 1978; Garg, 1973; Talsma *et al.*, 1978; Tayyab *et al.*, 1973). Most of these are either condenser humidifiers which have been reviewed frequently (Chalon *et al.*, 1984; Chamney, 1969; Ravenas and Lindholm, 1979; Shanks, 1974c; 1977; Steward, 1976), or provide water as vapour or nebulised droplets and these have also been reviewed (Chamney, 1969; Geevarghese *et al.*, 1976; Grant *et al.*, 1976; Hayes and Robinson, 1970; Shanks, 1977; Shanks and Gibbs, 1975). There is one which utilises the exothermic reaction of soda lime in a carbon dioxide absorber (Chalon and Ramanathan, 1974). Hygroscopic condenser humidifiers avoid the risk of excess humidity, bacterial contamination and of overheating (Gilston, 1984) though it is possible for fragments of the hygroscopic sponge to break off and be blown into the bronchi (James and Gothard, 1984).

There is the danger that the over-enthusiastic use of a number of these measures of preventing heat loss may in fact cause hyperthermia (Kirch and de Kornfeld, 1967; Lunn, 1969; Vale, 1973).

There is certainly a valid case for suppressing shivering in certain critically ill patients. This will decrease the caloric metabolic demand and decrease myocardial work, though at the expense of prolonging the rewarming period (Rodriguez *et al.*, 1983). This suppression can be done chemically (Rodriguez *et al.*, 1983) or by the use of airway warming which has been shown to suppress shivering (Pozos and Wittmers, 1983).

Conclusions

The fact, that many anaesthetics are given with no particular measures being taken to prevent heat loss and the patients seem to survive without any problems suggests that significant heat loss either does not occur very often or that most patients can restore their body temperature without difficulty. However, there are some patients and some operations where a drop in temperature might jeopardise survival or success and in these cases precautions should be taken. The measures selected will obviously depend on the particular surgical procedure and the theatre environment but warming and humidification of the inspired gases is one technique that can always be applied by the anaesthetist.

Burns

In patients with severe burns, the metabolic rate may be raised 100 to 150 per cent resulting in marked weight loss and protein catabolism. This increased metabolism is due to the loss of the normal protective skin layer which prevents heat and moisture loss, and in burned patients 60 to 80 per cent of the increased metabolism is to replace the loss of heat through evaporation and convection (Wilmore *et al.*, 1975). This heat loss can be prevented by adjusting the temperature and humidity of the environment to provide thermoneutrality. (The thermoneutral values of temperature and humidity will be higher for burned patients than for patients with an intact skin surface.) This measure reduces the metabolic response to injury (Barr *et al.*, 1968) and results in a marked improvement in patient comfort and speed of recovery. The high level of humidity and the raised temperature will also serve to reduce the respiratory heat loss, thus providing a further small reduction in the thermal load.

Drug Overdose

Many drugs depress metabolism as well as having specific depressant effects on particular organs, and this not only predisposes patients to develop hypothermia but it complicates the diagnosis of any injury or organ damage. Since hypothermia in turn depresses drug metabolism, recovery from an overdose will be delayed by hypothermia. Most cases require only general supportive measures and will rewarm spontaneously once they have been admitted to a warm hospital. There are, however, some cases where the combination of low body temperature and severity of overdose is sufficient to prevent any rise in temperature and in these cases active rewarming measures are necessary (Murray *et al.*, 1974). Peritoneal dialysis has obvious advantages in this situation since it can assist in drug removal as well as in rewarming. Airway warming has also been used successfully in these patients and can be used very easily if the patient's respiration is depressed and requiring mechanical assistance. As discussed in the section on airway warming, this measure is very simple to use and should be available in any hospital and may be invaluable through its potential to turn a static or cooling situation into one where there is a positive temperature rise.

Medical Problems

Some patients become hypothermic in hospital and for these the outlook is very poor because hypothermia in these circumstances usually denotes severe damage to the brain or spinal cord. Though it may be necessary to rewarm them to exclude any treatable cause for the hypothermia, death is almost inevitable (Hunter, 1971). However, acute illness may occasionally cause thermoregulatory failure (Whittle and Eates, 1979) and therefore all patients must be rewarmed before any irrevocable decision is taken. In these circumstances airway warming might be the method of choice because of its simplicity.

23 NEONATAL AND INFANT HYPOTHERMIA

The transition from an intra-uterine thermostable environment to the thermally hostile and variable extra-uterine environment (Hey, 1972) calls for profound adjustments in thermal physiology (Chiswick, 1978) and, as this occurs at a time when massive changes in circulatory and respiratory physiology are also occurring, it becomes a source of wonder that so many babies successfully make the transition. Maclean and Emslie-Smith (1977) have considered physiology, pathology, epidemiology and management of hypothermia in the child in great detail and have quoted other reviewers. It is interesting that hypothermia in the newborn could be considered a new syndrome as recently as 1955 (Mann, 1955).

Predisposing Factors and Prevention

There is a high incidence of hypothermia in infants among people with low socioeconomic conditions in countries with cold winters (Arneil and Kerr, 1963; Racini and Jarjoui, 1982) but neonatal hypothermia may also occur in countries considered hot, e.g. West Africa (Briend and de Schampheleire, 1981). Most cases of neonatal hypothermia occur at the start of a sudden cold spell and are due to the cold stress overwhelming rather than exhausting the thermoregulatory mechanisms (Hey, 1972) and are therefore of the 'immersion' type.

Cold stress with a normal core temperature is itself a hazard to the neonate even without the development of full-blown hypothermia (Hey, 1972). The cold stress may result in an increased metabolic acidosis (Gandy *et al.*, 1964) and a lower arterial oxygen tension (Stephenson *et al.*, 1970) or increased oxygen consumption (de Saintonge *et al.*, 1979; Kappacoda and Macartney, 1976). One of the signs of exposure to cold stress is unsatisfactory growth of a baby. If there is inadequate clothing, too much energy is being expended on thermogenesis and the correct treatment is to provide warmer clothing and not artificial feeding. In primitive countries the lack of hygiene means that artificial feeding is associated with an increased risk of gastroenteritis (Briend and de Schampheleire, 1981). As discussed earlier, there may be the risk of precipitating a 'cot death' through pulmonary hypertension or hypothermia. Hypothermia may be overlooked because of the good pink colour of the baby (Racini and Jarjoui, 1982) and the associated lethargy may be welcomed by a tired mother. Prevention of cold stress and hypothermia requires an awareness that the possibility exists and can exist in any walk of society. Large, poorly heated bedrooms are dangerous (Rogers *et al.*, 1971; Wigglesworth, 1973) and the room temperature should ideally not drop below 18 °C (Health Education Council, 1977), though Hey (1972) recommends higher temperatures. To take account of the individual variations of the child, a table has been developed (Young and Marks, 1983) which gives the neutral thermal environmental temperatures for the age and weight of the baby in the first six weeks of life. In the 1950s many cases of hypothermia occurred because the babies had been washed in an unheated bathroom and became chilled. The problem was compounded by the mothers wrapping them up well before returning to the warmer rooms and the babies therefore remained chilled because the blankets kept the environmental heat out (Wigglesworth, 1973). The baby should be warmed by bodily contact (Ebrahim, 1984) before being wrapped in pre-warmed blankets and put in the cot (Health Education Council, 1977). In the primitive areas of West Africa the most useful preventive measures were to prohibit unnecessary washing of the baby and for the baby to be put into bed with its mother and not nursed in a cot (Briend and de Schampheleire, 1981). Finally some old-fashioned beliefs may have to be overcome, namely that babies 'benefit' from cold fresh air by having a bedroom window permanently open or by being put into the open air in a pram regardless of the conditions (Hutchison, 1969; Wigglesworth, 1973). Any cot-nursed baby should be kept in a really warm room both day and night (Hey, 1972) and it is important to remember that a room which may feel very warm to an adult may be too cold for a baby (Ebrahim, 1984; Hey, 1972; Young and Marks, 1983). Even when the general environment is warm, a cold air current (even oxygen) across the baby's face will cause cold stress and result in an increased metabolic rate and therefore oxygen consumption (Young and Marks, 1983).

In the hospital a number of items of equipment have been introduced which raise the environmental temperature round the child to prevent inadvertent cold stress, and mortality has dropped as a result (Buetow *et al.*, 1964; Day *et al.*, 1964; Jolly *et al.*, 1962; Silverman and Sinclair, 1966; Silverman *et al.*, 1958). Adequate warmth also reduces the oxygen consumption of the neonate (Darnall and Ariagno, 1978). Incubators are designed to enable increased environmental warmth to be provided for the baby without heating the whole room, but with the current practice of nursing the baby naked in the incubator, the environmental control has had to become very precise with regards to both temperature and humidity (Hey *et al.*, 1970; Rashad and Benson, 1967). Even in an incubator pre-term infants may suffer cold stress if the atmosphere is too dry and even a minor change in incubator design may affect the baby (Hermansen *et al.*, 1984). Unfortunately, if the incubator is in a cold room, the perspex canopy will be cold and this will result in an increased radiant heat loss from the baby (Hey and Mount, 1966). It is possible to compensate for this by raising the air temperature inside the incubator but it may be impossible without increasing the air temperature above 35 °C, the highest air temperature allowable under current British standards (Hey and Mount, 1966). Sunlight and phototherapy lamps placed close to the incubator may heat the perspex and alter the radiant environment unpredictably (Hey, 1972). An attempt has been made to overcome the problem of variations in environmental heat and infant requirement by means of servo-control of the heat output by a sensing thermistor strapped to the baby's abdomen (Friedman *et al.*, 1967; Levison *et al.*, 1966). This is attractive in theory but has dangers in practice (Brydon, 1977b; Hey, 1972) and should not be used as a routine (Young and Marks, 1983). Other devices such as 'silver swaddler' (Baum and Scopes, 1968; Wauer, 1978) and 'baby bubble bag' (Besch *et al.*, 1971), designed to reduce radiant and convective heat loss, may not be as efficient as claimed and may in fact have dangers (Hey, 1972) (see 'Space Blanket', pages 168 to 171).

Hey (1972) suggests that there should be a return to the use of swaddling in the nursing of normal healthy babies. Not only will this provide a warm and stable environment almost free of the twin perils of serious cold stress and hyperthermia, but access is easy, the anxiety caused to the mother by obvious physical barriers can be minimised, and gentle swaddling has a subtle, soothing effect on the child. Clothing a child being nursed in an incubator would also tend to reduce the risks of extreme variations in temperature (Hey, 1972; Young and Marks, 1983). In addition small babies develop the ability to withstand cold stress better when nursed in cots rather than in incubators (Glass *et al.*, 1968; Perlstein *et al.*, 1970) and the risk of precipitating apnoea by excessively warm air over the face (Perlstein *et al.*, 1970) is avoided. As the brain is a major heat-producing organ in the newborn infant (Cross and Stratton, 1974) it seems logical to prevent heat loss from the head (Hey, 1972), and the use of a close-fitting gamgee-lined hat not only reduces the rate of fall in the core temperature of a naked neonate but it also reduces the oxygen consumption (de Saintonge *et al.*, 1979). The same gamgee insulation over the lower abdomen did not have a measurable effect. After birth a baby should be dried immediately and have adequate covering of the head as well as the body (Ebrahim, 1984).

Treatment

If hypothermia does develop, the recommended management, for those babies who have cooled slowly over more than six hours, is to place the baby in an environment just a few degrees warmer than the deep body temperature (Hey, 1972; Kennaird, 1973; Mann, 1967; Rogers *et al.*, 1971). This will avoid causing vasodilatation or burning and, by blocking all the major avenues of heat loss, will cause the baby to warm up from within at a speed dependent on the metabolic rate. The environmental temperature should be adjusted every two hours. As the incubators are humidified as well as heated, respiratory heat loss will also be reduced to a minimum. However, rewarming by this method may be slow with a prolonged rewarming period (12 to 18 hours) and there may be a high mortality (70 per cent) (Racini and Jarjoui, 1982). Setting the incubator thermostat at 37 °C from the start and giving additional core rewarming by stomach lavage and enemas with fluid at 37 °C resulted in rewarming in three to four hours and only 33 per cent mortality (Racini and Jarjoui, 1982). For the infant with hypothermia occurring in less than six hours, rapid rewarming is possible, and several children and babies have been rewarmed in a hot bath with good results (Anderson *et al.*, 1970; Mann, 1967). Rapid rewarming may reduce the degree of metabolic acidosis and hypoglycaemia (Young and Marks, 1983), but rapid rewarming increases oxygen consumption and may cause apnoea (Young and Marks, 1983), and fits may be triggered by too rapid rewarming (Maclean and Emslie-Smith, 1977). Possibly the use of moderate rewarming under total physiological control in an intensive care unit would avoid all these dangers. Because the neonate has such a small tidal volume in comparison with its surface area, active airway warming, either alone or to supplement the humidity of the incubator, would produce a negligible thermal benefit and in fact when airway warming was being used, it was found that there was no significant increase in radiant heat demand after airway warming was stopped (Soulski *et al.*, 1983). Any other physiological benefit would be far outweighed by the technical problems and dangers of the necessary equipment. However, if an infant requires oxygen, the gas should be warmed and humidified (Young and Marks, 1983). Finally the infants who become hypothermic in the Tropics are probably also suffering from malnutrition, and the provision of high calorie feeds can relieve the acute depletion of energy reserves and lead to a rapid restoration of normal body temperature (MacLean and Emslie-Smith, 1977).

In a baby the normal thermoregulatory mechanism breaks down if the core temperature drops below 32 °C, and it may not recover for several days, even after the temperature has been restored to normal (Hey, 1972). Therefore any hypothermic baby should be observed carefully for some days after rewarming.

24 ACCIDENTAL HYPOTHERMIA IN THE ELDERLY

Accidental hypothermia is now recognised as an important hazard for the elderly (Butler and Stalowitz, 1978; Carne, 1979; Collins, 1983a, b; Emslie-Smith, 1981; Horvath and Rochelle, 1977; Kurtz, 1982; MacLean and Emslie-Smith, 1977; NHS, 1974) though as recently as 1958, when Rees described four cases of hypothermia in the elderly, he could state in the introduction that 'In clinical medicine hypothermia is uncommon . . .' though Emslie-Smith (1958) considered it common.

Risk Factors

With increasing age there is a progressive impairment of thermoregulatory function (Cooper and Ferguson, 1983; Wagner *et al.*, 1974) shown by a reduction in the normal gradients between the core and the shell (Collins *et al.*, 1977) and this must result in increased heat loss. Those of the elderly who show no vasoconstrictor response to cold, have a decreased peripheral blood flow and an increased incidence of orthostatic hypotension are those with the greatest risk (Collins *et al.*, 1977). The elderly also have a lower metabolic rate than young people (Paton, 1983b). The thermoregulatory function may be further impaired by disease and/or by some of the drugs prescribed for illness or for other problems such as anxiety or insomnia. An additional problem, which may contribute to the occurrence of hypothermia in the elderly, is a desynchronisation of the diurnal cycles controlling heat loss and heat production (Moore-Ede, 1983).

Though the elderly person may succumb to any of the types of hypothermia, the common one is an acute episode superimposed on a pre-existing subclinical chronic hypothermia and though the core temperature may have been normal during the weeks preceding the acute episode, the cold stress has resulted in considerable shifts of the body fluids into the cells, and this fluid shift complicates the treatment of any superimposed episode of acute hypothermia.

As discussed earlier, cold stress can produce impairment of vital bodily functions even before there is a significant drop in the temperature of the body core. Therefore it can be appreciated that, since many of these functions are impaired among the elderly (Anderson, 1981), further deterioration may be critical and may result in falls, confusion or irrational behaviour resulting in illness or injury requiring hospital admission. Unfortunately since the official definition only allows the diagnosis of hypothermia to be made once the core temperature has dropped below 35 °C (35.1 °C is not hypothermic), the precipitating factor is always attributed to old age rather than cold stress. A low body temperature, which may be missed, increases the risk of ischaemic heart disease in the elderly (West *et al.*, 1973a, b).

One problem is the identification of the elderly who are at risk from the cold and there are many contributing factors, economic, environmental (Salvosa *et al.*, 1971) and social (Wicks, 1978). For example there may be mental confusion due to old age itself, or drugs, or problems with finance may lead to decisions having to be taken as to whether food or fuel should be purchased when both are required. Lack of food intake will increase the risk of hypothermia through reduced energy intake, and any loss of weight will result in a reduction in the insulating layer of fat and in lean body mass, and this last will produce a decrease in resting metabolism (Morgan and York, 1983). Clothing may be neglected, sometimes through financial stringency (Irvine, 1974), but also sometimes from loss of personal pride or from excessive thrift. The problem may be aggravated by the fact that some old people will not claim benefits to which they are entitled for a variety of reasons, e.g. independence, pride, unawareness of eligbility or lack of knowledge of the system (West, 1980). To save on fuel bills some old people spend the day in bed which, while it conserves fuel and avoids having to produce heat through the metabolism of scarce food, may result in decreasing mobility and a decrease in the ability to exercise. In cold weather there is then a greater risk of developing hypothermia because of the lack of the heat produced through eating food, as a result of a fall due to muscle weakness or because the unfit muscles can no longer produce sufficient heat. There is growing evidence that regular exercise for the elderly improves temperature regulation and maintains nutrition (Morris, 1983) with the secondary thermal gain from the consumption of food (Morgan and York, 1983). Lack of voluntary exercise has been shown to be a greater mortality risk factor in the elderly than hypertension (Hammond and Garfinkel, 1969). Hypothermia may also be a reflection of the disruption of normal circadian rhythms of which heat production is one (Moore-

Ede, 1983). The loss of routine which often accompanies the lifestyle of a single non-working person could increase the risk of circadian rhythm disruption, as would staying in bed for long periods of the day.

Isolation is one risk factor which has been aggravated by the increased mobility of the working population with young people moving further afield, even abroad, to live and work. The end result is that, while the young people can travel back to where they came from with relative ease, it may not be so easy for the elderly lacking personal and vehicular mobility to travel to the young. (For the young a ten-minute, comfortably protected car journey from a suburban house to a down-town flat may mean in reverse for the elderly a one-hour bus journey with waits at the bus stop and changes of bus, frequently at the mercy of the elements.) It is interesting, however, that surveys of isolation tend to restrict their enquiries to 'how often?' and 'how recently?' has the elderly person been visited by members of the younger generation. An enquiry as to when the old person last visited anybody would also give useful information, since an old person who is interested in others and has the physical ability to visit others has a very low risk of developing hypothermia.

Another factor in the prevention of hypothermia would be improved medical care since a high proportion of the cases reported suffer from endocrine disorders, e.g. hypothyroidism and diabetes, and a number of others have been prescribed drugs which are known to cause vasodilatation and therefore increased heat loss, e.g. phenothiazines and barbiturates. Malnutrition is also frequently associated with hypothermia (Howitt, 1971; Sadikali and Owor, 1974). This problem is once again easier to highlight than to treat, since the only way of overcoming it is for the old people themselves to consult their doctors, and any symptoms are frequently ascribed, by the person and the doctor, to increasing age. It has in fact been suggested that elderly patients seldom develop hypothermia unless they are already incapacitated or ill (Emslie-Smith, 1981) but as discussed earlier, exposure to cold may itself be a cause of incapacity or illness.

A fall is a factor frequently precipitating hypothermia with the person unable to rise and therefore lying in a cold room without any protection. There is an increased incidence of fractures of the femoral neck in the elderly in winter (Bastow *et al.*, 1983) which must be related to temperature. There was an 80 per cent increase in cases occurring outdoors but a 350 per cent increase in cases occurring indoors and this increase happened within days of a fall in environmental temperature (Allison and Bastow, 1983). It is at least possible that this statistic may be due to the effects of cold on sensory perception, co-ordination and muscle function as discussed earlier. The effects of cold would obviously aggravate the impairment of postural control common in old age (Overstall *et al.*, 1977). However, undernutrition also affects mortality, with the undernourished having a higher number of midwinter cases following falls indoors, a higher incidence of hypothermia and a higher mortality than the well nourished (Bastow *et al.*, 1983). However, a fall may also be due to a stroke, or may result in a fracture, either of which are sufficient to prevent the person rising again. Since some of the falls are due to loose flex or worn or torn linoleum or carpet, there is an obvious possibility for prevention. Despite the fact that a fall is such a common incident in the history of a hypothermic patient (Lloyd, 1973; Mills, 1973d; Simpson, 1974), in a list of hazards following a fall (Garland, 1978b) accidental hypothermia is not even mentioned, though the same author devotes a section to hypothermia in an earlier part of his review (Garland, 1978a).

Though the elderly prefer the same temperature for comfort as the young (Collins and Exton-Smith, 1981; Collins *et al.*, 1981) they show a slower awareness of change with poor temperature discrimination and a lack of precision when they do adjust the temperature. This makes them increasingly vulnerable to hypothermia and in fact many elderly people live in cold environmental conditions (Collins *et al.*, 1977; Fox *et al.*, 1973a; Primrose and Smith, 1981), though these may not be very cold for danger to be present (*Medical Tribune*, 1978). It has been calculated that an elderly person, who does not shiver when exposed to an environmental temperature of 5 °C, will become hypothermic in about five hours (Collins, 1983c). In many of the elderly, the body temperature is related to the environmental temperature and what is also worrying is the observation that those who are coldest appear to be the least aware of discomfort from the cold (Fox *et al.*, 1973b).

The health visitor using an age–sex register is the obvious person to assess the risk factors at regular intervals (Church, 1974), though it is important to remember that the air temperature in the room may be warm because the old person has switched on a fire in anticipation of the arrival of the health visitor. However, as a spot check, measuring the temperature of an internal wall of the house will give a more accurate estimate of the amount of heat being provided regularly in that room and therefore the person's normal thermal environment.

The situation of warm air/cold walls is one in which there is a significant but often overlooked risk of hypothermia (Lloyd, 1981b). The warm air gives a sensation of warmth (perceived warmth) and this may be sufficient to abolish any vasoconstrictor capacity that is still present in the old person without providing any real thermal input. However, there is still a marked radiant heat loss to the cold walls and the person may therefore become hypothermic while feeling warm, or at least not cold. It is possible that the elderly person at greatest risk from hypothermia is not in fact the one who has no heating anywhere in the house but the person who uses minimal intermittent heating, especially if only the living room is heated and not the bedroom. One possible source of chilling which is likely to be overlooked is the person undressing and washing, or bathing in an unheated bathroom in winter (Wigglesworth, 1973).

Prevention

The health visitor is probably the best person to organise preventive measures. The problem of preventing hypothermia among the elderly is merely the problem of reducing heat loss from the body to a level which can be replaced by the metabolic heat produced from the ingestion and metabolism of food. Adequate feeding will increase the metabolic rate, though not to the extent found in young people (Morgan and York, 1983), and the higher intake will provide more available energy and reduce the dangers of undernutrition. Reducing the heat loss is achieved by insulation, reducing the temperature difference between the person and the environment, and supplemental heating.

If the macroenvironment of the whole house is considered, suggestions for central heating, fuel subsidies, etc. (BMJ, 1980; *Social Work*, 1977; Wicks, 1978) are too expensive for the individual and the state, even with the maximum use of insulation and draught proofing. One recommendation frequently made is that the old person should move his or her bed into the room in which he or she cooks and lives. This reduces the volume requiring heating but some rooms in old houses may be large or have other disadvantages, and some people may find the suggestion unacceptable. It also takes a fair degree of organisation to be able to live entirely in one room and since this may be difficult even for a young, healthy and alert person it may be too much to ask of the group of elderly people for whom it would be of most thermal benefit.

The creation of a warmed microenvironment (BMJ, 1980; West and Lowe, 1976) or 'cosy corner' may be cheaper, simpler and more thermally efficient. Many Victorian habits made good thermal sense, though not the habit of having a bedroom window open at night whatever the weather. Full-length curtains on the windows and a curtain behind the door are simple measures to reduce draughts. A large screen around the back of a chair also keeps out the draughts and in addition reflects the heat, and a layer of aluminium foil on the screen would increase the amount of heat reflected. (This may be the only real value of a 'space blanket'?) The Victorian chairs themselves had high backs and occasionally wings for the same effect — traditional Orkney chairs often had a cowl over the top as well. These things created a small corner of the room usually heated by being placed facing a fire. A recent development has been the design of an electrically heated chair (Ledingham, 1983b) though the design will have to be safe, even in the presence of urinary incontinence.

The individual can reinforce the 'cosy corner' by using more personal insulation (BMJ, 1980), e.g. long underwear (BMJ, 1977a). Quilted anoraks or duvet jackets and trousers can keep people warm in the severest of outdoor environments, but, if these are not acceptable for the elderly, similar quilted material could be made in the form of a 'shawl', 'cape' or 'housecoat' (Church, 1974) and a simple hot-water bottle could supply a very useful quantity of heat under the insulation. Muffs would insulate the hands while sitting down and when sitting the feet could be insulated by wearing warm slippers with woollen ankle warmers. Foot muffs, especially double, would be very effective thermally (Lloyd, 1981a) but, if the elderly person has some sudden stimulus such as a ring at the door or a kettle boiling or the telephone ringing, he or she might forget the foot muffs and fall when trying to respond to the stimulus. The duvet housecoat could be worn while working around the house and old-fashioned gloves knitted without finger-tips would help to keep the hands warm with minimal restrictions. At night the same microenvironmental theme can be continued with a sleeping bag (Hails, 1973) or a low-wattage electric blanket (Questions in the Commons, 1973) under a Downie. Bowesman (1981) described a double-barrelled respiratory tube which would allow the person to breathe normally while having the Downie over his head. This would conserve the respiratory heat loss and would also allow total insulation of the heat loss from the head, though an easier way to achieve this latter benefit might be a return to the use of a Victorian night cap (BMJ, 1977a; Thompson, 1977a) or to cover the head with a cellular polyester/nylon blanket (Stephens, 1982). The rate of heat loss from the head is increased in the elderly since there is a loss of skin thickness and subcutaneous fat with increasing age (Thompson, 1977a) and the hair cover becomes thinner, sometimes progressing to varying degrees of baldness. (The author can vouch for the increase in comfort and warmth provided by wearing a woollen hat when trying to sleep in a cold environment.) A return to the fashion of wearing hats or caps during the day would also help personal insulation (BMJ, 1977a).

Prevention is difficult enough to achieve with the present generation of the elderly. However, the problem may become worse in the future since the present generation of young and middle-aged have been brought up with central heating at least at work and in public buildings. They are therefore conditioned to wearing lightweight summer clothing all year round and if the weather is cold their immediate reaction is to turn up the central heating (and complain of the expense). They often refuse to wear additional or warmer clothing because it is restricting or not fashionable. This aspect of hypothermia prevention requires a massive education programme which needs the collaboration of many bodies including the fashion industry and the media, e.g. if people in indoor scenes in TV plays wore warm jerseys more people would adopt the fashion themselves and the fashion industry could have a field day with Shetland, Arran, Fair Isle, etc.

Unfortunately in the present economic climate objections will be raised to implementing these ideas for prevention on the grounds of the cost of making improvements to the houses of the elderly, or of providing the equipment for producing the warmed microenvironment. However, cases of hypothermia are admitted to primary-cost beds at a time of maximum demand for the beds, and the savings achieved by preventing one admission with hypothermia would provide the funds for many sets of microenvironmental equipment.

One possible preventive measure is the compulsory removal of old people at risk from home to hospital but in practice this is not legally or morally possible (Cargill, 1982).

Identification

Every winter elderly people become hypothermic, and a high index of suspicion is required to spot when a person is not just at risk but is cooling towards hypothermia. This is because many of the symptoms of hypothermia mimic senility (Danzl, 1983) and one of the earliest symptoms of hypothermia in an old person is a change of personality. For example a garrulous and gregarious person becoming morose and monastic is often considered to be part of old age and therefore ignored. In the early stages, even if hypothermia is suspected, the core temperature will be above the 'magic' 35 °C and hypothermia will be 'excluded' as a definite diagnosis though the person may be sliding towards it. One possible solution would be to measure the total body heat which requires the measurement of some skin temperatures as well as the core temperature (Burton and Edholm, 1955; House and Vale, 1972). However, even measurement of the core temperature sometimes presents a problem. Rectal temperature, while accurate, is socially unacceptable as a routine screening procedure, though probably the best if the patient is unconscious. The mouth temperature, while not accurate in hypothermia, is socially acceptable and does give a reading which will never be higher than the true core temperature. The temperature of freshly voided urine is probably the most accurate practical measurement (Fox *et al.*, 1971) provided the patient is not incontinent and is capable of passing urine on request. The urine temperature measurement could be reserved for those patients with a low mouth temperature and a low mouth temperature with a normal urine temperature may be an indication that the old person is being subjected to cold stress (Lloyd, 1979c).

Management

If despite preventive measures and regular observation the old person has drifted into hypothermia, or been tipped into it by some other factor such as a fall, the first step is to stop the continuing loss of heat from the body by wrapping the patient in blankets, quilts or whatever is available, and the head should also be included. The 'space blanket' is frequently used but it is no more effective than the equivalent thickness of polythene or nylon (Marcus *et al.*, 1977) though it is much more expensive than either and it has the added disadvantage that it is noisy and this may make a hypothermic patient confused and restless. Once insulation has been completed the patient should be admitted to hospital for rewarming. It may be tempting to try airway warming in the patient's home since airway warming does accelerate the rate of rewarming but, in the elderly, unless airway warming is performed with intermittent positive pressure ventilation (IPPV) in an intensive care unit, the patient may die because of cerebral and/or pulmonary oedema. Even with spontaneous rewarming pulmonary oedema may develop if the rewarming becomes too rapid which tends to be if the rate becomes faster than 0.5 °C/hour. The cerebral or pulmonary oedema can be treated by IPPV or, if this is not available, the insulating covers should be removed to slow or reverse the rewarming.

Some elderly patients will always die after rewarming because of the pathological condition which precipitated the hypothermia, e.g. a cerebral haemorrhage, and it has been suggested that any underlying or associated disease is more important (in determining survival) than any physiological changes occurring as a result of hypothermia or any method of treatment (Simpson, 1974). If the hypothermia is secondary to some other cause the mortality is high (75 to 90 per cent) but if the hypothermia is primary the mortality is low (0 to 10 per cent) (Kurtz, 1982). However, the rewarming of hypothermic patients is justified because the diagnosis of any underlying pathology or even death is impossible while the patient is hypothermic, since the clinical features of any pathology are masked by the features of hypothermia (Ledingham and Mone, 1980; Maclean and Emslie-Smith, 1977). In many reported studies some of the patients have died while still hypothermic and the only way to avoid this is to use intensive-care monitoring and treatment (Ledingham and Mone, 1980). It wil be argued that the expense associated with intensive care is unjustifiable in the elderly even though accidental hypothermia is a benign condition. However, there seems to be a nihilistic attitude towards hypothermia in the elderly which is illustrated in a newspaper report of a coroner's inquest (*Daily Mail*, 1976). An elderly man living alone (a prime candidate for hypothermia (Simpson 1974)) was found, having been lying helpless on the floor all night after a fall (a common history in elderly patients with hypothermia (Mills, 1973d; Simpson, 1974)). The general practitioner found he was cold and sent him to hospital where his temperature was reported to be normal (was a low reading thermometer used correctly? (Mills, 1973d)) and since his other recordings were normal he was returned home. The next day his general practitioner sent him back to a different hospital. This time he was found to be extremely cold with slow respirations and pulse and an unrecordable blood pressure. He died (possibly during rewarming) and the pathologist said that he would have died within a few days anyway. By contrast, patients in the same age range who have severe illnesses, e.g. malignancies, dissecting aortic aneurysms or severe cardiorespiratory disease, have the services of all the diagnostic facilities of the National Health Service and may be subjected to expensive investigations followed by surgery — sometimes extensive and sometimes requiring intensive care in the post-operative period. This shows that age is not the reason for the nihilistic approach to the management of accidental hypothermia in the elderly. It is therefore reasonable to suggest that in the present state of knowledge, all elderly patients should be admitted to an intensive care unit (Emslie-Smith, 1981; Exton-Smith, 1973; Ledingham and Mone, 1980, 1982) and any hospital where this does not happen should admit that the care being provided is less than the optimum possible.

'Down and Outs'

Another urban group with a high hypothermia risk are the 'down and outs' who often have to sleep out of doors. It has been estimated that in Glasgow alone there are 2,000 'down and outs' and with insufficient night shelter beds the majority must sleep in the open. During the winter of 1977–78, 80 of these people died in the streets. Because of the common occurrence of a high alcohol intake among the 'down and outs', the person may be dead for several days before it is realised that he is not 'drunk' (*Sunday Post*, 1978). Malnutrition is likely to be an additional factor in this group and not only will this increase the risk of hypothermia developing (Howitt, 1971) but there is a high mortality during rewarming (Sadikali and Owor, 1974) and they should therefore be managed as for an elderly patient.

25 GENERAL ASPECTS OF HYPOTHERMIA OUTDOORS

Factors Leading to the Hypothermia Situation

Before considering individual measures which can be adopted to prevent the onset of hypothermia, it is useful to consider how the hypothermia risk situation may arise.

The risk of hypothermia in the outdoors could be markedly reduced by preventing people going to sea or into the mountains unless they were providing essential services. However, this is impractical in a free society, and the reasons for people going out are many and varied, e.g. caving may be an escape from an over-controlled society (Thomson, 1981) and reasons given for mountaineering include a sense of challenge and risk (Hillary, 1979; Hunt, 1977; Meldrum, 1972; Tunley, 1978; Ward, 1973). Unfortunately some attitudes will inevitably lead to an increased risk of death, e.g. climbing has been looked on as being 'about attempting the impossible' (White-Thomson, 1981), and the 'excelsior' spirit (Hunt, 1977) may lead to people taking unacceptable risks and it is probably this attitude which lead to the death of Mick Burke in 1975 on Everest and of Maurice Wilson 40 years earlier (Hunt, 1977). Also the old idea that pushing people to the limit is good for character development is almost suicidal in the Scottish mountains because of the subarctic nature of the climate (Stewart, 1972, 1981; Taylor, 1972) and people with experience now advise a party to 'go to ground' early (Andrew and Parker, 1978; Ogilvie, 1977) and this advice has saved many lives.

Selfishness, e.g. a party changing its plans without informing anyone (Cross and Stilling, 1976; Humble, 1972), or lack of thought (Dinwoodie, 1977) has exposed many rescue teams to the hazards of unnecessary call-outs. Accidents also happen when people ignore warning signs or barriers (Guest, 1977), and over-ambitious plans and a late start are other factors often contributing to tragedies. Even the wreck of the *Titanic* was precipitated by the fact that the captain was so determined to establish a transatlantic record that he ignored normal safe practices. Though there were indeed many icebergs in the vicinity, there was in fact a safe gap through which a cargo ship had passed just before the accident (Dowle, 1977). The cargo ship, however, had taken care and slowed down.

By their nature accidents are unpredicted and usually occur because of a number of factors which, while small in themselves, together lead to disaster. For example in one case (Elliott, 1967) not only did the aircraft's navigation aids fail, but so also did the radio and the emergency electrical locating devices, despite being on separate circuits. In another example, in the tragic 1979 Fastnet race, though at least one crew specifically checked on the weather forecast before leaving, there was no warning of a gale and the later gale warnings on the BBC were broadcast only at specific times and on certain wavelengths. Unfortunately this particular crew missed them because they were not transmitted on the usual band or at the times shipping normally use, and the crew were too busy fighting the wind to check other stations (O'Donnell, 1980). Sometimes accidents happen because of something entirely unpredictable and unavoidable such as avalanches (Gruner, 1979; Segantini, 1979), crevasses (Guest, 1977; Schell, 1978) or sudden weather problems (Cook, 1978; Fuller, 1977). Whatever the cause, accidents inevitably happen in awkward places, at awkward times and in bad weather conditions (Campbell, 1972).

Psychological Factors

There are many reports of incidents where a number of people have been precipitated together into a hypothermia risk situation but not all have survived or died. In these circumstances, though there may be obvious physical factors involved, psychological factors are also important (Hayward, 1982) and ultimate survival often seems to depend on the human spirit having some psychological reason for living, e.g. some other person present or absent, or just sheer determination (Cook, 1978; Elder and Streshinsky, 1978; Elliott, 1967; Lathrop, 1972; Lee and Lee, 1971; Lehrmann, 1982; Low, 1982). It is interesting that in 1912 in Antarctica, Henry Mawson struggled alone for three weeks after the deaths of his two companions, and managed to make it back to safety despite atrocious weather conditions of gales and blizzards and several accidental falls into crevasses (Bickel, 1977). At exactly the same time and in similar weather conditions, Scott and his party were failing to survive (Brent, 1974), and it is intriguing to speculate how much was due to the psychological blow of finding that Amundsen had reached the Pole before Scott.

Education and Training

Education is obviously extremely important and can be effective, e.g. the education of clubs and schools in one area led to a subsequent decrease in the incidence of deaths in cold water (Graham and Keatinge, 1978). There are indeed a growing number of productions — pamphlets, books, tapes/slides — all aimed at educating the public to the dangers and prevention of hypothermia. Training is also of vital importance (Cross, 1981) since panic during an emergency may cause people to take wrong or delayed actions, and therefore compromise their survival (Balfour and Underwood-Ground, 1980). Both training and education should relate to relevant situations, e.g. the tape/slide/booklet presentation by the US Coastguards (Bernhartsen *et al.*, 1980) relates to the immersion problem, and, following severe blizzard conditions which struck North America (Norberg *et al.*, 1979), specific survival measures were recommended for people to follow if they became trapped in a house or car (Gordon, 1979). In boating, education should include pressure on every participant to have and wear a flotation device (Hayward, 1982), and, if immersion occurs, to stay still (Keatinge, 1977) and hold on to any boat or equipment rather than try to swim for shore unless the water is warm.

Education should also include training in the assessment of the weather (Adam, 1981) and this should not only include listening to forecasts and observing the sky but, on land, observation of the vegetation and animal life which will indicate the general climate of the region, e.g. on the mountain tops in the Cairngorms the vegetation and bird life are the same as those found in the arctic tundra. Not only is the climate subarctic but the very rapidly changeable weather plus frequent wind and rain makes the Cairngorms more dangerous than the Arctic (Simpson, 1972). Observation of the vegetation and knowledge of wind flows round hills may enable a person or party in difficulties to select a place where the wind is minimal, even on a bare hillside.

Technical training and education, e.g. the ability to navigate by map and compass, is not however sufficient without commonsense, e.g. the knowledge of how to construct a snow hole is of no value if the expedition is too early in the season for enough snow to have fallen to provide a sufficient depth for its construction or if the wrong place is chosen or a start delayed until exhaustion is imminent. It should also be taught that, in the face of deteriorating weather conditions, to 'go to ground' or turn back from a climb or outing before the planned completion is a sign of strength of character and not weakness (Ogilvie, 1977).

Clothing, Shelter and Other Protection

These are obviously of vital importance and their correct use could go a long way towards preventing many cases of hypothermia but there are no general recommendations which can be applied in all situations and therefore each environment will be considered individually. However, in all cold stress situations it is important to remember that the head is a very important route for heat loss (Danzl, 1983; Froese and Burton, 1957) and adequate protection should be provided for the head.

Many cases of hypothermia in the outdoors occur because of clothing and equipment which has been grossly inadequate for the conditions (Atukorale, 1971; Cross and Stilling, 1976; Humble, 1972; Westmorland and Gate, 1972). However, it is also important to remember that too many clothes may also be dangerous. If there is an imbalance of clothing and exercise, this will result in sweating which will make the clothes wet. The exercise will also cause vasodilatation with the associated effects of cardiac stress and fatigue, and there will also be an increased respiratory heat loss because of the high ventilation volumes. When the person stops, the respiratory heat loss continues, the vasodilatation is still present and because the clothing is wet, hypothermia can develop rapidly (Dalgleish, 1969; Kaufman, 1983). To prevent this the amount of clothing should be reduced during the exercise and replaced when the exercise stops. There is an additional related problem (Kaufman, 1983). If the hands and feet are too well insulated, this may prevent cold stimulus reaching the body, and therefore vasoconstriction may not occur. This may result in the ironic position of a person having warm hands and feet but shivering and having a falling core temperature. If the hands and feet are kept cool or cold, the core temperature remains high and the person is comfortable (Kaufman, 1983). While the performance of specific items of clothing is often tested under particular situations, e.g. ice-water (Hayward, 1984), there are relatively few general studies on clothing and insulation (Cena and Clark, 1979; Houdas *et al.*, 1985; Newburgh, 1949). One difficulty is that while it is relatively easy to provide clothing which gives adequate protection when dry, this same clothing may become next to useless when wet (Hirvonen, 1982). The insulation value of clothing is reduced 30 to 40 per cent by wind and 50 per cent by wetting, but the combination of wind and wet causes a disastrous 90 per cent reduction in insulation (Pugh, 1968). Natural wool, because of its crimped fibre, retains 40 per cent of its insulation value when wet as compared with 10 per cent for wet cotton (Danzl, 1983). However, some synthetic fibres may be better because they are hydrophobic and do not retain moisture (Stephens, 1982).

Shelter is also important and this may take the form of bothies (Humble, 1969), tents, survival bags or the construction of snow holes. The insulating value of snow can be illustrated by an accident which happened in 1902 on one of Scott's early Antarctic expeditions. A young man went missing and a blizzard developed, but when the blizzard ceased 48 hours later, he walked back to the ship. He had in fact taken shelter from the wind, fallen asleep for 36 hours and been covered by the snow (Brent, 1974). In some areas there may be bothies in the hills and the knowledge of their locations as well as those of inhabited dwellings may be life-saving. Another item which may be life-saving is the ability to locate 'dead areas' — localised areas of calm — which exist in all hills whatever the wind strength or direction. Posture is also important in the survival situation. A person sitting fully flexed reduces the exposed surface area of the body by 30 to 40 per cent (Pugh, 1968) and is the basis for the heat escape lessening posture (HELP) recommended for water immersion (Hayward *et al.*, 1975b).

It must be remembered that hypothermia protection in the water requires special garments and, though the general requirements of survival suits can be easily stated (Leese and Norman, 1979), all the suits at present available carry some disadvantages which may result in them not being available when needed. They are expensive (Hayward, 1982) and some people may economise by not having a survival suit. When worn they are not flattering for the person (Hayward, 1982) and for example the bikini-clad girl on deck in warm sunshine will not thank anyone who insists on her wearing thermal protective clothing because the water is very cold. All protective garments are uncomfortable to a varying degree and may cause heat stress if worn before the immersion occurs (Hayward, 1982; White and Roth, 1979). In addition to the protection against hypothermia, the presence of protective clothing reduces the incapacitating effects of sudden immersion in very cold water (Hayward, 1983) and dry suits with added insulation have the capability of allowing a person to survive for 24 hours even in 1 °C water, but the person has to remain inactive and rough water may cause drowning at an early stage (Hayward, 1984). Suits should be brightly, luminously coloured to aid rescue (BMJ, 1978a) and it is suggested that the suits should not incorporate buoyancy, and buoyancy aids should be provided separately (BMJ, 1978a). Unfortunately if the two elements necessary for survival are separate this will result in increasing the time needed to prepare for immersion and an increased chance that one or other of the elements will be missing. Before any recommendations are made, survival suits should be assessed in practical use (Hampton, 1981; Marcus and Richards, 1978; Veghte, 1972; White and Roth, 1979) because the suit which is theoretically best may be easily damaged, which will make it ineffective. Nor is price alone an adequate guide (Hampton, 1981).

In many situations there is insufficient time to don survival suits when the emergency occurs, e.g. a boat can capsize suddenly (Lehrmann, 1982; Low, 1982) and a fisherman working on the deck of a trawler will get no warning of a freak wave or a fall which may precipitate him into the water. Similarly if a helicopter has to ditch, there will be no time or space for the passengers to put on their survival suits before the plane hits the water. In a review of this latter problem (BMJ, 1978a) it was suggested that though the provision of immersion suits may be the easy answer, it might be better to prevent immersion, and therefore the best solution to the problem of a helicopter ditching would be for the passengers to be transferred directly to covered rafts. The modern covered rafts are extremely effective at raising the temperature of the internal environment (Gavshon and Rice, 1984; Pugh, 1968) but if the doors cannot be closed properly (Pugh, 1968) most of the protective effect is lost, and if a raft has many fewer people than the intended number, the thermal benefit can be reduced. After the sinking of the Argentine cruiser *General Belgrano* off the Falklands Islands in 1982, the rafts which had the intended 20 men preserved life well whereas most of the deaths from cold and exposure occurred in the rafts which had only three or four men, and these rafts were also the most easily capsized (Gavshon and Rice, 1984). There are other practical problems with life-rafts (Pugh, 1968), including the inability to launch the rafts because of the ship capsizing too fast (Low, 1982) or because of problems caused by the ship listing or fire damage to rafts and boats. Even with ideal conditions of calm weather when fire started on the cruise ship *Lakonia* only 75 per cent of the lifeboats could be launched even though there was plenty of time available (Keatinge, 1965). Therefore in the true emergency situation, where the weather is likely to be bad, cold immersion is almost inevitable.

When immersion occurs there are a number of measures which will increase the chance of survival. The people should stay near the wreck as long as possible, especially if the boat is still afloat, because not only will this save energy but it is also easier for the rescue services to find a wreck rather than bodies in the water (Lehrmann, 1982). If the wreck is in coastal waters, the survivors should never waste energy by swimming against the tide because the coastal currents will always wash a person ashore, the only doubts being as to when and where (Lehrmann, 1982). The survivors must resist the temptation to swim to get somewhere or just to keep warm, because physical activity in cold water increases the surface area of warm skin exposed to the cold water (Wade and Veghte, 1977) and increases the heat loss by 30 to 50 per cent (Hayward, 1982). Exercise will only reliably raise body temperature if the water temperature is above 24 °C (Goode and McDonald, 1982; Hirvonen, 1982) and in cold water there are no conditions in which activity would prolong survival, and under most conditions exercise will accelerate hypothermia (Keatinge, 1969). Deliberate inactivity markedly decreases cooling rates (Hayward and Eckerson, 1984) and may increase the survival time by up to an hour (Hayward, 1982) which gives the rescuers more time. Drown-proofing is a measure sometimes recommended as a measure to prolong survival. In this the person lies relaxed and motionless in the water only moving when a breath is needed. However, while less energy is expended than during treading water, the rate of cooling is greater in drown-proofing than in treading water. This is because the head is under water during drown-proofing with the resulting great increase in heat loss (Goode and McDonald, 1982). The adoption of a fetal position or the heat escape lessening posture (HELP) (Hayward, 1982; US Coastguard, 1980) will decrease the body heat losing surface area by 20 to 30 per cent (Hayward *et al.*, 1975b). If there are a number of people in the water, by huddling together (Hayward *et al.*, 1975b) they will decrease the heat loss by trapping water between them. This keeping together will be aided by the survivors being roped together, though the rope should be long enough to allow the survivors some movement (Lehrmann, 1982). Roping would also mean that if one person becomes unconscious he does not drift away and get lost.

One final danger is that prolonged immersion results in dehydration which increases the risk of hypothermia.

Food

Many cases of exposure in walkers are associated with some restriction of food intake, either accidental or by intention (Andrew and Parker, 1978). A restriction of calories results in a low core temperature in a cold environment (Iampietro and Bass, 1962), and by depleting the body's glycogen stores makes the person more sensitive to fatigue (Guezennec and Pesquies, 1985). Maintaining a high blood sugar level, even after the consumption of alcohol, prevents the onset of problems with hypoglycaemia and reduces the rate of cooling (Graham and Dalton, 1980) and it has also been found in canoeists (Green and Bagley, 1972) that, if the blood glucose level can be kept above normal fasting levels, this prevents any deterioration of performance during severe exercise and also prevents prolonged post-exercise exhaustion. This is obviously of great importance in outdoor activities such as climbing, since deterioration of performance will increase the risk of accidents. In addition an exhausted person is unable to increase his heat production in response to cold and the rate of heat loss is maximal when a person is exhausted (Witherspoon *et al.*, 1971). This necessity for food has been translated into practical recommendations for Arctic survival (Rogers, 1971).

Rescue

The resuce services all have their own individual problems and therefore the equipment to be carried has to fit the individual needs. In most rescue situations the medical aid will be limited to a person trained in first aid though in some parts of the world radio links will allow the first aider to get advice from the base or hospital.

In the hills of Britain, most equipment is carried by parties on foot and should therefore be lightweight, waterproof and wind resistant. It should also be relatively cheap, any controls should be capable of being manipulated with gloved hands, it should be simple enough to be used without needing a lot of training (Jones in Marcus, 1979a) and it should be robust (Norman in Marcus, 1979a). If the equipment needs to be transported by motorised vehicles its usefulness will be greatly reduced (Jones in Marcus, 1979a). In the Alps, on the other hand, there is an extensive helicopter service which carries people and equipment up the mountains and surivors back. This means that most groups will have generators which can power equipment as well as lights (Legrand, 1984), and radio communication has been more extensively developed (Dubas, 1980).

The use of helicopters, when the weather permits, shortens the time between rescue and arrival at hospital (Barwood in Marcus, 1979a) but there are specific problems associated with their use. During the resuce there is a tremendous wind-chill effect from the downdraught of the rotors over and above the wind-chill present in the rescue situation (Golden in Marcus, 1979a) and in those helicopters where the stretcher is carried outside the cabin, some means must be adopted to prevent this killing the patient during transport. Even where the stretchers can be accommodated in the cabin, there is still a tremendous wind-chill while the door is open and the patients should be wrapped in blankets and plastic bags for protection (Barwood in Marcus, 1979a).

Lifeboat rescue has its own particular problems with the inevitability that in most instances there will be heavy seas, strong winds and severe ship motion. The rescues are likely to be prolonged, lasting from 1 to 24 hours and longer in some of the newer, bigger boats coming into service with the Royal National Lifeboat Institution, and any equipment must therefore be simple and robust (Guild in Marcus, 1979a).

The state of Alaska has issued a booklet which contains guidelines for the management of hypothermia and near-drowning. The guidelines are divided into sections so that each level of expertise knows what is expected at any particular situation from a lay member of the public to a fully equipped hospital (Doolittle *et al.*, 1982; Samuelson *et al.*, 1982). These guidelines were prepared with the particular situation of Alaska in mind in that they have three grades of emergency medical technicians and small bush hospitals as well as members of the public and large hospitals. However, these guidelines could be adapted to fit the knowledge and training schemes found in any part of the world.

26 EXPOSURE IN MOUNTAIN AND CAVING ACCIDENTS

General

Exposure in the mountains is a non-technical term which usually includes aspects of exhaustion as well as a dropping body temperature (Ogilvie, 1977) and hypothermia in the outdoors has even been called the 'Killer of the unprepared' (Lathrop, 1972). Deaths from accidental hypothermia appear to have increased with the increasing popularity of hill climbing, hill walking and mountaineering (Mountain Rescue, 1968; Freeman and Pugh, 1969). Reports from mountain rescue organisations all indicate a high level of activity which, even in a mild winter, may involve thousands of man hours for the teams on the ground and for helicopters (Harper, 1981). In the Four Inns Walk disaster in 1964 (Pugh, 1964) there were many cases of exposure and three deaths and Pugh (1966) also reported on 25 deaths occurring in Wales, the Lake District and Scotland. In 1967 (Rawlins, J., personal communication) two army cadets died on Dartmoor and in 1971 on a charity walk many walkers became hypothermic but fortunately there were no deaths. Unfortunately in the November of the same year a party of school-children were lost in the Cairngorms during a school expedition and six out of the eight people in the party died.

Even in a small island like Britain, hazards may vary between different mountainous regions, e.g. conditions in Scotland are materially different from those in England (Pugh, 1966): the country is more rugged and longer distances must be covered on foot whilst inhabited dwellings in mountainous districts are few. Weather conditions are more unreliable and severe; even in the summer months, blizzards of sleet and snow may occur above 2,500 feet, and in winter, snow storms may reach arctic severity (Mountain Rescue and Cave Rescue, 1972). Mist can also suddenly cover the tops of the mountains and the temperature can then drop by up to 20 to 30 °C and a level plateau becomes a featureless death trap surrounded by cliffs. Therefore experience gained only in England and Wales can be misleading.

Accidental hypothermia from exposure is a problem which may be met by many people and organisations. The predisposing conditions are well described (Dalgleish, 1969; Mountain Resuce, 1968; Pugh, 1964, 1966, 1967 and 1968) and the review by Freeman and Pugh (1969) is summarised below:

> Most cases of accidental hypothermia occur on trips that would be considered easy in fine weather. Groups of young people walking together are not always well matched physically and, when conditions are such that the mean skin temperature falls to 25 °C, there is a strong inclination to walk faster thereby raising the core temperature to a value that makes the low skin temperature tolerable. In this way the less fit persons may become exhausted. The extra effort involved in progressing against gale-force winds, the elevation of metabolism associated with shivering, and the effect of pain and discomfort may also cause premature fatigue and exhaustion. Exhausted parties who fail to take shelter before nightfall seldom survive.

Another common feature of exposure cases is being wet through and it was pointed out that people caught out with wet clothing might as well be naked at a slightly higher environmental temperature.

When a group is out on the hills, it is not always easy to recognise early or mild cases of hypothermia, but it is most important to be on the watch for it (Mountain Rescue, 1968). The usual sequence of events preceding a tragedy is as follows (Freeman and Pugh, 1969; Ogilvie, 1977): The affected person begins to lag behind and to fall down repeatedly. Commonly there are mental changes consisting of apathy, aggressiveness or unco-operative behaviour, and speech becomes slurred. There are sometimes other mental changes with irrational behaviour and hallucinations. Muscular weakness, cramp, ataxia and collapse soon follow, then stupor and rigidity. Death occurs in a variable period, sometimes as short as one to two hours. Even an expert on hypothermia in a high-risk situation can fail to recognise the symptoms and signs of hypothermia developing in himself (Dalgleish, 1969). As soon as incipient hypothermia is suspected the party should 'go to ground'. A sheltered spot should be found and after putting on all available spare clothing, the victim should be put in a heavy duty polythene bag (Andrew and Parker, 1978).

On the mountain the rescue party is faced with many problems, not the least being the same environmental conditions which caused the victim to become hypothermic, i.e. snow, sleet or rain and wind (Earnshaw, 1978; Jones in Marcus, 1979a; Norman in Marcus, 1979a). The instinct of a rescue team is to remove the victim and themselves immediately from such a hazardous situation. There is also the problem that if one member of the party has become hypothermic, the other members are probably verging on it and may have slipped into definite hypothermia before the rescue team arrives. However, patients have died during the evacuation, others have had convulsions through being carried in a head-up position (Pugh, 1966) and sudden death has also occurred on moving a patient from a stretcher (Freeman and Pugh, 1969). In many cases the correct procedure is to set up camp and revive and stabilise the condition of a patient on the spot (Andrew and Parker, 1978; Earnshaw, 1978; Frankland, 1981; Freeman and Pugh, 1969; Mountain Rescue, 1968; Pugh, 1966). The first aid treatment relies heavily on insulating the patient to prevent further heat loss from the skin though in the past the heat loss from breathing (Burton and Edholm, 1955; Pugh, 1968) was neglected. The only traditional means of supplying heat were by hot food and drink (Lilja, 1983) if the patient was conscious, via a companion's body heat (Mountain Rescue, 1968) and by the use of heated packs (Neureuther, 1979) but all these methods are relatively inefficient. Warming clothing and/or blankets to wrap round a victim (Lilja, 1983) may be logistically difficult and, as discussed elsewhere, may be dangerous. The only major source of heat is the body's own metabolism which is itself depressed in the hypothermic situation (Burton and Edholm, 1955).

The use of airway warming is being investigated in the field since most other recommended methods of treatment are impossible till after evacuation (Berkley, 1972) and the evidence so far is favourable. It has been suggested that in mild hypothermia airway warming produces a rise in temperature equal to that produced by continuing exercise (Kaufman, 1983) and airway warming is probably safer. It must be emphasised, however, that airway warming is only an extra measure to complete and supplement the insulation of the body and, if the body is completely insulated and the respiratory heat loss is also insulated, the victim will rewarm (Ogilvie, 1977). This has been seen in practice (Pugh, 1966) and it is therefore difficult to accept the statement that 'not even polar clothing will prevent a normal person in a cold room from losing heat if he remains sedentary' (BMJ, 1977a).

As well as treatment airway warming has a potential as a

preventive measure and the benefit increases with the increasing vigour of the exercise (Kaufman, 1983). Condenser humidifiers prevent the loss of respiratory heat and moisture with the best reaching 75 to 80 per cent efficiency. These condenser humidifiers are very lightweight, weighing only a few grams even when combined with a face mask (Lloyd, 1986; Lloyd and Croxton, 1981). They could therefore be carried as first aid equipment by climbers and could then be used as soon as a member of the group started to develop signs of hypothermia. This, as an addition to putting him or her in a shelter in a sleeping bag, would mean that he or she either rewarmed without assistance or if a rescue team was called, his or her state would not be critical when the team arrived. In an emergency a polo-neck sweater (Guest, 1977) or a scarf wrapped round the mouth and nose would provide some condenser humidifier action.

High Altitude

When climbers reach high altitudes the added danger that immediately comes to mind is hypoxia with the partial pressure of oxygen falling to 35 mm Hg at 6,500 metres (21,300 feet), after which with increasing altitude there is no further reduction of the partial pressure of oxygen (West, 1984). There are other dangers. The higher the altitude the lower the environmental temperature (1 °C per 150 metres) and therefore the greater exposure to cold. However, cold air is dry air with a low total moisture content. In addition because of the lower barometric pressures at altitude, which is latitude-dependent (West, 1984), the water vapour content of the air is also very low (Heath and Williams, 1981). Both hypoxia and exercise will markedly increase minute ventilation volumes and, since the humidity of the air is very low at altitude through the combination of low barometric pressure and low temperature, there is a very high respiratory water loss. In fact the respiratory moisture loss at altitude may be sufficient to cause dehydration (Heath and Williams, 1981; West, 1984) and dehydration is a major factor in the development of frostbite and hypothermia (Mills, 1983a, b and c). There is a final worrying point about expeditions to extremely high altitudes. There is now evidence of impairment in central nervous system function after return to sea level and in some instances this impairment has persisted for over a year (West, 1984).

Crevasses

In many parts of the world crevasses are an additional hazard faced by climbers, and not only may the fall into a crevasse cause death or injury but even people who are uninjured may die from hypothermia. If the person lands on a large ledge he is probably reasonably safe but if he is trapped with his body in direct contact with the ice he will cool very rapidly (Foray and Cahen, 1981). There are many cases recorded where a climber has been trapped in a crevasse and, though he was alive and conscious when the rescue team found him, he has died from hypothermia before he could be freed. There may only be two to three hours available for the rescue (Foray and Cahen, 1981). The rescue team may have to chip an approach route out of the ice and then evacuate the victim. To overcome this problem, Foray (Legrand, 1984) has developed a system for providing airway warming which can be used while the victim is still in the crevasse. The evidence so far suggests that this measure will either stop or at least slow the fall in the victim's temperature and thus allow more time for the rescue service to extricate the victim from the crevasse. Because of the clinical effects Foray has called his device a 'thermal parachute'.

Avalanches

There are three main types of avalanche (Legrand, 1984):

(1) Powder snow. This usually follows a fresh fall and travels at speeds up to 300 km/hour. It tends to cause multiple injuries and pulmonary damage through blast injury or suffocation and the aerosol state of the snow can fill the respiratory passages and will infiltrate the clothing, producing a marked chilling.
(2) Plaque or slab snow. This is the type which occurs when an overhanging corniche breaks away and it travels at 20 to 50 km/hour. It may cause injury, hypothermia or asphyxia through lack of air, compression of the thoracic cage or the inhalation of snow.
(3) Wet snow. This usually happens during the afternoon in spring when the sun has raised the temperature and it is the slowest mover at 10 to 20 km/hour.

The number of avalanche accidents is increasing (Legrand, 1984) but 80 per cent of victims are alive when the avalanche stops (Dubas,

1980). The main cause of death in avalanches is asphyxia (Dubas, 1980; Hossli, 1979; Legrand, 1984) which may be due to:

(1) The air around the victim's face being used up.
(2) Inhalation of snow, aggravated by reflex laryngospasm.
(3) Rupture of the lungs due to barotrauma.
(4) Compression of the thorax making respiratory movement impossible.
(5) Airway obstruction because of unconsciousness.
(6) Brain damage causing ventilatory depression.

Because a person is totally covered by the snow does not mean that he will automatically asphyxiate because there is a variable permeability of air and carbon dioxide through snow, depending on the type of snow (de Quervain, 1979), and it is because of air permeability through snow that rescue dogs are able to scent buried victims (Legrand, 1984). It has been known for people to survive for prolonged periods buried under the snow. One survived for four days under 1.5 metres of snow because his rucksack had created an air pocket round his head and another survived for seven days because he was buried at the base of a tree which created an air pocket (Legrand, 1984). However, there is always the problem that the work of breathing may be increased (Hossli, 1979). There is another possible explanation for some of the survivals since there have been cases which have survived prolonged apnoea after being buried in snow (Harries, 1982) through the rapid development of hypothermia similar to the so-called diving reflex cases which occur in very cold water.

However, even though a person is buried in an avalanche hypothermia is not inevitable because of the low heat conductivity of snow, about matching that of wood (de Quervain, 1979) and because under the avalanche there is no wind (Legrand, 1984). If the person's clothing is of good insulating value it will stay dry and the person may remain normothermic. If, however, the clothing is poor, the temperature gradient across the clothing to the snow will be sufficient to melt the snow and this will soak the clothing, further reducing the insulating value of the clothing and the person will cool more rapidly. The average rate of cooling is 3 °C per hour, depending on the clothing (Dubas, 1980) and on any accompanying injuries (Legrand, 1984). However, the greatest risk of hypothermia, even with poor clothing, comes when the victim is removed from the protection of the snow and is exposed to the wind on the surface. The rate of cooling may then rise to 6 to 9 °C (Dangel and Hossli, 1979; Dubas, 1980) and therefore the urgent priority is to get the person into shelter from the wind. It should not be forgotten that avalanches may cause physical as well as thermal injury (Matter, 1979; Umach and Unterdorfer, 1979b), and these may require specific management.

If a person is unconscious after rescue from an avalanche and respirations are feeble, the patient should be intubated after pre-oxygenation with mouth-to-mouth ventilation, and given oxygen (Dubas, 1980).

Caving

The problems of hypothermia among cavers are very similar to those among hill walkers and climbers for while caving is less exposed to wind, there are cave systems and spots in which there may be a considerable draught even deep underground. Caves are frequently cold even in summer and it is almost impossible to explore caves without being immersed in cold water, sometimes ice-melt water. Because of this most cavers wear neoprene wet suits underground to reduce the risk of hypothermia. The weather influences cavers in a different way, too. Whereas climbers fear mist or snow with the resulting loss of visibility, cavers fear rain which may suddenly fill an underground stream and trap or drown the party. Darkness is also the norm. This hostile environment has been well described (Frankland, 1975; Glanvill, 1980; Thomson, 1981). Factors of adequate food and clothing and leadership in the prevention of hypothermia apply with equal force to cavers as to climbers, and the symptoms of developing hypothermia are also similar. Evacuation, however, may mean hauling the victim through narrow awkward passages with the limitations of space making it impossible to keep the victim in a head-down position. Further immersion during rescue is likely (Frankland, 1977; Lloyd, 1964) causing a further acceleration of cooling and this or the carrying position may be sufficient to cause death. While rapid evacuation to the surface is the ideal solution for any injured caver, it is often necessary to 'hospitalise' the patient underground (Frankland, 1975). This may be necessary while a constricted exit is widened, if the patient is physically trapped, e.g. by a fallen rock, or to improve the condition of the patient before evacuation. However, any delay increases the risk of hypothermia. This is another field in which airway warming is being evaluated and the clinical experience so far is that the cave rescuers feel that it is an effective method of treatment and that mild cases can be successfully treated underground. They can then make their own way to the surface without needing physical assistance (Frankland, J., personal communication, 1984).

27 WATER (IMMERSION)

Death from immersion is one of the leading causes of accidental death in the UK especially among the young (Golden, 1980) but there is a complex interrelation of possible factors which, either singly or together, can contribute to any particular death.

Effects of Immersion

Immersion, even in warm water, affects fluid and electrolyte balance (Greenleaf *et al.*, 1981) and both immersion and cold cause a rise in catecholamines (Weihl *et al.*, 1981). Immersion also produces a hydrostatic squeeze (Golden, 1980). On transition from air to 'head-out' immersion in thermoneutral (35 °C) water the pressure squeeze on the peripheral tissues of man increases the venous return and produces a rise in cardiac output of 35 per cent (Arborelius *et al.*, 1972; Begin *et al.*, 1976). Nevertheless in spite of the increased cardiac output there is a net rise in the intrathoracic pooling of blood (about 0.7 litres). This, together with the cephalic movement of the diaphragm caused by the hydrostatic squeeze on the abdomen, reduces the functional residual capacity by 30 to 60 per cent (Craig and Dvorak, 1975), altogether producing a small increase in pulmonary shunting and a small but consistent fall in the PaO_2. These physiological adjustments are not likely to be of any significance in a fit young adult but may prove incapacitating in an elderly person with poor cardiorespiratory reserves. It has also been claimed (Shulzenko *et al.*, 1979) that immersion reproduces many of the physiological changes of weightlessness.

Initial Entry into Water

If water enters the nose and/or ears it may cause a vagal reflex with instantaneous cardiac and respiratory arrest (Elsner and Gooden, 1983; Goode and McDonald, 1982; Wells, 1973). It has also been suggested that the sudden entry of very cold water into the ear may cause a caloric labyrinthitis with complete disorientation and death especially if underwater (Bernhartsen and Schlenker, 1981). In addition, on immersion in cold water (less than 15 °C) the initial cardiorespiratory responses exhibited by most people may have disastrous consequences for individuals with arterial disease or hypertension (Goode and McDonald, 1982). The sympathetic mediated reflex increase in heart rate and the surge in arterial blood pressure may result in a myocardial infarct or a cerebrovascular accident which in turn may cause death or at least a degree of incapacity that will lead to drowning. The cold-induced hyperventilation, and decrease in arterial CO_2, may reduce cerebral blood flow, thus causing impaired consciousness. In addition, even young fit people may be disabled by tetany due to hyperventilation within the first few minutes of immersion and either incapacity may cause drowning. Even very competent swimmers are unable to swim for very long (e.g. 90 seconds) in very cold (5 °C) water (Balfour, 1983; Keatinge *et al.*, 1969) if they are not accustomed to it, and the possible causes for this include cold affecting the neuromuscular co-ordination or muscular activity, or joint stiffness, as well as the increased viscosity of very cold water. In addition, in very cold water, a person tends to swim with the face and head out of the water. This increases the energy requirement by being a non-streamlined position, and by decreasing buoyancy (Goode and McDonald, 1982). However, it is certain that the incapacity cannot be explained by general hypothermia.

Drowning — Inhalation of Water

For terminological exactness the term 'drowning' means death by suffocation under water (Conn *et al.*, 1983) and therefore refers to incidents with a fatal outcome, and for people who survive the term used is 'near-drowning'. Drowning causes 140,000 deaths each year in the world (Conn *et al.*, 1983) and the clinical features of drowning and near-drowning have been well described (Rivers, 1972; Rivers *et al.*, 1970) and the close interrelation between hypothermia and drowning has also been emphasised (Conn, 1979a; Golden and Rivers, 1975; Miles, 1975).

The standard description of the sequence of events leading to drowning is totally irrelevant to the clinical situation since it describes what happens when conscious dogs were forcibly held with their heads under water. This is not the usual scenario for human drowning where the heads are held above water for as long as possible. A great deal of research has also been carried out into the different effects of drowning in fresh water as compared with drowning in salt water (Modell, 1971; 1976) but the differences tend to be largely of academic interest (Rivers *et al.*, 1970) since in both, water is rapidly transferred across the alveolar membrane to the bloodstream (Pearn, 1980). One problem is that in the original experimental work, which was done on dogs (Swann and Spafford, 1951), the researchers used pure distilled water as fresh water and pure normal saline as the salt water. This is a far cry from the situation found in clinical work. In clinical experience it has also been found that, even in fatal accidental drowning in humans, if the accident has occurred in fresh water the volume of water inhaled is usually considerably less than that necessary to produce haemolysis (Modell and Davis, 1969) and similarly no significant differences have been found in the serum electrolyte levels or serum haemoglobin concentrations whether the drowning occurred in fresh, salt or brackish water (Hasan *et al.*, 1971; Modell *et al.*, 1976). Even though sufficient fluid may be aspirated to produce detectable changes in the blood, in the majority of cases such changes are so small that they do not contribute directly to the death of the person (Golden, 1980).

In 10 to 15 per cent of all drownings no water is found in the lungs at postmortem (Elsner and Gooden, 1983; Stoddart, 1976) — so-called dry drowning — and the mechanism may be that hypothermia has caused death before the person has become totally submerged, or that the initial contact of water with the larynx has caused laryngospasm (Elsner and Gooden, 1983) with death occurring due to hypoxia before respiration restarts, or death has occurred from asystole caused either through direct vagal stimulation of the larynx or through an exaggeration of the bradycardia observed in the diving reflex (Elsner and Gooden, 1983). Ventricular ectopics can be produced by spraying cold water over the head (Balfour, 1983). In people with cardiovascular disorders 'dry' drowning may be due to cardiac arrhythmias (Balfour, 1983) and even in one young person swimming in cold water, death was due to ventricular fibrillation (Keatinge and Hayward, 1981). Another possible cardiovascular cause for 'dry' drowning is the intense vasoconstriction caused by sudden immersion in cold water. This produces an increase in venous and arterial pressure and therefore cardiac output. The response is greater in the elderly and may therefore cause death through acute cardiac failure before hypothermia or drowning can develop. Anaphylaxis in a person with hypersensitivity to cold may be another cause of 'dry' drowning.

Death from drowning may occur despite the use of a life-jacket (Golden, 1980) because, except in very calm water as in the *Lakonia* (Keatinge, 1965) and *Titanic* disasters (Mersey, 1912) waves will break over the face and inhalation will occur as soon as any incoordination or loss of consciousness develops. A special spray shield fitted to protect the face will be of some benefit (Golden, 1980) but even then steep or breaking waves or surf may lead to a relative lack of buoyancy with temporary submersion despite the life-jacket. It is possible for a person to swallow, and possibly inhale, large quantities of water despite being fully conscious and wearing a life-jacket because in a severe storm the air may be filled with spray and the head may be surrounded by froth and in inshore waters the land configuration may cause chopping and changing seas (Lehrmann, 1982). In this condition even small waves can project water into the airways (Hirvonen, 1977) and the person is unable to prevent drowning (Balfour, 1983). The colder the water the greater the respiratory drive, especially during the first two minutes following immersion (Hayward, 1983), and the maximal breath-hold time in water at 0 to 15 °C is reduced to 15 to 25 seconds (Goode and McDonald, 1982; Hayward, 1983; Hayward *et al.*, 1984b). This respiratory drive will also facilitate the inhalation of water and therefore drowning (Hayward, 1983). For aircrews there is the additional hazard that having safely ejected they may drown through the parachute not collapsing properly and causing dragging. This leads to a bow wave breaking over the helmet and forcing the head under water despite efforts to raise it and this can happen even at slow speeds of drag, e.g. 5 knots (Balfour and Underwood-Ground, 1980).

Treatment must start immediately on rescue using expired air resuscitation and external cardiac massage, in the water if necessary, and continued till the hospital is reached (Conn and Barker, 1984). Victims should have their neurological categories assessed in the emergency room and graded: A — awake, B — blunted or C — comatose. Categories A and B have a good prognosis and C is subdivided into C1 — decorticate, C2 — decerebrate, C3 — flaccid and C4 — ?deceased (Conn and Barker, 1984). It is difficult to predict the outcome of group C following near-drowning (Conn *et al.*, 1983; Conn and Barker, 1984; Young and Marks, 1983) even though initial resuscitation has been achieved. It appears that if spontaneous ventilation is re-established the prognosis is good whereas the absence of spontaneous respiration after the initial resuscitation means severe brain damage and a poor prognosis even if the heart has restarted (Jacobsen *et al.*, 1983). It is worthwhile adopting an aggressive therapeutic approach to all comatose near-drowning victims (Conn *et al.*, 1983) and the HYPER regimen has been shown to be of value but it should only be started after the circulation has remained stable for one hour and should be maintained for two to four days (Conn and Barker, 1984). This tries to treat the five main problems following near-drowning:

(1) Hyperhydration is treated by restricting fluids to 30 to 50 per cent of normal while giving frusomide 0.5 to 1.0 mg/kg intravenously and the frusomide is repeated till there is an adequate diuresis.
(2) Hyperventilation using high oxygen levels with positive end expiratory pressure (PEEP) is adjusted to maintain the $PaCO_2$ at 30 mm Hg. Any problem with a decrease in cardiac output caused by the PEEP is due to relative hypovolaemia and can be overcome by giving increased fluids.
(3) Hyperpyrexia is counteracted and normothermia maintained, though if the intracranial pressure is difficult to maintain, the temperature should be lowered to 30 °C.
(4) Hyperexcitability, as shown by spasms and convulsions, are treated with sedation and relaxants as necessary.
(5) Hyperrigidity is treated by complete muscular paralysis.

It is impossible to diagnose drowning at postmortem (BMJ, 1981; Hansen, 1977) since there is no one autopsy test or chemical test which is diagnostic (Thompson, 1977b) and diagnosis must therefore be after exclusion of other causes though this may be difficult if the body has been mauled by fishes after death (Keatinge, 1965; Thompson, 1977b).

Inhalation of Substances Other Than Water

In a fire the inhalation of smoke and other chemicals is a very important cause of immediate death and of late, sometimes fatal, pulmonary complications (Lloyd and MacRae, 1971) and there seems to be no logical reason why the inhalation of chemicals dissolved in water should be any less damaging to the lungs than the inhalation of chemicals carried in the air. Since most inland and coastal waters are polluted to some extent there may be aspiration of mineral debris, aquatic flora and fauna (Fuller, 1963; Pearn, 1980) as well as chemicals or bacteria (Pearn, 1980). The outcome of any immersion incident is therefore liable to be prejudiced, e.g. a case was reported of a man trapped in a car in a flooded culvert (Barr and Taylor, 1976). He inhaled water but never enough to cause loss of consciousness and when he died of secondary drowning ten days later, the question was raised as to a possible chemical cause for the fulminating pneumonitis. Bacterial pollution of the water may result in bronchopneumonia.

Secondary Drowning

The utmost vigilance for secondary effects is required in all cases of near-drowning and indeed in any patients who may have inhaled water even if they appear to have made a complete recovery or have never been unconscious (Barr and Taylor, 1976). An acute pulmonary oedema may develop 15 minutes to 72 hours after the drowning incident (Pearn, 1980; Rivers *et al.*, 1970; Theilade, 1977) and this is one time when it is useful to know the type of water in which the incident occurred. This is because secondary drowning following sea-water near-drowning is much more lethal than that following fresh-water near-drowning (Rivers *et al.*, 1970; Pearn, 1980) even though the onset is more rapid after fresh-water near-drowning (Pearn, 1980). The clinical picture (Golden, 1980) is not unlike that following the inhalation of smoke (Lloyd and MacRae, 1971) and at least some elements of secondary drowning are probably due to bacterial or chemical pneumonitis (Pearn, 1980; Rivers *et al.*, 1970). Some cases may be due to pulmonary barotrauma or damage during resuscitation, or secondary to central neurological damage or oxygen toxicity (Pearn, 1980).

Hypothermia

Water conducts heat ten to twenty-five times better than air and therefore the cooling rate in water is two to four times greater than in air (Hirvonen, 1982). It has been said that water of 21 °C is unlikely to cause hypothermia (Miles, 1974), but Beckman and Reeves

(1966) found that, even in water as warm as 23.8 °C, some subjects became hypothermic in less than twelve hours. There are therefore very few areas of water in the world where hypothermia will not occur. (Unfortunately sharks also prefer water of over 21 °C (Miles, 1974).) Hypothermia may not be present alone since, when consciousness is lost, the face will fall forward and the person will inhale water and drown. Equations have been produced for heat loss and heat production in cold water to produce a prediction as to the rate of cooling in any given situation (Hayward *et al.*, 1975a; 1977) but to produce this equation the authors presuppose a steady rate of cooling on immersion, a concept which is challenged by White and Roth (1979) who postulate three phases of cooling, viz. a phase during which the core temperature is maintained followed by a linear rate of cooling to 34.5 °C at which there is a levelling off before the final drop starts. Recent investigations have shown that survival times for humans in ice-water are twice those found in the Dachau experiments (Hayward and Eckerson, 1984), probably because the Dachau prisoners were emaciated with a very small amount of subcutaneous fat.

Diving Reflex

The ability of diving mammals to remain submerged for prolonged periods (30 minutes plus) with breath-hold diving is dependent on a peculiar reflex shunting of the circulation. The peripheral circulation is virtually shut down and the animal becomes to all intents and purposes a heart/lung/brain preparation. There is also a profound bradycardia, which may be as low as two or three beats per minute and which decreases cardiac output thus preventing a rise in systemic pressure. The reflex is triggered by the trigeminal nerves and is independent of either chemoreceptor or baroreceptor function (Daly *et al.*, 1977; Elsner *et al.*, 1977). In man cold-water stimulation of the trigeminal area on the face also produces a bradycardia and vasoconstriction in the forearm (Elsner and Gooden, 1970) and one suggestion is that this phenomenon is a vestigial diving reflex. It has been postulated that the explanation why some individuals are capable of being resuscitated after periods of up to 40 minutes of submersion (Kvittingen and Naess, 1963; Nemiroff *et al.*, 1977; Siebke *et al.*, 1975; Theilade, 1977) is due to this vestigial diving reflex, which is most marked in children and young adults, together with generalised hypothermia (Harries, 1982). This hypothesis gains credence when one considers that nearly all of these accounts of survival refer to small children. It is usually stated that a decrease in water temperature produces a more profound bradycardia (Elsner and Gooden, 1983) and that a pronounced diving response can trigger such an intense parasympathetic response that cardiac arrest results (Elsner and Gooden, 1983), but while this may explain some cases of 'dry' drowning, it cannot explain the diving reflex cases. Many of these have occurred in ice-water which would be expected to have a maximum effect on the diving reflex but an explanation for the clinical findings must include the presence of an intact circulation (Harries, 1982) to maintain cerebral perfusion during the apnoea. Other studies have found the effect of reducing the water temperature to be slight (Kawakami *et al.*, 1967; Hayward, 1983), with there being no further slowing of the heart as the water temperature was lowered below 25 °C (Hayward, 1983; Hayward *et al.*, 1984b). Fear certainly potentiates the bradycardia (Elsner and Gooden, 1983) and this fact alone may explain many of the related observations. The use of a general anaesthetic reduces the response from 29 per cent to 3.6 per cent (Elsner and Gooden, 1983) and there is also less response if the facial immersion is carried out without breath-holding (Elsner and Gooden, 1983) and a similar effect occurs if a thin plastic sheet is interposed between the face and the water (Elsner and Gooden, 1983), none of which have any effect on the temperature impinging on the face. Even in diving mammals it has been observed that, when they are held underwater, there is a profound bradycardia which is absent when they are underwater voluntarily (Blix, 1985; Butler, 1985; Kanwisher *et al.*, 1981). In all these instances the reduced response could be explained by a reduction in fear, and since a decrease in water temperature might increase subjective fear, this may explain the variable findings in relation to water temperature. However, there are difficulties in accepting this explanation in its entirety. In diving mammals there are, in addition, other complex circulatory and metabolic adjustments as well as specific anatomical and physiological features which are only found in diving mammals and in birds which dive (Elsner and Gooden, 1983; Hochachka and Murphy, 1979; Kanwisher and Gabrielsen, 1985). There is no evidence that any terrestrial mammals have the ability to make the complex metabolic adjustments made by seals immediately on diving and on surfacing again. Also the diving reflex in diving mammals appears to occur, irrespective of the water temperature, whereas in man submersion accidents in warm water result in death, and therefore survival in man is entirely due to the development of hypothermia and the more rapid the development of hypothermia the greater the chance of survival.

Vasoconstriction reduces heat loss from the periphery and, if the almost complete peripheral shutdown found in diving reflex cases was present as an initial effect immediately on entry to the cold water, this would be expected to reduce the heat loss to a negligible quantity, even in children with their large surface area to body mass ratio. This physiological theory does not tally with the clinical picture of the children resuscitated from the diving reflex where in the instance where temperatures have been measured and the time of submersion known the rate of cooling has been fast (Harries, 1982), up to a phenomenal rate of 36 °C an hour (Conn, 1981). This rate of cooling is impossible without the presence of an intact circulation. When the rates of cooling achieved in experiments with volunteers (Golden and Hervey, 1972) are compared with the victims of the diving reflex it is found that the average rate of cooling in the diving reflex is double the maximum rate achieved with the volunteers despite the absence of clothing in the latter (Harries, 1982). There must therefore be some significant factor to cause this difference. One factor must be the parts of the body in the water. In the experiment the volunteers would have their heads and some of the neck out of the water whereas the diving reflex victims are totally submerged. The neck is one of the regions of the body which retains a high level of heat loss even when the body is immersed in cold water (Hayward *et al.*, 1973; Reed *et al.*, 1984; Wade *et al.*, 1979) and the head is a major route for heat loss even in adults with 50 per cent of the body's metabolic heat production (at −4 °C with the person at rest in air) being lost through the head (Froese and Burton, 1957). The younger the child the larger the head in proportion to the body and therefore the greater potential heat loss from the head and this reaches its extreme in the neonate where gamgee around the head decreases the risk of a fall in core temperature whereas the same quantity of gamgee wrapped round the abdomen has no measurable effect (de Saintonge *et al.*, 1979). Finally not only is there very little subcutaneous fat on the head, especially in young people, but there is an extensive vascular network in the scalp (Edwards and Burton, 1960) and the vessels appear to have a very poor vasoconstrictor response (Froese and Burton, 1957). It has also been shown that facial temperatures stabilise well above freezing (Steegman, 1979), which means that though the face may be resistant to frostbite it is always an important route for heat loss. The importance of the head as a route for heat loss even in adults is illustrated by a number of observations. The fact that in drown-proofing the head is under water resulted in cooling rates faster than when the head is kept out of the water by treading water (Goode and McDonald, 1982). Also it has proved possible to selectively cool the brains of dogs by immersing their heads in ice-water and perfusing the nasopharynx with the same ice-water while at the same time maintaining the rest of the body at normothermia by warm-water blankets (White *et al.*, 1984). The experimental situation with the anaesthetised dogs is remarkably similar to the clinical situation in which the diving reflex cases are found with the victims being unconscious and the head submerged in ice-cold water probably with the ice-water also bathing the nasopharynx. It has also been suggested that the victim inhales the cold fresh water. In animal experiments this water is quickly absorbed and rapidly cools the brain and heart before the circulation stops (Conn and Barker, 1984). It has also proved possible to stabilise the core temperature of a person in a hyperthermic climatic chamber by applying cooling to the head alone (Brown and Williams, 1982).

The phenomenon of the diving reflex in man might be better called 'rapid or acute submersion hypothermia' (Conn *et al.*, 1983). Most of the clinical findings can be explained by the rapid heat loss from the head, face and neck and the features of the diving reflex would act in a manner opposite to the known features of human clinical cases. It is suggested that the bradycardia might, however, have some survival value by preventing a massive hypertension following the rapid vasoconstriction which in turn would reduce the oxygen consumption in the periphery. However, the bradycardia found in victims at rescue may be due to the hypothermia rather than to the diving reflex (Hayward *et al.*, 1984b) and there may be a similar explanation for the profound vasoconstriction.

It is known that the colder the water the greater the respiratory drive (Hayward *et al.*, 1984b) but this may be overcome by the apnoeic effect of sudden facial immersion which can be present even though the subject is able to breathe through a snorkel (Elsner and Gooden, 1983). Cardiac activity may persist for ten to fifteen minutes after respiratory arrest (Harries, 1982) and during this time the vital heart and brain will therefore receive adequate oxygenation during the rapid development of hypothermia. Similar cases of survival following prolonged apnoea have been reported following burial in snow, or intoxication with alcohol or barbiturates (Harries, 1982). A more satisfactory explanation for the cases of so called diving reflex is that the person was suddenly precipitated into cold water producing a reflex apnoea. Because of absence of fear due to alcohol or lack of warning, there was no initial bradycardia and the circulation remained intact maybe even in the limbs initially. The sudden cold immersion may also have prevented physical activity thus preserving the oxygen content of the body, and the total immersion would accelerate the rate of cooling thus further reducing the oxygen demand.

The importance of recognising the diving reflex phenomenon lies in the fact that people, especially children and young adults, can be successfully revived after prolonged periods of submersion in cold water. All cases who survived from this type of submersion hypothermia were given emergency resuscitation with expired air resuscitation (EAR) (mouth-to-mouth) immediately on rescue and it is likely that the benefit came as much from the airway warming effect of the warmth and moisture in the expired air as from the oxygen supplied. Another benefit of EAR is that inflation of the lungs reflexly abolishes any vagal-induced bradycardia (Elsner and Gooden, 1983). Therefore, if there is to be any hope of success, resuscitation must start immediately and be continued during transport (Conn *et al.*, 1983), because if resuscitation is delayed while the patient is being transferred to hospital, death is the inevitable outcome. Before a diagnosis of death can be made in these cases cardio-pulmonary resuscitation must be continued for one to two hours (Conn *et al.*, 1983).

Exhaustion

If the water temperature is not sufficiently cold to induce hypothermia rapidly, the person may struggle or swim around or shiver for prolonged periods and this will eventually result in exhaustion or cramps (Beckman and Reeves, 1966; Low, 1982), with an inability of the person to maintain his position in relation to waves and the water. In addition, when the person becomes exhausted, his rate of heat loss reaches a maximum and, since exhaustion also means that there is no more available fuel for exercise or heat, it is obvious that the exhausted person will rapidly become hypothermic. Exhaustion also causes loss of co-ordination and strength and this will inevitably increase the possibility of drowning.

Hypoglycaemia

This may occur before the person becomes hypothermic and will cause increased heat loss, an inability to continue exercise and unconsciousness leading to an increased risk of hypothermia and drowning.

Injury

Injuries are common during entry into the water (Golden, 1980; Keatinge, 1965) or while in the water (Glennie, 1969). An injury may also be the reason for the immersion and diagnosis may be difficult because of the associated hypothermia or near-drowning (Golden, 1980).

Other Factors

Alcohol is an important factor in immersion deaths (BMJ, 1979), especially where the person submerges suddenly and unexpectedly (Hirvonen, 1977). Some victims fall in because they are drunk and then drown because of lack of co-ordination and sense. Others drown because the alcohol has increased the bravado to a level where they try things beyond their abilities, and alcohol impairs temperature regulation and they then become hypothermic and drown.

Death may also occur in underwater swimming if the person hyperventilates before diving into the water. Having eliminated the carbon dioxide element of the respiratory drive, the person may lose consciousness from hypoxia before the carbon dioxide has built up again and he will then drown (Craig, 1976; Elsner and Gooden, 1983; Fuller, 1963).

Muscular cramp as a cause of incapacity leading to drowning is also a possibility (McCrone, 1978) and a heavy meal just prior to immersion may cause incapacity and drowning by diverting blood into the splanchnic area, and the full stomach may obstruct the diaphragm (Hirvonen, 1977).

Rescue

A victim should ideally be handled gently and kept horizontal while being removed from the water (Harnett *et al.*, 1983a) but in an emergency situation it is more important that the person is removed from the water by any means available, especially if the weather conditions are very bad. In one case the only way an unconscious person could be removed from the water was to haul him up twelve feet of vertical height by a rope which had accidentally become looped round his neck. The man was successfully resuscitated and the only residual damage was a circumferential rope burn round the neck (Frankland, 1983). It has been recommended that triage should be applied to immersion victims in the same way as it is applied to victims of a mass land disaster. In this scheme (Keatinge, 1973, 1977; Keatinge in Marcus, 1979a) the quietest, thinnest and youngest people should be rescued first, and the older, larger and fatter later, and males before females. Though these are indications of the different rates of cooling, in practice rescue craft will pick up victims as they are reached since the survival of any individual is improved by removal from the water, and, if a person is bypassed for any reason, he may not be in the same place when the rescuers return, because of tides, currents or wind, and he may be lost (Guild in Marcus, 1979a). If a large number of casualties are in the water, it may be necessary for triage to be carried out once the survivors are on board ship (Steinman, 1982) but the procedure is exactly the same as for mass casualties on dry land. Once the person is out of the water resuscitate and insulate and in practice resuscitation is the same whether the water is salt or fresh (Fraser-Darling, 1981).

All immersion casualties should be admitted to hospital for observation (Maclean and Emslie-Smith, 1977; Pearn, 1980). If water has been inhaled and there are clinical signs in the chest, they should be admitted to an intensive care unit (Pfenninger and Sutter, 1982). This is necessary not only because of the possibility of secondary drowning but because there may be other complications such as cerebral oedema, pulmonary infection or renal failure which can best be treated in hospital. If high-dose barbiturates are used to reduce brain swelling and protect against brain damage, artificial ventilation will be needed (Pearn, 1980). Acid base status can be corrected and if there is any evidence of secondary drowning developing, positive end expiratory pressure ventilation (PEEP) should be instituted early since this reduces the incidence of severe secondary drowning effects (Theilade, 1977). Even if the use of PEEP is delayed it can produce a marked improvement in the blood gases while having a minimal adverse effect on the cardiovascular system (Lindner *et al.*, 1983). Any decrease in cardiac output occurring following the start of PEEP is due to relative hypovolaemia and therefore giving additional fluids improves the cardiac output (Tabeling and Modell, 1983). Dopamine infusion in this situation produces no consistently beneficial effect (Tabeling and Modell, 1983).

28 HYPOTHERMIA AND COLD STRESS DURING WORK

There are many situations where men are exposed to cold stress while working (Green, 1978; Kinnersley, 1974), but cold as a hazard is often ignored (Health and Safety Executive, 1978; Waldron, 1976). There is in fact no generally acceptable definition of what constitutes cold working (Hassi, 1982), though cold can affect people who work outside, people who work inside and people whose jobs involve inside and outside work (Hassi, 1982).

In the fishing and timber industries, and on building sites and farms, workers are obviously exposed to all weathers, and with the growth of deep-freeze storage there are an increasing number of workers exposed to temperatures of −20 °C to −40 °C, sometimes with an additional fan-produced wind-chill. People who are employed to work in a cold-store environment should be carefully selected on certain physical and psychological criteria (Andrew, 1963). The population at risk are not just workers in large food storage depots but those in individual shops, e.g. butchers often have large deep-freeze rooms which people enter, and maintenance engineers may be trapped after an accident (Cohen, 1968; *Sun*, 1977). Many lorries now transport food in refrigerated containers and a driver may become trapped inside if the wind blows the door shut. Some medical facilities, e.g. blood transfusion products, also need deep-freeze rooms and because of the unpredictable nature of medical emergencies staff will frequently have to enter the cold room at night or at the weekend, times when the number of people on the premises is at a minimum and there may be no one in the room with the alarm.

The North Sea is one of the most hostile environments in the world (Golden, 1976; Green, 1980) with waves up to 24 metres in height (Faulkner, 1977) and winds up to 160 kph (Wilkinson, 1975). With fishing boats, oil supply vessels, helicopters, oil rigs and merchant and naval vessels there is a large population at risk, though because of the wide range of facilities and living environments protection and prevention have to be tailored to each situation.

Fishing is a very hazardous occupation with the accident rate being five times greater than the most dangerous land-based transport industry (Vanggaard, 1977). It is often suggested that seamen are heavy alcohol drinkers and that accidents and losses at sea are a result of the skipper being drunk. This is one of a number of myths about alcohol consumption. One often-stated myth is that there is a greater consumption and a greater incidence of alcohol-related problems in Scotland, especially in the north, compared with the south-east of England. However, when a study was made, it was found that there was no difference in the amount of alcohol consumed (Crawford *et al.*, 1984), and the reason for the higher number of hospital admissions with alcohol-related problems especially in the north of Scotland was entirely due to the fact that, because of distance and geographical problems, cases in the north of Scotland were admitted to hospital, whereas those in the south-east of England were treated as outpatients (Latcham *et al.*, 1984). Similarly when the actual consumption was studied it was found that the total alcohol consumption of seamen is similar to that of industrial and office workers, and alcohol abuse was as prevalent among factory employees as fishermen (Helgason, 1977). As far as accidents at sea are concerned, it is usually forgotten that the symptoms and signs of alcohol intoxication are similar to those of hypothermia (Pugh, 1968) and hypothermia, or the other effects of cold stress, may be more important than alcohol as causes of accidents and death among fishermen.

The risks of work in the cold are not only from the obvious dangers of frostbite and hypothermia, but also from the insidious effects of cold discussed earlier on skin sensation, muscle function, manual dexterity, on the cardiovascular and respiratory systems, and on higher cerebral function. Cold can cause apathy (Enander, 1984), which can be dangerous in the working environment, but some environmental stress is needed to provide optimal performance, and large, slow swings of temperature have been shown to improve performance (Enander, 1984). Much can be done to prevent problems by education (Andrew, 1963), but training must be specific to the conditions in which the work is to be done (Enander, 1984). With continued exposure there is a degree of physical adaptation, e.g. the person learns to use movements of the arms and shoulders to compensate for the impairment caused by cold hands (Enander, 1984). The duration of exposure to cold, insufficient protective clothing and low or intermittent physical activity may produce cooling of the body and hands, and this can have a great effect on manual performance (Enander, 1984), and unfortunately the effect cannot be assessed by monitoring ambient temperature and other climatic variations, or even by measurement of skin temperature.

The provision of protective clothing (Newburgh, 1949) for people working in the cold is an obvious precautionary measure (Enander, 1984) but, when a particular series of fishing losses were investigated, it was noted that despite icing conditions and high winds, all the crew members of one particular boat were wearing light clothing and there was only sufficient waterproof clothing for 12 out of the crew of 19 (Pugh, 1968). However, it is difficult to provide protection and maintain flexibility and satisfactory function, especially of the hands (Enander, 1984). An additional problem is human nature. Being what it is, if the person is just 'nipping in' to the cold room for one item he/she may not bother to put on the available clothing. This situation is also the one where the person will fail to ensure that the door is properly wedged open and a draught may blow it shut, leaving the person trapped.

Where applicable, special measures, such as heated cabs for crane operators and tractor drivers, can allow work to continue safely in the cold (Andrew, 1963). Since adequate gloves impair manual function (Enander, 1984), an attempt has been made to provide local auxiliary heating to the hands (Lockhart and Keiss, 1971). A more practical measure is that controls on equipment should be large enough to be operated with gloved hands and all knobs, levers, handles and seats should be made of materials with low thermal conductivity (Andrew, 1963).

After a spell of work in a cold room the standard procedure is for the person to have a hot drink in a warm room before returning to the cold room. This unfortunately is the worst possible method of rewarming (Enander, 1984), because the sensation of warmth, which can be produced by temperatures around 0 °C, overcomes the cold-induced vasoconstriction, and return to the cold room results in an acceleration of the rate of heat loss (see under the heading 'Symptomless Cooling' in Chapter 4).

Some cold rooms can be opened from the inside but the door may still be jammed and therefore there should also be an alarm system so that a person trapped inside a cold room can call for help. However, the alarm system may fail or there may be no one present to notice the alarm. In the case of the driver of a refrigerated lorry who becomes trapped in the refrigerated section the alarm is likely to be in the cab and it is conceivable that it will either not be noticed or the significance will not be understood. To cover this contingency emergency protective gear should be kept inside the cold room. This equipment should include an arctic quality sleeping bag with an integral insulated hood, a large polythene bag of the type used by climbers to keep out the wind and a face mask with a condenser humidifier device (Lloyd and Croxton, 1981) since this will not only provide insulation to reduce or eliminate the heat lost through breathing but will also trap the exhaled moisture and prevent it wetting the inside of the sleeping bag.

29 COLD STRESS IN SPORT

Water Sports

On the Surface of the Water

For water sports there are special problems because of the close association with wind and cold water.

Windsurfing is a relatively new sport which is quickly gaining a large number of participants. One of its attractions is that the board and sail are relatively cheap, at least as compared with other sailing craft, are easy to store in any garage, can easily be carried on the roof rack of a car and are easy to launch without assistance. These factors, however, cause some of the dangers because the equipment can be bought by a novice and then launched without any training or supervision. As the number of windsurfers increase so do the number of emergencies. In the UK more than 300 windsurfers were rescued in 1984 by the Royal National Lifeboat Institution (Ayers, 1985) and 80 per cent of all rescues carried out by the Federal German Lifeboat Service are for windsurfers (Duesberg, 1982).

One of the greatest dangers for a windsurfer is an off-shore wind because a windsurf board cannot head as close into the wind as does a dinghy or keelboat. Because of the windshadow produced by the land and buildings, the sailor is unaware of the true wind strength until he is some distance out from shore and even expert sailors can be caught out. Windsurfing needs strength as well as expertise to haul a sail out of the water and to keep it up against the wind. As the person becomes fatigued, not only is he or she less able to keep the sail up, but he or she is also more likely to fall off the board, and after each fall, the sail has to be hauled up again, causing more fatigue and a vicious circle is started. At this stage the surfer is in trouble especially with an off-shore wind because of the inevitable drift downwind during each fall and raising of the sail. Hypothermia is then a real hazard.

For thermal protection windsurfers, like scuba divers, wear wet suits, but because of the need for more rapid and flexible movement the wet suits are thinner (3 to 5 mm). In addition the windsurfer tends to be repeatedly in and out of the water. Now a wet suit is very warm while it remains dry, and while the surfer is in the water the trapped layer of water preserves the body heat. However, as soon as the person is out of the water the surfer starts to lose heat from evaporation and the stronger the wind the greater the evaporative heat loss. A wet suit is therefore very inefficient if the wearer is in and out of the water a lot. This is liable to be the case for beginners, for better sailors in stronger winds and for those who are becoming exhausted. All windsurfers need wind and once past the beginners stage, 'fun' for windsurfers means strong wind. The better the surfer the stronger the wind he likes and for experts 'fun' really starts with a storm warning (Schonle, 1982). When the weather starts to get cold there are several things that the windsurfer can do for protection. A neoprene hood increases the area protected. A good fitting wet suit is much warmer than a poorly fitting one (Schonle, 1982) and beginners tend to skimp on price spent on wet suits (Duesberg, 1982) and therefore frequently end up with a poorly fitting one. Any incompatibility between the shape of the wet suit and the shape of the person inside allows spaces in which water collects and then pours out, taking away heat. Many wet suits are loose round the waist and a neoprene kidney belt eliminates this looseness and by trapping the water increases the heat saving for the surfer (Duesberg, 1982; Schonle, 1982). In one comparison during a regatta in which the physical work involved would normally cause a rise in core temperature, two surfers who were not wearing the kidney belt had core temperatures just above 35 °C, and their pale cold fingers and bluish colouring of the tongue and mouth showed incipient hypothermia. On the other hand, two surfers who did have kidney belts had warm peripheries and core temperatures above 37.5 °C (Schonle, 1982). The advertised claim that the kidney belt protects the kidneys from damage due to cooling is nonsense. The use of windproof cagoul and trousers over the wet suit reduces evaporation and has a marked thermal benefit. However, for really cold weather the windsurfer needs a dry suit. This has very little insulation value itself but the surfer wears enough clothes to keep warm on land and the dry suit on top keeps them dry.

As the sailors move through *dinghies* to *larger boats* the risk of immersion drops fast. For 'Laser' sailors the immersion is fairly frequent and a wet suit with windproof overgarments is probably required as for windsurfers, while on the big yachts all the sailor needs is warm clothing with overgarments which keep out the wind and spray. For in-between craft the needs of protective clothing must be assessed and tailored to the craft and the conditions.

Water skiers and *canoeists* also have to balance mobility with thermal protection but in both the activity requires a high energy (heat) output but is of relatively short duration. Canoeists have a special hazard in the cold. During a capsize or roll the sudden shock of cold water may cause disorientation (Baker and Atha, 1981) which may be the result of a caloric labyrinthitis from cold water entering the ears (Bernhartsen and Schlenker, 1981).

Most competitive and leisure *swimming* now takes place in warmed indoor pools but there is still a fair amount of swimming done in the open sea and inland lochs, especially during the summer months. In one incident, of 49 competitive swimmers who took part in a race in 19 °C water, 30 had a fall in core temperature, with 10 being hypothermic, i.e. below 35 °C, and 5 could not complete the swim and had to be helped out of the water (Horvath, 1981). The fact that the waters round the British Isles are colder than 18 °C even on the south coast of England during the summer should provide warning of the dangers. Many holiday swimmers become mildly hypothermic every year by being chilled in the cold water and then when they come out of the water, there is the wind-chill plus evaporation. However, most recover without specific treatment by drying, putting on warm clothes and taking shelter.

Sports Diving

Scuba divers usually wear 6 mm-thick closed-cell foam neoprene suits which keep the diver warm by trapping a layer of water between the suit and the body and this gives adequate protection against the cold water for sporting divers who do not dive too deep. The subject of cold and diving is dealt with in the next chapter.

Sports on Land

Winter Sports

Surprisingly most sporting activities classed as winter sports are not at great risk from hypothermia. Curling, skating and ice hockey are usually done in indoor rinks and even speed skating, tobogganning, luge, ski jumping and downhill piste skiing are done in safe areas and are abandoned if the weather conditions deteriorate. The people at risk are those who indulge in cross-country skiing if the weather conditions deteriorate (Renstrom, 1982), and where skating and curling are being done on outdoor ponds there is obviously a great danger if the ice breaks. If a person suffers an injury there is also a danger of hypothermia if the situation is such that the victim has to remain exposed to adverse weather for any length of time.

Other Sports

The greatest risk of harm for these groups is muscle and ligament damage occurring while the limbs are still cold. Protective clothing should be worn initially while the athlete is warming up. This should be taken to the point where sweating is about to start and once this stage had been reached, the athlete can shed his protective clothing, and he will remain warm in minimal clothing provided he is exercising vigorously. The warm-up is also of value since the performance of muscle is improved by raising the muscle temperature (Horvath, 1981).

In *team games* the players usually come out of a warm changing room and either have a kick-about period or start playing before they have had time to cool down. Also during the early stages the game tends to be slow as the teams size each other up and this allows time for the muscles to warm up. Once started some players may become almost too warm, e.g. the steam arising from a rugby scrum. However, some players are still at risk, and therefore the goalkeeper wears track suit trousers, a sweater and gloves to try to keep warm so that he can move quickly when required. A rugby wing threequarter is also a player at risk since he has less constant activity than most of the rest of the team, but, when required, he is expected to move suddenly and fast and this is the main reason why pulled muscles in rugby are common among wing threequarters.

Athletes participating in *cross-country running* in winter leave the changing rooms some time before their race to look round the course and the race starts fast and continues hard, and the cold athlete will not only perform badly but is also at risk from pulled muscles. To avoid this athletes make a deliberate effort to warm up. Once the event is under way, cold is no longer a problem and as long as the athlete is running or active he/she will stay warm. When the race is over, the athlete puts on warm clothes and needs to warm down. This not only eases the stiffness out of the muscles, but also allows the body to adjust the rate of heat production and by preventing sweating will help to prevent hypothermia developing. *Track* athletes have a similar problem and the shorter and more explosive the event the greater the risk of muscle damage. *Field* athletes have an even greater problem in that their events tend to involve sudden explosive effort with periods of complete inactivity between the rounds of the competition.

The *marathon* is an event which provides special thermal problems in that it is possible in the same race for some runners to collapse from hyperthermia while others in a similar state of collapse may be suffering from hypothermia (Maughan, 1984). The climatic conditions are more important for distance events than in almost any other situation. If the weather is very cold with rain and wind there is an obvious danger of hypothermia, while if the weather is hot and humid the danger of heatstroke increases rapidly and it is suggested that no distance race should start if the wet bulb temperature is over 28 °C (Porter, 1984). There is the added problem with the 'people's' marathons that, since the slowest participants may take six hours or more, there is sufficient time for there to be major changes in the weather during the race (Maughan, 1984). In addition each runner is different in respect of mechanical efficiency, and body size, shape and weight, and other thermal mechanisms, e.g. rate of sweating, also differ between individuals (Maughan, 1984; Porter, 1984), thus making each person uniquely susceptible to changes in body temperature, either up or down. Each runner therefore has to assess the weather conditions and decide on the clothing to be worn during the race while taking into account his own particular physiology. Unfortunately knowledge of this last point is only likely to be acquired through practical experience of running distances. One problem is that before the start the runner is standing in a cold environment and therefore needs extra clothing. However, once the race starts the person is producing heat, and clothing which provided comfort before the race will result in overheating during the race. The ideal is for the runners to remove the extra clothing just before the race starts, and in races with limited numbers, e.g. championship marathons, it is possible for arrangements to be made so that the clothing can be collected and is available for the runners at the end of the race. In the mass marathons this is impossible because of sheer numbers, and another complication is that runners have to be at the start for much longer than for other races. A warm-up is impractical because of numbers and is probably unnecessary since, because of the nature of the event, runners tend to start relatively slowly. Even top-class athletes tend to limit themselves to mobility exercises. The only practical solution in the mass marathon is for runners to cut arm and head holes in a large polythene bag and wear this over their running gear before the start. A polythene bag has the advantages that it is wind proof and water proof and is cheap and readily available. The bag can be retained during the race until the runner is thoroughly warm and then discarded, and in very bad weather some runners have worn the bag till the finish.

During the race most runners remain in thermal equilibrium but if the runner goes too fast and the heat production exceeds the heat loss, heatstroke will develop, and this can happen even in cold climates (Nilsson, 1984). (There is a suggestion that some cases of heatstroke may be due to the genetic condition of malignant hyperpyrexia (Ellis and Campbell, 1983) and, if this is true, it may have important implications with the growth of popular marathons, since there is specific treatment with dantrolene.) Overheating may occur in the middle of a race if the runners increase the pace and symptoms can develop within five to ten minutes of increasing the pace (Porter, 1984). Some runners develop a hyperventilation before becoming hyperthermic (Oakley, H., personal communication, 1985). This may be an indication that the core temperature is starting to rise, and the hyperventilation may be an attempt to increase the rate of heat loss through the respiratory tract, akin to the panting adopted by dogs and other hairy animals. Panting, however, involves the rapid passage of air over the mucosa to increase evaporation and panting in animals is rapid and shallow. Unfortunately in man the hyperventilation involves rapid and deep breathing, and this may be counterproductive since, if it results in lowering the CO_2 level, it may produce vasoconstriction and therefore reduce the rate of heat loss from the skin. Hyperthermia has also been recorded in a runner who was taking an antipyretic for a sore throat (Whitworth and Wolfman, 1983) and runners are advised not to participate if they feel unwell, since any viral infection increases the risk of hyperthermia and heatstroke (Oakley, H., personal communication, 1985). Hypothermia is likely to occur towards the end of the event as the runner is becoming fatigued and the pace is slowing or the runner stops. If the weather is cold and/or wet and/or windy the heat loss will exceed heat production and the body temperature may drop rapidly.

One additional problem is that fluid is lost through sweating (Maughan, 1984), and the person may be unaware of this because a runner is never running in still air (Porter, 1984). If the runner is running at an average 14 to 17 kph this is equal to a force 3 wind and the wind of movement will convert an air temperature of 10 °C to a wind-chill equivalent of 4 °C (Porter, 1984). The person also loses moisture during the respiration and the volume is proportional to the respiratory minute volume (Brebbia *et al.*, 1957). Despite the presence of many 'watering stations' on the course, it is almost impossible to maintain adequate hydration (Maughan, 1984; Porter, 1984) and dehydration will increase the risk of both hypothermia and heatstroke.

The literature was reviewed for thermal problems in marathons (Maughan, 1984; Porter, 1984) and there were 26 cases where the recorded rectal temperature was over 40 °C and of these four developed renal failure (Porter, 1984). A low body temperature at the end of a race is relatively common, especially if the weather is cold (Maughan *et al.*, 1982; Porter, 1984) but most of these are mild. The claim that there is no certain record of death from hypothermia in road racing (Porter, 1984) is not correct (Sutton, 1983) but that particular race was very abnormal in that it started in a mild temperature at low altitude and the runners ran up a mountain into snow at the top (Sutton, 1983). In the one case in the UK where a runner collapsed 30 metres from the finishing line and was thought to have died from hypothermia (Ledingham *et al.*, 1982) this was on the basis of a rectal temperature of 34.2 °C recorded 75 minutes after the collapse. This diagnosis seems unlikely not only because the rectal temperature recorded is not normally considered dangerous, but the same runner, who was also experienced over shorter distances, had successfully completed a marathon a few weeks earlier in what were very much worse weather conditions, and in a respectable time (Lloyd, 1983b).

The problem in differential diagnosis is that hypothermia and hyperthermia have similar symptoms (Maughan, 1984) and not only may the hyperthermic person be shivering and dry (Whitworth and Wolfman, 1983) but a hypothermic person is unlikely to be shivering and may not be aware of feeling cold (Maughan *et al.*, 1982). Temperature measurement is the only certain way of differentiating between the two conditions. The treatment of hypothermia is relatively easy in that all that is needed is for the runner to put on more clothes and to be removed from the cold environment into shelter.

Heatstroke is a condition in which there are many problems in addition to a raised body temperature (Guezennec and Pesquies, 1985; Khogali and Hales, 1984). Detailed discussion of the pathophysiology of heatstroke is beyond the scope of this book, and there are some extensive reviews of the subject (American College of Sports Medicine, 1984; Khogali and Hales, 1984; Shibolet *et al.*, 1976). The immediate management problem is to reduce the body heat. The traditional method of ice baths, ice packs and even cold sponging plus blowing cold air over the person, may be counter-productive since the cold stimulus to the skin will produce vasoconstriction, thus reducing the rate of heat loss, and may cause shivering, thus increasing the heat production (Khogali *et al.*, 1983).

The most effective management appears to be to spray the body with 15 °C water and blow warm air at 45 °C over the person (Khogali *et al.*, 1983). (Warming 1 litre of cold water from 4 °C to 34 °C requires 30 kcal, while evaporating 1 litre of water requires 580 kcal (Kaufman, 1983).) The perceived warmth on the skin inhibits shivering and maintains vasodilatation with a high flow of blood, and therefore heat, through the skin to be dissipated by evaporation (Khogali *et al.*, 1983). A special unit has been designed for this purpose (Weiner and Khogali, 1980). The other emergency problem is dehydration accompanied by electrolyte disturbances. Rehydration is essential to allow the vascular heat loss mechanisms to work, but most sufferers from heatstroke have normal or low serum sodium levels (Guezennec and Pesquies, 1985; Gumaa *et al.*, 1984), and when the patient is rehydrated the hyponatraemia is aggravated (Gumaa *et al.*, 1984). Emergency rehydration should therefore be done with a sodium-rich fluid such as normal saline, but the electrolytes must be checked as soon as the person reaches hospital. Treatment in hospital should be done in an intensive care unit because of the other problems and dangers. If the runner has been hyperventilating, rebreathing into a paper bag may be necessary to restore the carbon dioxide levels to normal (Oakley, H., personal communication, 1985).

There is, however, another risk factor for runners in the cold. Exercise causes catecholamine secretion (Hartung *et al.*, 1984; Keatinge *et al.*, 1984; Northcote and Ballantyne, 1983) and the levels may remain high for some time after the exercise stops (Northcote and Ballantyne, 1983). Cold stress also causes catecholamine secretion (Danzl, 1983; Keatinge *et al.*, 1984; Mager and Francesconi, 1983; Maclean and Emslie-Smith, 1977; Weihl *et al.*, 1981) in order to increase heat production. Adrenaline is an antidote to muscular fatigue (Hilton, 1965), and the observation of a tachycardia occurring in the latter stages of a sporting event (Northcote and Ballantyne, 1983) may be clinical evidence of this. Stress also causes increased catecholamine secretion (Rosch, 1983; Taggart *et al.*, 1972) and the stress response to exercise is increased by facial cooling (Riggs *et al.*, 1983). In the death described by Ledingham *et al.* (1982) there could have been very high levels of catecholamines from the cold and the exercise, which would be increased by cold on the face. Since the runner had been in a state of physical exhaustion for some time prior to his collapse (Ledingham, I. McA., personal communication, 1982) there could have been a superimposed increase from counteracting the fatigue. Finally there would be the stress of wanting to finish, and, since he was only 30 metres from the finishing line when he collapsed, this effect would have been accentuated by the encouragement from the crowd. There is therefore the possibility of very high levels of catecholamines being present in the circulation. High levels of catecholamines may cause cardiac damage and death (Rosch, 1983) and may have been implicated in the myocardial necrosis found in patients with phaeochromocytoma (Ricci *et al.*, 1979). In one young woman the accidental intravenous injection of adrenaline produced severe myocardial ischaemia which required admission to a coronary care unit. Despite the fact that she was later shown to have a normal ECG, normal risk factors and a normal effort stress test, the pain and ECG ischaemia persisted for several hours and required an intravenous infusion of nitroglycerine to produce control (Horak *et al.*, 1983). The fact that the runner was in ventricular fibrillation when treatment was first started (Ledingham *et al.*, 1982) would tend to support the idea that catecholamines were the cause of death and not cold. There is one further possibility in that cold causes a release of free fatty acids (FFA) into the circulation (Hanson and Johnson, 1965), and there is also an increase in FFA after exercise (Northcote and Ballantyne, 1983) and FFA are liable to produce arrhythmias (Northcote and Ballantyne, 1983).

Other endurance type of activities, such as the half-marathon, orienteering, cycle touring, cycle distance races or time-trials, and hill walking, may have similar thermal problems and this should be considered by organisers and participants. Members of the armed forces also have to face the same problems of thermal balance during prolonged exercises outdoors.

30 DIVING

Though a diver is both working and in water, the environment is sufficiently unique to require special consideration. Diving is now being used for many purposes including sport, marine biology, marine archaeology, oil exploration and many other activities. Some of these are unexpected to the outsider, e.g. in mountain lakes to inspect and repair dams, and in this situation there may be additional complications since these dams may be at altitude (Rey, 1985). Diving, as work, takes place in all parts of the world, even under the ice in polar regions, and for this last there are particular operational requirements (Rey, 1985). It is important to remember that in arctic diving, there may be greater cold stress for the support staff than for the divers themselves (Kuehn, 1985). Diving is certainly a high-risk occupation but the mortality has decreased over recent years so that the risks are now on a par with very-high-risk land-based occupations (Bradley, 1984). In diving, man enters a very hostile environment where cold is a very important cause of death (Rawlins, 1981), being a major factor in 11 per cent of North Sea diving deaths (Bradley, 1984). Other common causes of diving accidents are decompression sickness, pulmonary barotrauma, gas poisoning (Hirvonen, 1977), oxygen toxicity and carbon dioxide variations (Leitch, 1981). The deep diver on oxyhelium is in an almost unique situation in that, because of the very narrow safety limits, he is in danger of becoming unconscious from either hypoxia or hyperoxia (Levack, 1983).

Whilst it is true that the colder the weather the more rapid the onset of hypothermia, many of the fatalities occur in relatively warm water. For example in the National Underwater Accidents Data Center (NUADC) study of scuba diving fatalities in the USA, 33 per cent of the cases of hypothermia occurred in Californian waters (McAniff, 1980), an area commonly assumed to have warm water. The diver is also exposed to all the systemic hazards of cold stress and when the specific stresses imposed on the cardiovascular system by cold stress are superimposed on what is strenuous physical exercise, sometimes accompanied by mental stress, it is not surprising that the NUADC survey in the USA found that of those over the age of 35 who had died in diving accidents, 22 per cent had died of a heart attack, and 7 per cent of the deaths among commercial divers were due to heart disease

(Bradley, 1984). In addition the risk of decompression sickness ('bends') rises if the body is cold (Belaud and Barthelmy, 1979), especially if the diver is warm at depth and cools during decompression (Kuehn, 1985), and there are sufficient dangers and uncertainties in compression and decompression (Bennett and Elliott, 1969; Lambertsen, 1976) without adding to them. Cold injury has also been misdiagnosed as decompression sickness (Leitch and Pearson, 1978). One other practical problem is that after a dive the diver may feel comfortable even though he still has a heat debt. If he then dives again this heat debt is carried over and further exposure to cold may result in the diver quickly becoming incapacitated (Hayes, 1985). To prevent this the diver should ensure that he is completely rewarmed between dives (Hayes, 1985). Even if the diver is not in the water he may be at thermal risk in a heliox atmosphere because the higher the pressure the higher the ambient temperature for comfort and the narrower the tolerable temperature range (Hayes, 1985; Raymond, 1975). In addition divers in heliox have difficulty in discerning accurately whether discomfort is due to heat or cold (Bennett and Elliott, 1969) and in fact some divers have died from hyperthermia while in a decompression chamber.

The temperature of the North Sea is a constant 4 °C below 100 metres depth (MDC, 1982), and the same is true throughout most of the world (Vanggaard, 1985) but it drops to −2 °C in the Arctic (Kuehn, 1985; Vanggaard, 1985). Protective clothing is therefore needed for all divers. As discussed in the previous chapter, scuba divers tend to wear 6 mm neoprene foam wet suits. However, the increasing pressure at depth reduces the insulating power of the normal wet suit by compressing the neoprene closed-cell foam (Hayes, 1985; Raymond, 1975) and the use of dry suits becomes necessary. With increasing pressure there is also the problem of nitrogen narcosis and helium is substituted in the breathing mixture. However, helium has a far greater thermal transport capacity and this, plus the fact that at increased pressures all gases have an increased capacity to transfer heat (MDC, 1982), means that at depth the rate of heat loss with helium can be as great as the heat loss which occurs on immersion in water (Raymond, 1975). As a result, if helium is circulating within a dry suit, the thermal protection provided is severely impaired. A dry suit is normally inflated with the breathing gas but, if the oxyhelium mixture could be replaced by a gas with low thermal conductivity such as air, the body heat loss would be greatly reduced even without additional heating (Lippitt and Nuckols, 1983).

Because of the severity of the cold stress additional heat has to be supplied, and though there are different methods (Hughes, 1976; Kettle, 1975; Rawlins, 1981; SUT, 1976) the most common method actually employed is to have a free flow of hot water from the surface over the diver, the rate of flow being regulated by the diver (Lippitt and Nuckols, 1983; MDC, 1982; SUT, 1975b). Because of the inefficiency and cost when this system is used with deep diving, electrically heated underwear is now being developed for use under a dry suit (Virr, 1985).

With increasing depth there is an increasing respiratory heat loss, and this is the subject of much investigation (Craig and Dvorak, 1976; Hoke *et al.*, 1976; Lippitt and Nuckols, 1983; Moore *et al.*, 1976; Varene *et al.*, 1976; Webb, 1976). Eventually not only will the respiratory heat loss, with the 100 per cent relative humidity of the exhaled gas, equal or exceed the total maximum metabolic heat production (Kettle, 1975; MDC, 1982) but the respiratory heat loss can become so great that the diver will become hypothermic even if the temperature of the water flowing over the body is raised to a level which will cause severe burns to the skin (Hughes, 1977). There is therefore a limiting depth/temperature factor (Kettle, 1975) and heating the inspired heliox is not only essential (Hughes, 1977; MDC, 1982; Rawlins, 1981) but is now mandatory (SUT, 1976) though the methods so far employed, which utilise hot water from the surface to warm the breathing loop (MDC, 1982), are inefficient (Hayes, 1985; Lippitt and Nuckols, 1983). The respiratory gas heater, in which the hot water heats the gas in line on the pipe supplying the gases, is satisfactory to a depth of 180 metres, but for deeper dives it is better to use the more efficient heater which is incorporated in a shroud on the diving helmet (Hayes, 1985). In commercial diving, certainly at the depths approached in operations in the North Sea, there is an additional reason for warming the inspired gases since cold dry helium can cause such an outpouring of the secretions of the respiratory tract (Hayes *et al.*, 1982) that the victim can virtually drown in his own secretions. Unfortunately if the gas is dry and heated too much it can also cause discomfort. If the respiratory gas heating is suddenly withdrawn during deep diving, the diver may collapse suddenly and too rapidly for the collapse to be due to hypothermia (Vanggaard, 1985).

The control of the respiratory heat loss becomes even more urgent in the 'lost bell' situation in deep diving because all heat from the surface is lost and the survival time for an unprotected diver is three to four hours (MDC, 1982). The rescue services consider they need 24 hours to be certain of retrieving a lost bell, but, even in an arctic-type sleeping bag, a diver in a totally unheated bell (equivalent to −90 °C) would not survive 24 hours unless the loss of heat and moisture, which normally occurs during breathing, was also prevented (Tonjum *et al.*, 1980). In case of failure of the power supply from the surface, all diving bells are equipped with accumulators supplying auxiliary power for lighting and for the carbon dioxide scrubbers, but the power capacity is not sufficient for heating (MDC, 1982). Even the self-contained submersible craft with its own power (Busby, 1976; SUT, 1975a) is not without risk. The people in the compressed lock-out section are at greater risk than those in the atmospheric driving section (Rawlins, 1981) but even the drivers are at risk if the submersible becomes trapped. In an experiment where a submersible lay in water at 4 °C (Kuehn *et al.*, 1977), after 25 hours the power failed rendering the carbon dioxide scrubbers inoperable and the carbon dioxide levels started to rise to near-toxic levels. By the same time the cold stress was causing a drop in core temperatures. In the experiment the submersible started with full power available whereas in the real situation some of the power will be exhausted before the problem arises and the accident is liable to disrupt some of the remaining power so that the experiment merely tested the best possible situation.

There must therefore be personal survival systems for divers operating out of bells or submersibles. The active systems, which have a chemical or electrical heating mechanism, tend to be too complex or too energy consuming and are susceptible to damage, especially since some items have to be mounted on the outside of the bell to save space (MDC, 1982). A passive system is the obvious solution and this must incorporate personal carbon dioxide scrubbers, which save the respiratory heat loss as well as the humidity from the exhaled gas, in addition to insulated clothing and sleeping bag (MDC, 1982). A series of experiments have been carried out simulating the lost bell situation in Norway (Brubakk *et al.*, 1982; Tonjum *et al.*, 1980), in Britain (Hayes *et al.*, 1981) and in Sweden (MDC, 1982), and from the progressive information gained some practical recommendations have been made (MDC, 1982).

There is a list of survival equipment which is kept in the bell, and a net, on which the divers lie, which is stretched across the bell to prevent direct contact with the cold walls of the bell, and to prevent a sleeping, exhausted or unconscious diver from blocking the hatch

(Hayes *et al.*, 1981). When a lost bell emergency occurs, the divers do all the strenuous physical work, such as fitting the net and stowing the diving gear, before drying themselves and putting on dry underclothes (MDC, 1982). If the thermal protective equipment is put on before doing the hard work, the perspiration soaks the garments and markedly reduces the insulation value (Hayes *et al.*, 1981). In addition to the thermal underwear, the rest of the equipment includes a hood, a quilted jacket with hood, synthetic fur gloves, quilted socks and a quality sleeping bag which has a zip down one side and a hood with a neck seal. Respiratory heat loss is prevented by a canister with the carbon-dioxide-absorbent soda lime. This not only acts as a condenser humidifier, trapping the heat and moisture lost when the victim breathes out to be returned to him on the next inspiration, but the carbon dioxide breathed out by the diver reacts with the soda lime gradually producing heat and moisture and resulting in a positive heat input (Hamilton, 1981 a, b; Lloyd, 1979 d). There are three spare soda lime canisters kept in the sleeping bag along with all the other emergency gear. The soda lime in use is inside the sleeping bag, which prevents it cooling and retains the maximum amount of heat. The canister is changed every seven hours without the diver having to open the sleeping bag. For a similar reason, plastic urine bags with liquid-absorbent material are kept in the bag and there is the secondary benefit that the heat voided with the urine is retained within the sleeping bag. The only time a diver has to open or leave the bag is to check the oxygen partial pressure every five hours and make appropriate adjustments (MDC, 1982). One slight but probably temporary problem is the rapid build-up of carbon dioxide while the divers are dressing in their protective clothing (Hayes *et al.*, 1981). The evidence suggested that this system could buy up to 24 hours' survival, the time considered to be sufficient for the rescue services to retrieve the bell. In a test continued over 24 hours, the fact that the core temperature remained above the hypothermic level of 35 °C for the whole period (Tonjum *et al.*, 1985) means that with these current methods the divers could be expected to survive longer than 24 hours if necessary.

It is undoubtedly true that the development of equipment to warm the inspired gases is going to be a major factor in preventing diving deaths and in allowing diving to take place at even greater depths than at present.

The diver, underwater because of work or leisure, may suffer injury as on land, but underwater the slightest mistake, accident or error or judgement carries a high risk of producing death from drowning. Another problem for divers is that they can cool to hypothermic levels without being aware of the cold and without shivering (Keatinge *et al.*, 1980) and the hot water flowing over the body surface may merely suppress the sense of cold and the impulse to shiver (Hong and Nadel, 1979). Even scuba divers may persist in a task despite cooling to hypothermic levels. In one study the men were unaware of cooling and resisted instructions from the surface, where their core temperature was being measured with a radiopill, that they should abandon the task and surface (Davis, 1979; Davis *et al.*, 1975). Since hypothermia can develop without any recognisable symptoms it is a possible cause of the 'sudden death syndrome' (McAniff, 1980) in which, though the victim has appeared to be all right, he is observed a few seconds or minutes later lying face down in the water with no physical responses. The victim has shown none of the classic signs of drowning such as thrashing about or cries for help but appears to have collapsed without warning. The 'buddy' system, with two divers responsible for keeping an eye on each other, is a safety measure but buddies may become parted due to inexperience or poor visibility and even with the buddy system it is possible to miss cases who have become hypothermic. It is certainly known that behavioural dysfunction — panic, anxiety, 'poor judgement' — contribute to death in between 20 and 40 per cent of diving fatalities, with experience and good training reducing the risks (Bradley, 1984; Rey, 1985). However, some of the pre-fatal actions of the divers are inexplicable and part of the answer may be through the effects of cold on the higher cerebral functions or through misinterpretations or even hallucinations. This is the only possible explanation for the diver, known to be cold before and during a dive, who severed his own life-line (Rawlins, 1981).

As an extra complication, visual recognition thresholds are impaired by increasing pressure (Banks *et al.*, 1979) which may be superimposed on the impairment due to cold and when it is considered that in many dives the environment is in darkness there is obviously a great potential for disaster. Powers of judgement are also affected by cold and in a study of scuba divers (Baddeley, 1966) the ability to judge or estimate the passage of time was significantly affected by the cold, resulting in slow time counts and underestimates of the passage of time, with the obvious risk of the diver running out of air. Free swimming divers face the additional hazard of currents which may be unknown and may carry them a long way from the support ship

(Anton, 1979).

In diving the hands are particularly exposed to cold and, as was discussed earlier, cold has a profound effect on the functions of the hand. For divers therefore special protection is needed for the hands (Hayes, 1985) and a special three-fingered glove has been found to be the most useful (Adolfson *et al.*, 1985).

Scuba divers face their own particular hazard from the cold. As the person cools he has to increase his heat production and this increases the oxygen requirement (Lippitt and Nuckols, 1983), and he therefore uses more air (Anon, 1974), which obviously increases the risk of running out of air while underwater. To get the increased air needed he has to breathe harder on the regulator and since this increases the work of breathing he may begin to think that he is low on air. Shivering aggravates the increased breathing requirement as also does any anxiety or panic and the combination of factors may lead to irrational decisions, resulting eventually in death (McAniff, 1980).

In arctic diving there is an additional hazard not present in other parts of the world. Because the water is saline it can still be liquid at −2 °C, and this may cause freezing of any fresh water present in the diver's equipment (Kuehn, 1985). If this freezing is of the water vapour from breathing and occurs in a diving gas regulator, the consequences may be disastrous (Kuehn, 1985).

APPENDIX: CONVERSION FACTORS FOR HEAT

1 cal = 4.18 joule
1 watt = 1 joule/s

BIBLIOGRAPHY

Aas, K. (1975) 'The effect of climate on respiratory allergy and bronchial asthma.' *Nordic Council Arct. Med. Res., Rep. No. 12*, pp. 48–50.

Achar, M.V.S.; Agarawala, I.P. (1972) 'Autonomic nerves and their transmitters in hypothermia.' *Indian J. Med. Sci.*, *26*, 467–9.

Adam, J.M. (1981) 'Cold weather; its characteristics, dangers and assessment.' In J.M. Adam (ed.) *Hypothermia Ashore and Afloat.* Aberdeen University Press, Aberdeen, pp. 6–14.

Adams, R.D. (1970) 'Sleep and its abnormalities.' In *Harrison's Principles of Internal Medicine, 6th Ed.* McGraw Hill, New York, pp. 157–63

Adelstein, A.M. (1973) 'Certification of hypothermia deaths.' *Br. Med. J.*, *i*, 482.

Admiralty Papers (1946) *Talbot Committee Report on Naval Lifesavings.*

Adolfson, J.A.; Sperling, L.; Gustavsson, M. (1985) 'Hand protection.' In L. Rey (ed.) *Arctic Underwater Operations.* Graham & Trotman, London, pp. 237–54.

Adolph, E.F. (1950) 'Oxygen consumption of hypothermic rats and acclimatisation to cold.' *Am. J. Physiol.*, *161*, 359–73.

Adriani, J.; Rovenstine, E.A. (1941) 'Experimental studies on carbon dioxide absorbers for anesthesia.' *Anesthesiology*, *2*, 1–19

Aldrete, J.A.; Cubillos, P. (1981) 'Humidity and temperature changes during low flow and closed system anaesthesia.' *Acta. Anaesth. Scand.*, *25*, 312–14

Alexander, G. (1979) 'Cold thermogenesis.' In D. Robertshaw (ed.) *Environmental Physiology III.* University Park Press, Baltimore, pp. 43–155.

Alexander, L. (1945) 'The treatment of shock from prolonged exposure to cold, especially in water.' *Combined Intelligence Objective Subcommittee, Item No. 24*, File No. 26–37.

Alexander, S. (1974) 'Effect of cold on the cardiovascular system." *Practitioner*, *213*, 785–9.

Allan, J.R.; Marcus, P.; Saxton, C. (1974) 'Effect of cold hands on emergency egress procedures.' *Aerospace Med.*, *45*, 479–81.

Allison, S.P.; Bastow, M.D. (1983) 'Undernutrition and femoral fracture.' *Lancet*, *i*, 933–4.

Althaus, U.; Aeberhard, P.; Schupbach, P.; Nachbur, B.H.; Muhlemann, W. (1982) 'Management of profound accidental hypothermia with cardiorespiratory arrest.' *Ann. Surg.*, *195*, 492–5.

——— ; Clerc, L.; Aeberhard, P.; Muhlemann, W. (1978) 'Treatment of profound accidental hypothermia with circulatory arrest.' *Praxis*, *67*, 1919–24.

American College of Sports Medicine (1984) 'Position statement; prevention of illness during distance running.' *The Physician and Sports medicine*, *12*, 43–51.

Andersen, P.K.; Hall, K.V.; Rasmussen, N.J.; Seerup, K. (1977) 'Burns after peroperative use of heated mattresses.' *Ugeskr. Laeger.*, *139*, 2568–70.

Anderson, F. (1981) 'Hypothermia in the elderly.' In J.M. Adam (ed.) *Hypothermia Ashore and Afloat.* Aberdeen University Press, Aberdeen, pp. 177–88.

Anderson, K.L.; Hellstrom, B.; Lorentzen, F.V. (1963) 'Combined effect of cold and alcohol on heat balance in man.' *J. Appl. Physiol.*, *18*, 975–82.

Anderson, S.; Herbring, B.G.; Widman, B. (1970) 'Accidental profound hypothermia; case report.' *Br. J. Anaesth.*, *42*, 653–5.

Andjus, R.K.; Smith, A.U. (1955) 'Reanimation of adult rats from body temperature between 0 and +2°C. *J. Physiol. (Lond.)*, *128*, 446–72.

Andrew, H.G. (1963) 'Work in extreme cold.' *Trans. Ass. Indust. Med. Off.*, *13*, 16–19.

Andrew, P.J.; Parker, R.S. (1978) 'Treating accidental hypothermia.' *Br. Med. J.*, *ii*, 1641.

Angelakos, E.T. (1959) 'Influence of pharmacological agents on spontaneous and surgically-induced ventricular fibrillation. *Ann. N. Y. Acad. Sci.*, *80*, 351–64.

Angus, R.G.; Pearce, D.G.; Buguet, A.G.C.; Olsen, L. (1979) 'Vigilance performance of men sleeping under arctic conditions.' *Aviat. Space Environ. Med.*, *50*, 692–6.

Anon (1974) 'Does a diver use more air in cold water?' *Nav. Res. Rev.*, *27*, 30.

Anton, Y. (1979) 'Drifting towards death.' *Readers' Digest, July*, 61–5.

Apps, M.C.P. (1983) 'Sleep-disordered breathing.' *Br. J. Hosp. Med.*, *28*, 339– 47.

Arborelius, M.; Balldin, U.I.; Lilja, B. Lundgren, C.E.G. (1972) 'Haemodynamic changes in man during immersion with head above water.' *Aerospace Med.*, *43*, 592–8.

Armstrong, H.G. (1936) 'The loss of tactical efficiency of flying personnel in open cockpit aircraft due to cold temperatures.' *Military Surgeon*, *79*, 133–40.

——— ; Heim, J.W. (1940) 'Medical problems of high altitude flying.' *J. Lab. Clin. Med.*, *26*, 263–71.

Arneil, G.C.; Kerr, M.M. (1963) 'Severe hypothermia in Glasgow infants during winter.' *Lancet*, *ii*, 756–9.

Aromaa, A.; Maatela, J.; Pyorala, K. (1977) 'Prevalence and incidence of hypertension in Finland, the social insurance institution's study on Finnish population groups.' *Nordic Council Arct. Med. Res.*, *Rep. No. 19*, pp. 88–94.

Aschoff, J.; Wever, R. (1958) 'Kern und Schale im Warmehaushalt des Menschen.' *Naturwissenchaften*, *20*, 477–85.

——— ; Biebach, H.; Heise, A.; Schmidt, T. (1974) 'Day-night variation in heat balance.' In J.L. Monteith and L.E. Mount (eds.) *Heat Loss from Animals and Man.* Butterworth, London, pp. 147–72.

Ashton, H. (1984) 'Benzodiazepine withdrawal: an unfinished story.' *Br. Med. J.*, *i*, 1135–40.

Atukorale, D.P. (1971) 'Accidental hypothermic coma at Adam's Peak.' *Ceylon Med. J.*, *17*, 100–3.

Auld, C.D. (1977) 'The oxygen requirements associated with shivering during hypothermia.' *Scot. Soc. Anaesth. Newsletter*, *18*, 28.

——— ; Light, I.M.; Norman, J.N. (1979) 'Accidental hypothermia and rewarming in dogs.' *Clin. Sci.*, *56*, 601–6.

Ayers, S. (1985) 'Survival.' *On Board*, *6*, *No. 2*, 59.

Back, O.; Larsen, A. (1978) 'Delayed cold urticaria.' *Acta Der. Venereol.*, *58*, 369–71.

Backman, C.; Linderholm, H. (1984) 'Effect of cold exposure on exercise tolerance and exercise ECG in patients with effort angina.' *Presentation at Sixth International Symposium on Circumpolar Health. May 13–18, 1984. Anchorage, Alaska.* Abstracts p. 101.

Baddeley, A.D. (1966) 'Time estimation and reduced body temperature.' *Am. J. Physiol.*, *70*, 475–9.

——— ; Cuccaro, W.J.; Egstrom, G.H.; Weltman, G.; Willis, M.A. (1975) 'Cognitive efficiency of divers working in cold water.' *Hum. Factors*, *17*, 446–54.

Bain, A.D.; Bartholemew, S.E.M. (1985) 'A review of the sudden infant death syndrome in south-east Scotland.' *Health Bull.*, *43*, 51–9.

Bain, J. (1984) 'Visual hallucinations in children receiving decongestants.' *Br. Med. J.*, *i*, 1688.

Bainton, D.; Moore, F.; Sweetnam, P. (1977) 'Temperature and deaths from ischaemic heart disease.' *Br. J. Prev. Soc. Med.*, *31*, 49–53.

Baker, S.; Atha, J. (1981) 'Canoists' disorientation following cold immersion.' *Br. J. Sports Med.*, *15*, 111–15.

Balfour, A.J.C. (1983) 'No drowning mark upon him.' *Aviat. Space Environ. Med.*, *54*, 1021–2.

——— ; Underwood-Ground, K.E.A. (1980) 'An unsuccessful ejection.' *Aviat. Space Environ. Med.*, *51*, 1050–1.

Balsvik, P-D.; Strass, P. (1975) 'The monthly incidence of respiratory tract infections (RTI) in Tromso 1969–73, related to meteorological variables.' *Nordic Council Arct. Med. Res., Rep. No. 12*, pp. 9–18.

Banks, W.W.; Berghage, T.E.; Heaney, D.M. (1979) 'Visual recognition thresholds in a compressed air environment.' *Aviat. Space Environ. Med.*, *50*, 1003–6.

Banssillon, V. (1985) 'Summary of the sessions on pathology.' In J. Rivolier, P. Cerretelli, J. Foray, P. Segantini (eds.) *High Altitude Deterioration.* Karger, Basel, pp. 216–20.

Barber, S.G. (1978) 'Drugs and doctorings for trans-Saharan Travellers.' *Br. Med. J.*, *ii*, 404–6.

Barbour, H.E.; Mackay, E.A.; Griffith, W.P. (1943) 'Water shifts in deep hypothermia.' *Am. J. Physiol.*, *140*, 9–19.

Barnard, C.N. (1956) 'Hypothermia: a method of intragastric cooling.' *Br. J. Surg.*, *44*, 296–8.

Barnes, P.J. (1984) 'Nocturnal asthma: mechanisms and treatment. *Br. Med. J.*, *i*, 1397–8.

Barone, R.P.; Caren, L.D. (1984) 'The immune system: effects of hypergravity and hypogravity.' *Aviat. Space Environ. Med.*, 55, 1063–8.

Barr, A.M.; Taylor, P. (1976) 'A case of drowning.' *Anaesthesia*, *31*, 651–7.

Barr, P.O.; Birke, G.; Liljedahl, S.O.; Plantin, L.O. (1968) 'Oxygen consumption and water loss during treatment of burns with warm dry air.' *Lancet*, *i*, 164–8.

Barrie, H. (1983) 'What you should know about SIDS.' *World Med.*, *July 9*, 38–40.

Bastow, M.D.; Rawlins, J.; Allison, S.P. (1983) 'Undernutrition, hypothermia, and injury in elderly women with fractured femur: an injury response to altered metabolism?' *Lancet*, *i*, 143–5.

Basycharov, Y.P.; Bozhedonov, V.V.; Klintsevich, C.M.; Popov, V.G. (1978) 'Acute renal insufficiency in cold trauma.' *Vestn. Khir.*, *121*, 78–80.

Baum, J.D.; Scopes, J.W. (1968) 'The silver swaddler. Device for preventing hypothermia in the new born.' *Lancet*, *i*, 672–3..

Bay, J.; Nunn, J.F.; Prys-Roberts, C. (1968) 'Factors influencing arterial PO_2 during recovery from anaesthesia.' *Br. J. Anaesth.*, *40*, 398–407.

Beart, P.M. (1982) 'Multiple dopamine receptors – new vistas.' In J.W. Lamble (ed.) *More About Receptors.* Elsevier Biomedical, Amsterdam, pp. 87–92.

Beavers, W.R. (1959) 'Hypothermia: effects of hypertonic solutions on incidence of ventricular fibrillation.' *Am. J. Physiol.*, *196*, 709–10.

——— ; Covino, B.G. (1959) 'Relation of potassium and calcium to hypothermic ventricular fibrillation.' *J. Appl. Physiol.*, *14*, 60–2.

——— ; Rogers, J.T. (1959) 'Hypothermia; alterations in cardiac and skeletal muscle electrolytes.' *Am. J. Physiol.*, *196*, 706–8.

Beckman, E.L.; Reeves, E. (1966) 'Physiological implications as to survival in water at 75 °F.' *Aerospace Med.*, *37*, 1135–42.

Bedford, T. (1946) *Environmental Warmth and its Measurement.* HMSO, London.

Beesley, L. (1912) *The Loss of the 'Titanic'*. Philip Allan, London.

Begin, R.; Epstein, M.; Sackner, M.A.; Levinson, R.; Dougherty, R.; Duncan, D. (1976) 'Effects of water immersion to the neck on pulmonary circulation and tissue volume in man.' *J. Appl. Physiol.*, *40*, 293–9.

Behnke, A.R.; Bauer, R.W. (1970) 'Cold injury and hypothermia.' In *Harrison's Principles of Internal Medicine, 6th Ed.* McGraw Hill, New York, pp. 700–3.

Belaud, A.; Barthelmy, L. (1979) 'Influence of body temperature on nitrogen transport and decompression sickness in fish.' *Aviat. Space Environ. Med.*, *50*, 672–7.

Belleau, R.; Durand, P.; Tremblay, N.; Duval, B.; Foggin, P. (1984) 'Respiratory health of an Inuit population.' *Presentation at Sixth International Symposium on Circumpolar Health. May 13–18, 1984. Anchorage, Alaska.* Abstracts p. 93.

Belopavlovic, M.; Buchtal, A. (1980) 'Cardiac arrest during moderate hypothermia for cerebrovascular surgery.' *Anaesthesia*, *35*, 368–71.

Benazon, D. (1974) 'Hypothermia.' In C.Scurr and S. Feldman (eds.) *Scientific Foundation of Anaesthesia.* Heinemann, London, pp. 344–57.

Bennett, P.B.; Elliott, D.H. (1969) *The Physiology and Medicine of Diving and Compressed Air Work.* Ballière, Tindall & Cassell, London.

Bentley-Phillips, C.B.; Eady, R.A.J.; Greaves, M.W. (1978) 'Cold urticaria; inhibition of cold induced histamine release by doxantrazole.' *J. Invest. Dermatol.*, *71*, 266–8.

Benton, W. (1973) 'Illusions and hallucinations.' *Macropaedia, Vol. 9. Encyclopaedia Brittanica*, London.

Benumof, J.L.; Wahrenbrock, E.A. (1977) 'Dependency of hypoxic pulmonary vasoconstriction on temperature.' *J. Appl. Physiol.*, *42*, 56–8.

Benveniste, D.; Pedersen, J.E.P. (1977) 'An attachment for the delivery of humidified gas.' *Anaesthesia*, *32*, 798–800.

Benzinger, T.H.; Kitsinger, C.; Pratt, A.W. (1963) *Temperature – Its Measurement and Control in Science and Industry. Part 3.* Reinhold, New York.

Beran, A.V.; Sperling, D.R. (1979) 'An improved method for inducing hypothermia and rewarming.' *Aviat. Space Environ. Med.*, *50*, 844–6.

Berger, P.A.; Barchas, J.D. (1981) 'Studies of β-Endorphin in patients with mental illness.' In C.H.Li (ed.) *Hormonal Proteins and Peptides. Vol. X, β-Endorphin*, Academic Press, London, pp. 293–311.

Berkeley, J.S. (1972) 'Treatment after exposure to cold.' *Lancet*, *i*, 378.

Bernbaum, J.C.; Russell, P.; Sheridan, P.H.; Gewitz, M.H.; Fox, W.W.; Peckham, G.J. (1984) 'Long-term follow-up of newborns with persistent pulmonary hypertension.' *Crit. Care Med.*, *12*, 579–83.

Bernhard, W.F. (1956) 'The effect of hypothermia on the peripheral serum levels of free 17-hydroxycorticoids.' In R.D. Dripps (ed.) *The Physiology of Induced Hypothermia.* Nat. Acad. Sci., New York, pp. 175–82.

Bernhartsen, J.C.; Schlenker, R. (1981) 'Cold water fatalities: an overview of physiological responses.' *Current/the Journal of Marine Education*, *2*, 6–9.

——— ; Reichle, M.N.; Davis, M.W. (1980) 'Hypothermia and cold water survival.' Tape/slide presentation. The Recreational Boating Institute Inc.

Berry, F.A.; Hughes-Davies, D.I.; di Fazio, C.A. (1973) 'A system for minimizing respiratory heat loss in infants during operation. *Anesth. Analg. (Cleve.)*, *52*, 170–5.

Besch, N.J.; Perlstein, P.H.; Edwards, N.K.; Keenan, W.J.; Sutherland, J.M. (1971) 'The transparent baby bag. A shield against heat loss.' *N. Engl. J.Med.*, *284*, 121–4.

Best, C.H.; Taylor, N.B. (1966) *The Physiological Basis of Medical Practice, 8th Ed.* Williams & Wilkins, Baltimore.

Bickel, L. (1977) *This Accursed Land.* Macmillan, London.

Biersner R.J. (1976) 'Motor and cognitive effects of cold water immersion under hyperbaric conditions.' *Hum. Factors*, *18*, 299–304.

Bigelow, W.G. (1959) 'Methods for inducing hypothermia and rewarming.' *Ann. N. Y. Acad. Sci.*, *80*, 522–32.

———; Hopps, J.A.; Callachan, J.C. (1952) 'Radio-frequency rewarming in resuscitation from severe hypothermia.' *Can. J. Med. Sci.*, *30*, 185–93.

———; Lindsay, W.K.; Harrison, R.C.; Gordon, A; Greenwood, W.F. (1950) 'Oxygen transport and utilisation in dogs at low body temperature.' *Am. J. Physiol.*, *160*, 125–37.

Bittel, J.; Marichy, J.; Henane, R.; Boussillon, V. (1977) 'Comparison of indirect calorimetry and direct heat flow discs. Results in measuring R + C heat loss in burned patients.' *Aviat. Space Environ. Med.*, *48*, 637–9.

BJA (1976) 'The effect of anaesthetic gas humidification on body temperature.' *Br. J. Anaesth.*, *48*, 504–5.

Bjerregaard, P. (1984a) 'Socio-economic conditions and infectious disease in Upernavik, Greenland.' *Presentation at Sixth International Symposium on Circumpolar Health. May 13–18, 1984, Anchorage, Alaska.* Abstracts p. 41.

——— (1984b) 'Regional variation in mortality from infectious disease in Greenland.' *Presentation at Sixth International Symposium on Circumpolar Health. May 13–18, 1984. Anchorage, Alaska.* Abstracts p. 87.

Blades, B.; Pierpont, H.C. (1954) 'A simple method of inducing hypothermia.' *Ann. Surg.*, *140*, 577–81.

Blair, E. (1964) 'Physiology of hypothermia.' In F. Blair, *Clinical Hypothermia.* McGraw Hill, New York, pp. 8–107.

——— (1969) 'Physiologic and metabolic effects of hypothermia in man.' In X.J. Mussacchia (ed.) *Depressed Metabolism.* Saunders, Elsevier, New York, pp. 525–68.

Bligh, J. (1973) 'Temperature regulation in mammals and other vertebrates.' In A. Neuberger and E.L. Tatum (eds.) *North-Holland Research Monographs, Vol. 30.* North–Holland Publishing, Amsterdam, pp. 80–4.

———; Chauca, D. (1978) 'The effects of intracerebroventricular injections of carbachol and noradrenaline on cold-induced pulmonary artery hypertension in sheep.' *J. Physiol. (Lond.)*, *284*, 53P.

———; Chauca, D. (1982) 'Effects of hypoxia, cold exposure and fever on pulmonary artery pressure, and their significance for arctic residents.' In B. Harvald and J.P. Hart Hansen (eds.) *Circumpolar Health '81.* Nordic Council for Arctic Medical Research, Report 32, Copenhagen, pp. 606–7.

———; Johnson, K.G. (1973) 'Glossary of terms for thermal physiology.' *J. Appl. Physiol.*, *35*, 941–61.

Blix, A.S. (1985) 'Diving response of mammals and birds.' In L. Rey (ed.) *Arctic Underwater Operations.* Graham & Trotman, London, pp. 73–80.

Bloch, J.H.; Dietzman, R.H.; Pierce, C.H.; Lillehei, R.C. (1966) 'Theories of the production of shock. A review of their relevance to clinical practice.' *Br. J. Anaesth.*, *38*, 234–50.

Bloch, M. (1965) 'Re-warming following prolonged hypothermia in man.' M.D. Thesis, University of London.

——— (1967a) 'Cerebral effects of rewarming following prolonged hypothermia; significance for the management of severe cranio-cerebral injury and acute pyrexia.' *Brain*, *90*, 769–84.

——— (1967b) 'Accidental hypothermia.' *Br. Med. J.*, *ii*, 376–7.

BMJ (1973) 'Sleep and metabolism.' *Br. Med. J.*, *iii*, 650.

——— (1975) 'Cold hypersensitivity.' *Br. Med. J.*, *i*, 643–4.

——— (1977a) 'The old in the cold.' *Br. Med. J.*, *i*, 336.

——— (1977b) 'Immersion and drowning in children.' *Br. Med. J.*, *ii*, 146–7.

——— (1978a) 'Preventing immersion hypothermia.' *Br. Med. J.*, *ii*, 1662–3.

——— (1978b) 'Treating accidental hypothermia.' *Br. Med. J.*, *ii*, 1383–4.

——— (1979) 'Drinking and drowning.' *Br. Med. J.*, *i*, 70–1.

——— (1980) 'Blows from the winter wind.' *Br. Med. J.*, *i*, 137–8.

——— (1981) 'Immersion or drowning.' *Br. Med. J.*, *i*, 1340–1.

Bodey, A.S. (1978) 'Changing cold acclimatization patterns of men living in Antarctica.' *Int. J. Biometeorol.*, *22*, 163–76.

Bonington, C. (1977) *Everest the Hard Way.* Appx 10 'Medicine' by C.R.A. Clarke. Arrow Books, London, p.337.

Bonnabeau, R.C.; Sterns, L.P.; Bilgutay, A.; Tkahashi, U.; Lillehei, C.W. (1963) 'Cardiac temperature gradients with various types of cardioplegia during cardiopulmonary bypass. *Surg. Gyn. Obs.*, *116*, 569–75.

Bonser, R.S.A.; Knight, B.H.; West, R.R. (1978) 'Sudden infant death syndrome in Cardiff, association with epidemic influenza and with temperature – 1955–1974.' *Int. J. Epidemiol.*, *7*, 335–40.

Booda, L.L. (1973) 'Tragedy in the Johnson-sea-link.' *Sea Technol.*, *14*, 17, 28, 58.
Bourke, D.L.; Wurm, H.; Rosenberg, M.; Russell, J. (1984) 'Intraoperative heat conservation using a reflective blanket.' *Anesthesiology*, *60*, 151–4.
Bowesman, R. (1981) 'Urban hypothermia.' *Br. Med. J.*, *i*, 474.
Boyan, C.P.; Howland, W.S. (1963) 'Cardiac arrest and temperature of bank blood.' *J. Am. Med. Ass.*, *183*, 58–60.
Bradbury, P.A.; Fox, R.H.; Goldsmith, R.; Hampton, I.F.G. (1964) 'The effect of exercise on temperature regulation.' *J. Physiol. (Lond.)*, *171*, 384–96.
Bradley, J.; Luff, D; Vallverdu, R.; Roberts-Thomson, P. (1984) 'Immunology.' *International Biomedical Expedition to the Antarctic.* Poster abstracts presented at 6th International Symposium Circumpolar Health, Anchorage, May 1984, pp. 70–1.
Bradley, M.E. (1984) 'Commercial diving fatalities.' *Aviat. Space Environ. Med.*, 55, 721–4.
Braestrup, C; Nielsen, M. (1983) 'Anxiety.' In *Neurotransmitters and CNS Disease. Lancet*, London, pp. 11–15.
Brash, J.C. (ed.) (1951) *Cunningham's Textbook of Anatomy*, Oxford University Press, London, p. 1235.
Braun, P. (1982) 'Hypothermia and primary internal diseases.' In P. Koch; M. Kohfahl (eds.) *Unterkuhlung im Seenotfall. 2nd Symposium.* Deutsche Gesellschaft zur Rettung Schiffbruchiger, Cuxhaven, pp. 100–11.
——— (1985) 'Pathophysiology and treatment of hypothermia.' In J. Rivolier, P. Cerretelli, J. Foray, P. Segantini (eds.) *High Altitude Deterioration.* Karger, Basel, pp. 140–8.
Brebbia, D.R.; Goldman, R.F.; Buskirk, E.R. (1957) 'Water vapor loss from the respiratory tract during outdoor exercise in the cold.' *J. Appl. Physiol.*, *11*, 219–22.
Brennan, P.J., Greenberg, G., Miall, W.E., Thompson, S.G. (1982) 'Seasonal variation in arterial blood pressure.' *Br. Med. J.*, *ii*, 919–23.
Brent, P. (1974) *Captain Scott and the Antarctic Tragedy.* Weidenfeld and Nicolson, London.
Briend, A.; de Schampheleire, I. (1981) 'Neonatal hypothermia in West Africa.' *Lancet*, *i*, 646–7.
Bristow, G. (1978) 'Treatment of accidental hypothermia with peritoneal dialysis.' *Can. Med. Ass. J.*, *118*, 764.
———; Smith, R.; Lee, J.; Auty, A.; Tweed, W.A. (1977) 'Cardiopulmonary arrest during hypothermia due to exhaustion and exposure.' *Can. Med. Ass. J.*, *117*, 247–9.
Bristow, G.K. (1981) 'Core rewarming by peritoneal lavage in accidental hypothermia.' *Cyrobiology*, *17*, 607.
British Mountaineering Council (1974) *Mountain Hypothermia.*
Brock, Lord (1975) 'Observations on peripheral and central temperatures with particular reference to the occurrence of vasoconstriction.' *Br. J. Surg.*, *62*, 589–95.
———; Skinner, J.M.; Manders, J.T. (1977) 'The importance of peripheral vasoconstriction in influencing body temperatures and the part played by certain environmental factors: the effect of inhaled gases.' *Br. J. Anaesth.*, *49*, 755–9.
Brooke, O.G. (1972a) 'Hypothermia in malnourished Jamaican children.' *Arch. Dis. Child.*, *47*, 525–30.
——— (1972b) 'Influence of malnutrition on the body temperature of children.' *Br. Med. J.*, *i*, 331–3.
——— (1972c) 'Malnutrition and body temperature.' *Br. Med. J.*, *ii*, 164.
———; Collins, J.E.; Fox, R.H.; James, S. (1973) 'Evaluation of a method for measuring urine temperature.' *J. Physiol. (Lond.)*, *231*, 91–3.
Brooks, C.J. (1984) 'Loss of cabin pressure in Canadian forces ejection seat aircraft.' *Aviat. Space Environ. Med.*, 55, 1154–63.
Brotherhood, J.R. (1975) 'Fitness and the relation of terrain and weather to fatigue and

accidental hypothermia in hill walkers.' In C. Clarke; M. Ward; E. Williams (eds.) *Mountain Medicine and Physiology.* Alpine Club, London, pp. 111–17.

Brown, E.B.; Miller, F.A. (1952) 'Ventricular fibrillation following rapid fall in carbon dioxide concentration.' *Am. J. Physiol.*, *169*, 56–60.

Brown, G.A.; Williams, G.M. (1982) 'The effect of head cooling on deep body temperature and thermal comfort in man.' *Aviat. Space Environ. Med.*, *53*, 583–6.

Brubakk, A.O.; Tonjum, S.; Holand, B.; Peterson, R.E; Hamilton, R.W.; Morild, E.; Onarheim, J. (1982) 'Heat loss and tolerance time during cold exposure in heliox atmosphere at 16 ATA.' *Undersea Biomed. Res.*, *9*, 81–90.

Brydon, J. (1977a) 'Making heated water beds work.' *Br. J. Clin. Equip.*, *2*, 39.

——— (1977b) 'Infant warmers under scrutiny.' *Br. J. Clin. Equip.*, *2*, 96.

Budd, G.M. (1965) 'Effect of cold exposure and exercise in a wet, cold Antarctic environment.' *J. Appl. Physiol.*, *20*, 417–22.

——— (1984) 'Daily fluid balance.' *International Biomedical Expedition to the Antarctic.* Poster abstracts presented at 6th International Symposium on Circumpolar Health, Anchorage, May 1984; pp. 59–60.

———; Brotherhood, J.R.; Thomas, D.W.; Beasley, F.A.; Hendrie, A.L.; Jeffrey, S.E.; Lincoln, G.J.; Porter, H.G.; Solaga, A.T.; Pidcock, L.M.; Baker, M.M. (1984) 'Infusion of noradrenaline.' *International Biomedical Expedition to the Antarctic.* Poster abstracts presented at 6th International Symposium on Circumpolar Health, Anchorage, May, 1984, pp. 30–1.

———; Hicks, K.E.; Macpherson, R.K. (1971) 'Death from exposure.' *Med. J. Aust.*, *2*, 1342.

Buetow, K.C.; Klein, P.H.; Klein, S.W. (1964) 'Effect of maintenance of "normal" skin temperature on survival of infants of low birth weight.' *Paediatrics*, *34*, 163–70.

Buguet, A.G.C.; Livingstone, S.D.; Reed, L.D. (1979a) 'Skin temperature changes in paradoxical sleep in man in the cold.' *Aviat. Space Environ. Med.*, *50*, 567–70.

———; Livingstone, S.D.; Reed, L.D.; Limmer, R.E. (1967) 'Cold induced shivering in men with thermoneutral skin temperatures.' *J. Appl. Physiol.*, *41*, 142–5.

———; Roussel, B.H.E.; Watson, W.J.; Radomski, M.W. (1979b) 'Cold-induced diminution of paradoxical sleep in man. *Electroencephalogr. Clin. Neurophysiol.*, *46*, 29–32.

Buky, B. (1970) 'Effect of magnesium on ventricular fibrillation due to hypothermia.'; *Br. J. Anaesth.*, *42*, 886–7.

Bull, G.M.; Morton, J. (1978) 'Environment, temperature and death rates.' *Age & Ageing*, *7*, 210–24.

Burch, G.E.; Giles, T.D. (1974) 'Cold hypersensitivity.' *Arch. Intern. Med.*, *134*, 663–8.

Burch, P.R.J. (1984) 'End of static decade for coronary disease?' *Br. Med. J.*, *ii*, 1142.

Burgess, K.R.; Whitelaw, W.A. (1984) 'Effects of nasal breathing at different temperatures on CO_2 sensitivity dyspnea and alae nasi EMG activity.' *Presentation at Sixth International Symposium on Circumpolar Health. May 13–18, 1984. Anchorage, Alaska.* Abstracts p. 207.

Burks, T.F.; Rosenfeld, G.C. (1979) 'Narcotic analgesics.' In P. Lomax and E. Schonbaum (eds.) *Body Temperature: Regulation, Drug Effects, and Therapeutic Implications.* Marcel Dekker, New York, pp. 531–50.

Burton, A.C.; Edholm, O.G. (1955) *Man in a Cold Environment.* Edward Arnold, London.

Burton, R. (1981) 'Fighting hypothermia with new developments.' *Lloyd's List, Wed. June 10*, 6, cols. 1–4.

Busby, R.F. (1976) *Manned Submersibles.* Office of the Oceanographer of the Navy, Washington.

Buskirk, E.R. (1977) 'Temperature regulation with exercise.' *Exerc. Sport Sci. Rev.*,

5, 45–88.

Butler, P.J. (1985) 'The diving reflex in free-diving birds.' In L.Rey (ed.) *Arctic Underwater Operations.* Graham & Trotman, London, pp. 49–62.

Butler, R.N.; Stalowitz, A. (1978) 'A winter hazard for the old: accidental hypothermia. Nurs. Care, *11*, 16–17.

Cabanac, M.; Massonet, B. (1977) 'Thermoregulatory responses as a function of core temperature in humans.' *J. Physiol.*, *33*, 699–703.

Calderwood, H.W.; Modell, J.H.; Ruiz, B.C. (1975) 'The ineffectiveness of steroid therapy for treatment of fresh water near-drowning.' *Anesthesiology, 43*, 642–50.

Caldwell, F.T. (1962) 'Metabolic response to thermal trauma. II Nutritional studies with rats in two environmental temperatures.' *Ann. Surg.*, *155*, 119–26.

Caldwell, P.R.B.; Gomez, D.M.; Fritts, H.W. (1969) 'Respiratory heat exchange in normal subjects and in patients with pulmonary disease.' *J. Appl. Physiol.*, *26*, 82–8.

Callaghan, P.B.; Lister, J.; Paton, B.C.; Swan, H. (1961) 'Effect of varying carbon dioxide tensions on the oxyhaemoglobin dissociation curves under hypothermic conditions.' *Ann. Surg.*, *154*, 903–10.

Calverley, P.M.A.; Leggett, R.J.; McElderry, L.; Flenley, D.C. (1982) 'Cigarette smoking and secondary polycythaemia in hypoxic cor pulmonale.' *Am. Rev. Respir. Dis.*, *125*, 507–10.

Calvert, D.G. (1962) 'Inadvertant hypothermia in paediatric surgery and a method for its prevention.' *Anaesthesia*, *17*, 29–45.

Campbell, D.I.; Shanks, C.A.; Flachs, J.; Austin, P. (1975) 'Accurate volume ventilation of neonates with maintenance of humidification.' *Anaesth. Intensive Care*, *3*, 295–8.

Campbell, I.A. (1972) 'Mountain accidents.' *Br. J. Sports Med.*, 6, 108–10.

Campbell, R.M.; Cuthbertson, D.P. (1966) 'Effect of environmental temperature on the metabolic response to injury.' *Nature*, *210*, 206–8.

——; Cuthbertson, D.P. (1967) 'Effect of environmental temperature on the metabolic response to injury.' *Quart. J. Exp. Physiol.*, *52*, 114–29.

Caplan, L.R.; Neely, S.; Gorelick, P. (1984) 'Cold-related intracerebral haemorrhage.' *Arch. Neurol.*, *41*, 227.

Cargill, D. (1982) 'Are we failing in our duty? *World Med.*, *Jan. 23*, 19–20

Carlini, E.A.; Lindsey, C.J. (1974) 'Pharmacological manipulation of brain catecholamines and the aggressive behaviour induced by marihuana in REM-sleep deprived rats.' *Aggressive Behaviour*, *1*, 81–99.

Carlson, L.D.; Hsieh, A.C.L. (1965) 'Cold.' In O.G. Edholm and A.L. Bacharach (eds.) *The Physiology of Human Survival.* Academic Press, London, pp. 15–52.

Carlsson, C.; Hagerdal, M.; Seisjo, B.K. (1976) 'Protectvie effect of hypothermia in cerebral oxygen deficiency caused by arterial hypoxia.' *Anesthesiology*, *44*, 27–35.

Carne, J. (1979) 'Hypothermia in the elderly.' *Br. Med. J.*, *i*, 690.

Carson, J.; Postl, B; Schaefer, O.; Spady, D. (1984) 'Lower respiratory tract infections among Canadian Inuit children. *Presentation at Sixth International Symposium on Circumpolar Health. May 13–18, 1984. Anchorage, Alaska.* Abstracts p. 67.

Carstenson, E.L.; Li, K.; Schwan, H.P. (1953) 'Determination of the acoustic properties of blood and its components.' *J. Acoustical Soc. Am.*, *25*, 286–9.

Catford, J.C.; Ford, S. (1984) 'On the state of the public ill health: premature mortality in the United Kingdom and Europe. *Br. Med. J.*, *ii*, 1668–70.

Cena, K.; Clark, J.A. (1979) 'Transfer of heat through animal coats and clothing.' In D. Robertshaw (ed.) *Environmental Physiology iii.* University Park Press, Baltimore, pp. 1–42.

Cerretelli, P.; di Prampero, P.E. (1985) 'Aerobic and anaerobic metabolism during exercise at altitude.' In J. Rivolier, P. Cerretelli, J. Foray, P. Segantini (eds.) *High Altitude Deterioration.* Karger, Basel, pp. 1–19.

Chalon, J.; Ramanathan, S. (1974) 'Water vapour heated by the reaction of neutralisation by carbon dioxide.' *Anesthesiology*, *41*, 400–4.

———; Ali, M.; Turndorf, H.; Fischgrund, G.K. (1981) *Humidification of Anesthetic Gases.* Charles C. Thomas, Springfield, Ill.

———; Kao, Z.L.; Dolorico, V.N.; Atkin, D.H. (1973) 'Humidity output of the circle absorber system.' *Anesthesiology*, *38*, 458–65.

———; Loew, D.A.; Malebranche, J. (1972) 'Effects of dry anaesthetic gases on tracheobronchial abated epithelium.' *Anesthesiology*, *37*, 338–43.

———; Markham, J.P.; Ali, M.M.; Ramanathan, S.; Turndorf, H. (1984) 'The Pall Ultipor breathing circuit filter – an efficient heat and moisture exchanger.' *Anesth. Analg. (Cleve)*, *63*, 566–70.

———; Patel, C.; Ali, M.; Ramanathan, S.; Capan, L.; Tang, C–K.; Turndorf, H. (1979b) 'Humidity and the anesthetised patient. *Anethesiology*, *50*, 195–8.

———; Patel, C.; Ramnathan, S.; Turndorf, H. (1978) 'Humidification of the circle absorber system.' *Anesthesiology*, *48*, 142–5.

———; Ramanathan, M.A.S.; Turndorf, H. (1979a) 'The humidification of anaesthetic gases: its importance and control.' *Can. Anaesth. Soc. J.*, *26*, 361–6.

Chambers, J.J.; Saha, H.K. (1979) 'Case report. Electrocution during anaesthesia.' *Anaesthesia*, *34*, 173–5.

Chamney, A.R. (1969) 'Humidification requirements and techniques. *Anaesthesia*, *24*, 602–16.

Cherniak, R.M.; Cherniak, L.; Norimark, A. (1972) *Respiration in Health and Disease.* W.B. Saunders, Philadelphia.

Chernow, B.; Lake, C.R.; Zaritzky, A.; Finton, C.K.; Casey, L.; Rainey, T.G.; Fletcher, J.R. (1983) 'Sympathetic nervous system "switch off" with severe hypothermia.' *Crit. Care Med.*, *11*, 677–80.

Chinard, F.P. (1979) 'Hypothermia treatment requires controlled studies.' *Ann. Intern. Med.*, *90*, 990–1.

Chiswick, M. (1978) *Neonatal Medicine.* Update Publications, London.

Choi, W.W.; Gergis, S.D.; Sokoll, M.D. (1985) 'Controversies in muscle relaxants. *Seminars in Anesth.*, *4*, 73–80.

Church, M.A. (1974) 'Prevention of accidental hypothermia.' *Br. Med. J.*, *i*, 159.

Clark, R.E.; Jones, C.E. (1962) 'Manual performance during cold exposure as a function of practice level and thermal conditions of training.' *J. Appl. Physiol.*, *46*, 276–80.

———; Orkin, L.R.; Rovenstine, E.A. (1954) 'Body temperature studies in anesthetised man: effect of environmental temperature, humidity and anesthesia system.' *J. Am. Med. Ass.*, *154*, 311–19.

Clark, R.P.; Toy, N. (1975a) 'Natural convection around the human head.' *J. Physiol. (Lond.)*, *244*, 283–93.

———; Toy, N. (1975b) 'Forced convection round the human head.' *J. Physiol. (Lond.)*, *244*, 295–302.

———; Mullan, B.J.; Pugh, L.G.C.E. (1974a) 'Colour thermography in running.' *J. Physiol. (Lond.)*, *239*, 81–2.

———; Mullan, B.J.; Pugh, L.G.C.E.; Toy, N. (1974b) 'Heat loss from the moving limb in running: the "pendulum" effect.' *J. Physiol. (Lond.)*, *240*, 8–9.

Clarke, C. (1976) 'On surviving a bivouac at high altitude.' *Br. Med. J.*, *i*, 92–3.

Clarke, R.S.J.; Hellon, R.F.; Lind, A.R. (1958) 'The duration of sustained contractions of the human forearm at different muscle temperature.' *J. Physiol. (Lond.)*, *143*, 454–73.

Close, W.H.; Mount, L.E. (1978) 'The effects of plane of nutrition and environmental temperature on the energy metabolism of the growing pig: 1. Heat loss and critical temperature.' *Br. J. Nutr.*, *40*, 413–22.

Cohen, N.M. (1968) 'Severe cold injury in London.' *Practitioner*, *200*, 403–10.

Cole, P. (1953a) 'Some aspects of temperature, moisture and heat relationships in the upper respiratory tract.' *J. Laryng. Otol.*, *67*, 449–56.

——; (1953b) 'Further observations on the conditioning of the respiratory air.' *J. Laryng. Otol.*, *67*, 669–81.

—— (1954a) 'Recordings of respiratory air temperature.' *J. Laryng. Otol.*, *68*, 295–307.

—— (1954b) 'Respiratory mucosal responses, air conditioning and thermoregulation.' *J. Laryng. Otol.*, *68*, 613–22.

Coleshaw, S.R.; van Someren, R.N.M.; Wolff, A.H.; Davis, H.M.; Keatinge, W.R. (1983) 'Impaired memory registration and speed of reasoning caused by low body temperature.' *J. Appl. Physiol.*, 55, 27–31.

Colin, J.; Timbal, I.; Houdas, Y.; Boutelier, C.; Guieu, J.P. (1971) 'Computation of mean body temperature from rectal and skin temperatures.' *J. Appl. Physiol.*, *31*, 484–9.

Collins, K.J. (1983a) 'Urban hypothermia in the United Kingdom.' In R.S. Pozos and L.E. Wittmers (eds.) *The Nature and Treatment of Hypothermia.* Croom Helm, London/University of Minnesota, Minneapolis, pp. 235–7.

—— (1983b) *Hypothermia: The Facts.* Oxford University Press, Oxford.

—— (1983c) Discussion. In R.S. Pozos and L.E. Wittmers (eds.) *The Nature and Treatment of Hypothermia.* Croom Helm, London/University of Minnesota Press, Minneapolis, p. 257.

——; Exton-Smith, A.N (1979) 'Oral temperature and hypothermia. *Br. Med. J.*, *i*, 887.

——; Exton-Smith, A.N. (1981) 'Urban hypothermia: thermoregulation, thermal perception and thermal comfort in the elderly.' In J.N. Adams (ed.) *Hypothermia Ashore and Afloat.* Aberdeen University Press, Aberdeen, pp. 158–76.

——; Dore, C., Exton-Smith, A.N.; Fox, R.H.; MacDonald, I.C.; Woodward, P.M. (1977) 'Accidental hypothermia and impaired temperature homeostasis in the elderly.' *Br. Med. J.*, *i*, 353–6.

——; Exton-Smith, A.N., Dore, C. (1981) 'Urban hypothermia: preferred temperature and thermal perceptions in old age.' *Br. Med. J.*, *i*, 175–7.

Collis, M.L.; Steinman, A.M.; Chaney, R.D. (1977) 'Accidental hypothermia; an experimental study of practical rewarming methods.' *Aviat. Space Environ. Med.*, *48*, 625–32.

Colquohoun, W.P. (1984) 'Effects of personality on body temperature and mental efficiency following transmeridian flight.' *Aviat. Space Environ. Med.*, 55, 493–6.

——; Paine, M.W.P.H.; Fort, A. (1978) 'Circadian rhythm of body temperature during prolonged undersea voyages.' *Aviat. Space Environ. Med.*, *49*, 671–8.

Committee on Exercise (1972) *Exercise Testing and Exercise Training of Apparently Healthy Individuals: A Handbook for Physicians.* American Heart Association, New York.

Coniam, S.W. (1979) 'Accidental hypothermia.' *Anaesthesia*, *34*, 250–6.

Conn, A.W. (1979a) 'Near-drowning and hypothermia.' *Can. Med. Ass. J.*, *120*, 397–400.

—— (1981) 'Submersion hypothermia.' *Hypothermia and Hyperthermia in Anaesthesia and Intensive Care.* Faculty of Anaesthetists Scientific Meeting, Royal College of Surgeons, London. Nov. 5 and 6.

——; Barker, G.A. (1984) 'Fresh water drowning and near-drowning – an update.' *Can. Anaesth. Soc. J.*, *31*, S38–44.

——; Barker, G.A; Edmonds, J.F.; Bonn, D.J. (1983) 'Submersion hypothermia and near-drowning. In R.S. Pozos and L.E. Wittmers (eds.) *The Nature and Treatment of Hypothermia.* Croom Helm, London/University of Minnesota Press, Minneapolis, pp. 152–64.

Conn, M.L. (1979b) 'Evaluation of Inhalation Rewarming as a Therapy for Hypothermia'. M.Sc. Thesis, Simon Fraser University.

Cook, G. (1978) 'Ordeal in the Indian Ocean.' *Reader's Digest*, *June*, 54–9.

Cools, A.R. (1982) 'The puzzling "cascade" of multiple receptors for dopamine: an appraisal of the current situation.' In J.W. Lamble (ed.) *More About Receptors.* Elsevier Biomedical, Amsterdam, pp. 76–86.

Cooper, J.R.; Bloom, F.E.; Roth, R.H. (1982) *The Biochemical Basis of Neuropharmocology.* Oxford University Press, Oxford.

Cooper, K.E. (1961) 'The circulation in hypothermia.' *Br. Med. Bull.*, *17*, 48–51.

——— (1976) 'Mechanisms of human cold adaptation.' In R.J. Shephard and S. Itoh (eds.) *Circumpolar Health.* Toronto University Press, Toronto, pp. 37–46.

———; Ferguson, A.V. (1983) 'Thermoregulation and hypothermia in the elderly.' In R.S. Pozos and L.E. Wittmers (eds.) *The Nature and Treatment of Hypothermia.* Croom Helm, London/University of Minnesota Press, Minneapolis, pp. 35–45.

———; Kenyon, J.R. (1957) 'A comparison of temperatures measured in the rectum, oesophagus, and on the surface of the aorta during hypothermia in man.' *Br. J. Surg.*, *44*, 616–19.

———; Ross, D.N. (1960) *Hypothermia in Surgical Practice.* F.A. Davis, Philadelphia.

———; Cranston, W.I.; Snell, E.S. (1964a) 'Temperature in the external auditory meatus as an index of central temperature changes. *J. Appl. Physiol.*, *19*, 1032–5.

———; Hunter, A.K.; Keatinge, W.R. (1964b) 'Accidental hypothermia.' *Int. Anesth. Clin.*, *2*, 999–1013.

———; Lomax, P.; Schonbaum, E. (1977) *Drugs, Biogenic Amines and Body Temperature.* Karger, Basel.

———; Martin, S.; Riben, P. (1976) 'Respiratory and other responses of subjects immersed in cold water.' *J. Appl. Physiol.*, *40*, 903–10.

Coopwood, T.B.; Kennedy, J.H. (1971) 'Accidental hypothermia.' *Cryobiology*, *7*, 243–8.

Coppin, E.G.; Livingstone, S.P.; Kuehn, L.A. (1978) 'Cold-decreased grip strength: Effects on handgrip strength due to arm immersion in a 10 °C water bath.' *Aviat. Space Environ. Med.*, *49*, 1322–6.

Coudert J. (1985) 'High-altitude pulmonary edema.' In J. Rivolier, P. Cerretelli, J. Foray, P. Segantini (eds.) *High Altitude Deterioration.* Karger, Basel, pp. 90–102.

Coughlin, F. (1973) 'Heart warming procedure.' *New Engl. J. Med.*, *288*, 326.

Covino, B.G.; Hegnauer, A.H. (1955) 'Ventricular excitability cycle; its modification by pH and hypothermia. *Am. J. Physiol.*, *181*, 553–8.

Cox, B. (1979) 'Dopamine.' In P. Lomax and E. Schonbaum (eds.) *Body Temperature: Regulation, Drug Effects, and Therapeutic Implications.* Marcel Dekker, New York, pp. 231–56.

———; Lomax, P.; Milton, A.S.; Schonbaum, E. (1980) *Thermoregulatory Mechanisms and their Therapeutic Implications.* Karger, Basel.

Craig, A.B. (1976) 'Summary of 58 cases of loss of consciousness during underwater swimming and diving.' *Med. Sci. Sports*, *8*, 171–5.

———; Dvorak, M. (1975) 'Expiratory reserve volume and vital capacity of the lungs during immersion in water.' *J. Appl. Physiol.*, *38*, 5–7.

———; Dvorak, M. (1976) 'Heat exchanges between man and the water environment.' In C.J. Lambertson (ed.) *Underwater Physiology V. FASEB*, Bethesda, pp. 765–74.

Cranston, W.I. (1966) 'Temperature regulation.' *Br. Med. J.*, *ii*, 69–75.

Crawford, A.; Plant, M.A.; Kreitman, N.; Latcham, R.W. (1984) 'Regional variations in British alcohol morbidity rates: a myth uncovered? 11: population surveys.' *Br. Med. J.*, *ii*, 1343–5.

Crawford, J.P. (1979) 'Endogenous anxiety and circadian rhythms.' *Br. Med. J.*, *i*, 662.

Cremona-Barbaro, A. (1983) 'Propranolol and depression.' *Lancet*, *i*, 185.

Criley, J.M.; Blaufuss, A.J.; Kissel, G.L. (1976) 'Cough-induced cardiac compression.' *J. Am. Med. Ass.*, *236*, 1246–50.

Crino, M.H.; Nagel, E.L. (1968) 'Thermal burns caused by warming blankets in the operating room.' *Anesthesiology*, *29*, 149–50.
Cross, J.H. (1981) 'Survival and rescue at sea.' In J.N. Adams (ed.) *Hypothermia Ashore and Afloat.* Aberdeen University Press, Aberdeen, pp. 125–33.
Cross, K.W.; Stratton, D. (1974) 'Aural temperature of the newborn infant.' *Lancet*, *ii*, 1179–80.
Cross, S.H.; Stilling, J.B. (1976) *Mountain Accidents.* Terence Howarth, Kendal.
Crow, T.J. (1980) 'Molecular pathology of schizophrenia; more than one disease process?' *Br. Med. J.*, *i*, 66–8.
Cumming, R.P. (1975) 'Medical problems of oil development in Shetland.' *Scot. Med. J.*, *20*, 146–7.
Cundy, J.M. (1972) 'Hypothermia during surgery.' *Anaesthesia*, *27*, 105.
——— (1980) 'Metallized plastic sheeting.' *Br. J. Anaesth.*, *52*, 359.
Curley, J.; Almeyda, J.R. (1979) 'Ice age ulcers.' *Br. Med. J.*, *i*, 412.
Currie, J. (1798) *Medical Reports on the Effects of Water, Cold and Warm, as a Remedy in Fever and Other Diseases Whether Applied to the Surface of the Body or Internally.* Caddell & Davies, London, Appx 2, pp. 20–5.
Currie, M.A.; Currie, A.L. (1984) 'Ketamine: effect of literacy on emergence phenomena.' *Ann. Roy. Coll. Surg.*, *66*, 424–5.
Curtius, H. Ch.; Niederwieser, A.; Levine, R.A.; Lovenberg, W.; Woggon, B.; Angst, J. (1983) 'Successful treatment of depression with tetrahydrobiopterin.' *Lancet*, *i*, 657–8.
Cuthbertson, D.P.; Smith, C.M.; Tilstone, W.J. (1968) 'The effect of transfer to a warm environment (30 °C) on the metabolic response to injury.' *Br. J. Surg.*, *55*, 513–16.
Daily Mail. (1976) 'Dying man refused bed.' *Daily Mail, Dec. 2*, *3*, Col. 4.
Dalgleish, D.G. (1969) 'Treatment of exposure.' *J.R. Coll. Gen. Pract.*, *18*, 297–9.
Dalhamm, T. (1956) 'Mucus flow and ciliary activity in the trachea of healthy rats and rats exposed to respiratory irritant gases (SO_2, H_3N, HCHO).' *Acta. Physiol. Scand.*, *36*, Supp. 123, 1–161.
Daly, B.M.; Marks, J.M.; Heaney, M. (1984) 'Mast cells and the skin.' *Hospital Update*, *10*, 815–22.
Daly, M. deB.; Elsner, R.; Angell-James, J.E. (1977) 'Cardiorespiratory control by carotid chemoreceptors during experimental dives in the seal.' *Am. J. Physiol.*, *232*, H508–16.
Dangel, P.; Hossli, G. (1979) 'Medizinische Massnahmen nach Auffinden eines Lawinenverschutteten.' In P. Matter, P. Braun, M. deQuervain, W. Good (eds.) *Skifahren und Sicherheit III.* Buchdruckerei Davos AG, Davos, pp. 186–201.
Danzl, D.F. (1983) 'Accidental hypothermia.' In P. Rosen, F.J. Baker, G.R. Braen, R.H. Dailey, R.C. Levy (eds.) *Emergency Medicine, Concepts and Clinical Practice, Vol 2: Trauma*, Mosby, Boston, pp. 477–96.
Darim, F.; Reza, H. (1970) 'Effect of induced hypothermia and rewarming on renal haemodynamics in anaesthetised dog.' *Life Sci.*, *9*, 1153–63.
Darnall, R.A.; Ariagno, R.L. (1978) 'Minimal oxygen consumption in infants cared for under overhead radiant warmers, compared with conventional incubators.' *J. Paediatr.*, *93*, 283–7.
Davies, D.M.; Millar, E.J.; Miller, I.A. (1967) 'Accidental hypothermia treated by extracorporeal blood warming.' *Lancet*, *i*, 1036–7.
Davies, L.W. (1975a) 'Treatment of hypothermia.' *Lancet*, *ii*, 656.
——— (1975b) 'The deep domestic bath treatment for advanced cases of hypothermia. In C. Clarke, M. Ward, E. Williams (eds.) *Mountain Medicine and Physiology.* Alpine Club, London, pp. 14–16.
——— (1979) 'The deep bath treatment for accidental hypothermia.' In P. Matter, P. Braun, M. deQuervain, W. Good (eds.) *Skifahren und Sicherheit III.* Buchdruckerei Davos AG, Davos, pp. 183–5.

Davis, F.M. (1979) 'Diving and hypothermia.' *Br. Med. J.*, *ii*, 494.

——; Baddeley, A.D.; Hancock, T. (1975) 'Diver performance: the effect of cold.' *Undersea Biomed. Res.*, *2*, 195–213.

Day, R.; Hardy, J.D. (1942) 'Respiratory metabolism in infancy and in childhood.' *Am J. Dis. Child.*, *63*, 1086–95.

Day, R.L.; Caliguiri, L.; Kamenski, C.; Ehrlich, F. (1964) 'Body temperature and survival of premature infants.' *Paediatrics*, *34*, 171–81.

de Meirleir, K.; Arentz, T.; Hollman, W.; Vanhaelst, L. (1985) 'The role of endogenous opiates in thermal regulation of the body during exercise.' *Br. Med. J.*, *i*, 739–40.

de Pay, A.W. (1982) 'Medical treatment of hypothermic victims.' In P. Koch and M. Kohfahl (eds.) *Unterkuhlung im Seenotfall. 2nd Symposium.* Deutsche Gesellschaft zur Rettung Schiffbruchiger, Cuxhaven, pp. 146–53.

de Quervain, M. (1979) 'Physical principles of hypoxia and hypothermia in the avalanche.' In P. Matter, P. Braun, M. de Quervain, W. Good (eds.) *Skifahren und Sicherheit III.* Buchdruckerei Davos AG, Davos, pp. 137–42.

de Saintonge, D.M.C.; Cross, K.W.; Hathorn, M.K.S.; Lewis, S.R.; Stothers, J.K. (1979) 'Hats for the newborn infant.' *Br. Med. J.*, *ii*, 570–1.

de Villota, E.D.; Barat, G.; Peral, P.; de Miguel, J.M.F.; Avello, F. (1973) 'Recovery from profound hypothermia with cardiac arrest after immersion.' *Br. Med. J.*, *iv*, 394–5.

Deacon, E.L.; Williams, A.L. (1982) 'The incidence of the sudden infant death syndrome in relation to climate.' *Int. J. Biometior.*, *26*, 207–18.

Deal, E.C.; McFadden, E.R.; Ingram, R.H.; Breslin, F.J.; Jaeger, J.J. (1980) 'Airway responsiveness to cold air and hyperpnea in normal subjects and in those with hay fever and asthma.' *Am. Rev. Respir. Dis.*, *121*, 621–8.

——; McFadden, E.R.; Ingram, R.H.; Jaeger, J.J. (1978) 'Effects of atropine on potentiation of exercise-induced bronchospasm by cold air.' *J. Appl. Physiol.*, *45*, 238–43.

——; McFadden, E.R.; Ingram, R.H.; Jaeger, J.J. (1979a) 'Role of respiratory heat exchange in production of exercise-induced asthma.' *J. Appl. Physiol.*, *46*, 467–75.

——; McFadden, E.R.; Ingram, R.H.; Jaeger, J.J. (1979b) 'Esophageal temperature during exercise in asthmatic and non-asthmatic subjects.' *J. Appl. Physiol.*, *46*, 484–90.

Dembo, A.G. (1957) 'External respiratory failure.' *Medgiz.*, *15*, 229–312.

Dery, R. (1971) 'Humidity in anaesthesiology: IV. Determination of the alveolar humidity and temperature in the dog.' *Can. Anaesth. Soc. J.*, *18*, 145–51.

—— (1973a) 'The evolution of heat and moisture in the respiratory tract during anaesthesia with a non-rebreathing system.' *Can. Anaesth. Soc. J.*, *20*, 296–309.

—— (1973b) 'Water balance of the respiratory tract during ventilation with a gas mixture circulated at body temperature.' *Can. Anaesth. Soc. J.*, *20*, 719–27.

——; Peeletier, J.; Jaques, A.; Clavet, M.; Houde, J.J. (1967a) 'Humidity in anaesthesiology: II. Evolution of heat and moisture in the large carbon dioxide absorbers.' *Can. Anaesth. Soc. J.*, *14*, 205–19.

——; Peeletier, J.; Jaques, A.; Clavet, M.; Houde, J.J. (1967b) 'Humidity in anaesthesiology: III. Heat and moisture patterns in the respiratory tract during anaesthesia with the semi-closed system.' *Can. Anaesth. Soc. J.*, *14*, 287–98.

DHSS (1976) *Prevention and health: everybody's business.* HMSO, London.

Dill, D.B.; Forbes, W.H. (1941) 'Respiratory and metabolic effects of hypothermia.' *Am. J. Physiol.*, *132*, 685–97.

Dinwoodie, E. (1977) 'The suicide squads.' *Weekend Scotsman, March* 5, 1, Col. 3.

Doolittle, W.; Hayward, J.; Mills, W.; Nemiroff, M.; Samuelson, T. (1982) *State of Alaska, hypothermia & cold water near drowning guidelines.* Alaska Department of Health & Social Services, Pouch H-06C, Juneau, Alaska.

Doolittle, W.H. (1977) 'Disturbances due to cold.' In H.F. Conn (ed.) *Current Therapy 1977.* Saunders, Philadelphia, pp. 972–1045.

Dorsey, J.S. (1983) Letter *Ann. Surg.*, *198*, 668–9.

Dowle, H. (1977) 'Record attempt wrecked the 'Titanic'.' *Weekend Scotsman, July 23*, 2, Cols. 1–8.

Downey, J.A.; Chiodi, H.P.; Darling, R.C. (1967) 'Central temperature regulation in the spinal man.' *J. Appl. Physiol.*, *22*, 91–4.

Drennan, P.C. (1984) 'Visual hallucinations in children receiving decongestants.' *Br. Med. J.*, *i*, 1688.

Dressler, H. (1982) 'Hypothermia and drowning.' In P. Koch and M. Kohfahl (eds.) *Unterkuhlung im Seenotfall. 2nd Symposium.* Deutsche Gesellschaft zur Rettung Schiffbruchiger, Cuxhaven, pp. 232–7.

Drew, C.E.; Keen, G.; Benazon, D.B. (1959) 'Profound hypothermia.' *Lancet*, *i*, 745–7.

Dubas, F. (1980) 'Aspects medicaux de l'accident par avalanche: hypothermie et gelures.' *Z. Unfallmed. Berufskr.*, *73*, 164–7.

Duckworth, W.C.; Cooper, B.C. (1964) 'Accidental hypothermia in the Bantu.' *S. Afr. Med. J.*, *38*, 295–8.

Duesberg, F. (1982) 'Accidental hypothermia from the view of a wind-surfer.' In P. Koch and M. Kohfahl (eds.) *Unterkuhlung im Seenotfall. 2nd Symposium.* Deutsche Gesellschaft zur Rettung Schiffbruchiger, Cuxhaven, pp. 178–83.

Duguid, H.; Simpson, R.G.; Stowers, J.M. (1961) 'Accidental hypothermia.' *Lancet*, *ii*, 1213–21.

Dyde, J.A.; Lunn, H.F. (1970) 'Heat loss during thoracotomy: a preliminary report.' *Thorax*, *25*, 355–8.

Dyerberg, J.; Bang, H.O. (1982) 'Factors influencing morbidity of acute myocardial infarction in Greenlanders.' In B. Harvald and J.P. Hart Hansen (eds.) *Circumpolar Health 81.* Nordic Council for Arctic Medical Research, Copenhagen, pp. 300–3.

Eady, E.A.; Bentley-Phillips, C.B.; Keahey, T.M.; Greaves, M.W.N. (1978) 'Cold urticaria vasculitis.' *Br. J. Dermatol.*, *99*, Suppl. 16, 9–10.

Earnshaw, D. (1978) 'Hypothermia on the fells.' *Basics*, *1*, 41–6.

Ebrahim, G.J. (1984) 'Care of the newborn.' *Br. Med. J.*, *ii*, 899–901.

Eccleston, D. (1982) 'The biochemistry of affective disorders.' *Br. J. Hosp. Med.*, *28*, 627–30.

Eddy, T.P.; Payne, P.R.; Salvosa, C.; Wheeler, E.F. (1970) 'Body temperatures in the elderly.' *Lancet*, *ii*, 1088.

Edholm, O.G.; Lobstein, T. (1981) 'Indoor temperature.' In J.N. Adams (ed.) *Hypothermia Ashore and Afloat.* Aberdeen University Press, Aberdeen, pp. 187–206.

Edwards, M.; Burton, A.C. (1960) 'Temperature distribution over the human head especially in the cold.' *J. Appl. Physiol.*, *15*, 209–11.

Edwards, R.H.T. (1975) 'Physiology of fitness and fatigue.' In C. Clarke, M. Ward, E. Williams (eds.) *Mountain Medicine and Physiology*. Alpine Club, London, pp. 107–10.

Edwards, R.J.; Belyavin, A.J.; Harrison, M.H. (1978) 'Core temperature measurement in man.' *Aviat. Space Environ. Med.*, *49*, 1289–94.

Edwards, W.S.; Tuluy, S.; Reber, W.E.; Siegel, A.; Bing, R.J. (1954) 'Coronary blood flow and myocardial metabolism in hypothermia.' *Ann. Sur.*, *139*, 275–81.

Elder, L.; Streshinsky, S. (1978) *And I alone survived.* Collins, London.

Elliot, G.B. (1980) 'The grey man — an explanation?' *The Scots Magazine, Jan.*, p. 574.

Elliott, H.W.; Crismon, J.M. (1947) 'Increased sensitivity of hypothermic rats to injected potassium and the influence of calcium, digitalis and glucose on survival.' *Am J. Physiol.*, *151*, 366–72.

Elliott, L. (1967) 'The man who refused to die.' *Readers' Digest, Dec.*, 120–7.

Ellis, F.R.; Campbell, I.T. (1983) 'Fatal heat stroke in a long distance runner.' *Br. Med. J.*, *ii*, 1548–9.

———; Zwana, S.L.V. (1977) 'A study of body temperatures of anaesthetised man in the tropics.' *Br. J. Anaesth.*, *49*, 1123–6.

Ellis, H.D. (1982) 'The effects of cold on the performance of serial choice RT and various discrete tasks.' *Hum. Factors*, *24*, 589–98.

———; Wilcock, S.E.; Zaman, S.A. (1985) 'Cold and performance: The effects of information load, analgesics, and the rate of cooling.' *Aviat. Space Environ. Med.*, *56*, 233–7.

Elsner, R.; Gooden, B. (1970) 'Reduction of reactive hyperaemia in the human forearm by face immersion.' *J. Appl. Physiol.*, *29*, 627–30.

———; Gooden, B. (1983) *Diving and Asphyxia*, University Press, Cambridge.

———; Angell-James, J.E.; Daly, M. de B. (1977) 'Carotid body chemoreceptor reflexes and their interaction in the seal.' *Am. J. Physiol.*, *232*, H517–25.

Emslie-Smith, D. (1958) 'Accidental hypothermia: a common condition with a pathognomonic electrocardiogram.' *Lancet*, *ii*, 492–5.

——— (1979) 'The electrical activity of the heart in hypothermia.' In P. Matter, P. Braun, M. de Quervain, W. Good (eds.) *Skifahren und Sicherheit III, Lawinen.* Buchduckerei Davos, AG, pp. 155–9.

——— (1981) 'Hypothermia in the elderly.' *Br. J. Hosp. Med.*, *26*, 442–52.

——— (1982) 'Hypothermia in the elderly.' *Br. J. Hosp. Med.*, *27*, 317.

———; Lightbody, I.; Maclean, D. (1981) 'Conservative management of urban hypothermia.' In J.N. Adams (ed.) *Hypothermia Ashore and Afloat*. Aberdeen University Press, Aberdeen, pp. 147–50.

Enander, A. (1984) 'Performance and sensory aspects of work in cold environments — a review.' *Ergonomics*, *27*, 365–78.

Encyclopaedia Brittanica (1973a) 'Hippocrates.' *Micropaedia*, William Benton, Chicago. Vol. V, p. 55.

——— (1973b) 'Illusions and hallucinations.' *Macropaedia*, William Benton, Chicago. Vol. 9, pp. 240–7.

Englund, A.; Engholm, G.; von Schmalensee, G. (1977) 'Chest symptoms among construction workers in northern and southern Sweden.' *Nordic Council Arct. Med. Res.*, *Rep. No. 19*, pp. 143–7.

Evans, A.T.; Sawyer, D.C.; Krahwinkel, D.J. (1973) 'Effect of a warm water blanket on development of hypothermia during small animal surgery.' *J. Am. Vet. Ass.*, *164*, 147–8.

Evans, C.; Parsons, C.; Hunton, (1971) 'Near drowning.' *Br. Med. J.*, *i*, 47.

Exton-Smith, A.N. (1973) 'Accidental hypothermia.' *Br. Med. J.*, *iv*, 727–9.

Fairley, H.B. (1961) 'Metabolism in hypothermia.' *Br. Med. Bull.*, *17*, 52–5.

Faller, J.P.; Rauscher, M. (1978) 'Severe hypothermia: importance of temporary electrosystolic pacing until the end of the warming.' *Nouv. Presse Med.*, *7*, 33–66.

Fanger, P.O. (1970) *Thermal Comfort. Analysis and Applications in Environmental Engineering*. McGraw-Hill, New York.

Faulkner, D. (1977) 'Some thoughts on the nature of hazards affecting structures in deep waters.' *J. Soc. Underwater Tech.*, *3*, 16–21.

Faulkner, J.A.; White, T.P.; Markley, J.M. (1980) 'The 1979 Canadian ski marathon: a natural experiment in hypothermia.' In F.J. Nagle (ed.) *Balke Symposium Proceedings.* Charles C. Thomas, Springfield, Ill., pp. 373–82.

Fedor, E.J.; Fisher, B.; Lee, S.H. (1958) 'Rewarming following hypothermia of two to twelve hours. I Cardiovascular effects.' *Ann. Surg.*, *147*, 515–30.

Feldman, S.A. (1971) 'Profound hypothermia.' *Br. J. Anaesth.*, *43*, 244–7.

——— (1979) 'Hypothermia and neuromuscular blockade.' *Anesthesiology*, *51*, 369–70.

Felicetta, J.V.; Green, W.L. (1979) 'Hypothermia and adrenocortical function.' *Ann. Intern. Med.*, *90*, 855.

Fell, R.H.; Dendy, P.R. (1968) 'Severe hypothermia and respiratory arrest in diazepam and glutethimide intoxication.' *Anaesthesia*, *23*, 636–40.

———; Cunning, A.J.; Bardhan, K.D.; Triger, D.R. (1968) 'Severe hypothermia as a result of barbiturate overdose complicated by cardiac arrest.' *Lancet*, *i*, 392–4.

Ferchiou, A. (1972) 'Reanimation medical infantile en Tunisia. Une experience de trois annees.' *Tunis. Med.*, *50*, 79–96.

Fernandez, J.P.; O'Rourke, R.A.; Ewy, G.A. (1970) 'Rapid active external rewarming in accidental hypothermia.' *J. Am. Med. Ass.*, *212*, 153–6

Finnegan, M.J.; Pickering, C.A.C.; Burge, P.S. (1984) 'The sick building syndrome: prevalence studies.' *Br. Med. J.*, *ii*, 1573–5.

Firbank, T. (1940) *I Bought a Mountain*. New English Library, London.

Fischman, L.G. (1983) 'Dreams, hallucinogenic drug states, and schizophrenia: a psychological and biological comparison.' *Schizophrenia Bull.*, *9*, 73–94.

Fisher, B.; Russ, C.; Fedor, E.; Wilde, R.; Engstrom, P.; Happe, J.; Prendergast, P. (1955) 'Experimental evaluation of prolonged hypothermia.' *Arch. Surg.*, *71*, 431–48.

Fisher, J.; Vaghaiwalla, F.; Tsitlik, J.; Levin, H.; Brinker, J.; Weisfeldt, M.; Yin, F. (1982) 'Determinants and clinical significance of jugular venous valve competence.' *Circulation*, *65*, 188–96.

Fitzgerald, F.T.; Jessop, C. (1982) 'Accidental hypothermia: a report of 22 cases and review of the literature.' *Adv. Intern. Med.*, *27*, 128–50.

Flora, G. (1985) 'Secondary treatment of frostbite.' In J. Rivolier, P. Cerretelli, J. Foray, P. Segantini (eds.) *High Altitude Deterioration*. Karger, Basel, pp. 159–69.

Foldes, F.F.; Kuze, S.; Vizi, E.S.; Deery. A. (1978) 'The influence of temperature on neuromuscular performance.' *J. Neural. Transm.*, *43*, 27–45.

Folinsbee, L. (1974) 'Cardiovascular response to apnoeic immersion in cool and warm water.' *J. Appl. Physiol.*, *36*, 226–32.

Fonkalsrud, E. (1975) Discussion. *J. Ped. Surg.*, *10*, 590–1.

Foray, J. (1983) Letter. *Ann. Surg.*, *198*, 668.

———; Cahen, C. (1981) 'Les hypothermies de montagne.' *Chirurgie*, *107*, 305–10.

———; Salon, F. (1985) 'Casualties with cold injuries: primary treatment.' In J. Rivolier, P. Cerretelli, J. Foray, P. Segantini (eds.) *High Altitude Deterioration*. Karger, Basel, pp. 149–58.

———; Kalt-Binder, F.; Lanoye, P. (1979) 'The sequelae of frostbite.' *Chirurgie*, *105*, 37–46.

———; Stieglitz, P.; Koch, M. (1977) 'Hypothermia in mountaineering. Apropos of 18 cases.' *Clin. Obstet. Gynaecol.*, *103*, 1040–52.

Forrester, A.C. (1958) 'Hypothermia using air cooling.' *Anaesthesia*, *13*, 289–98.

Fox, G.R.; Hayward, J.S.; Hobson, G.N. (1979) 'Effect of alcohol on thermal balance of man in cold water.' *Can. J. Physiol. Pharmacol.*, *57*, 860–5.

Fox, R.H. (1961) 'Local cooling in man.' *Br. Med. Bull.*, *17*, 14–18.

Fox, R.H.; Solman, A.J. (1970) 'A new technique for measuring deep body temperature in man from the intact skin surface.' *J. Physiol. (Lond.)*, *212*, 8–10.

———; Brooke, O.G.; Collins, C.J.; Bailey, C.S.; Healy, F.B. (1975) 'Measurement of deep body temperature from the urine.' *Clin. Sci. & Mol. Med.*, *48*, 1–7.

———; MacDonald, I.C.; Woodward, P.M. (1973a) 'A hypothermia survey kit.' *J. Physiol. (Lond.)*, *231*, 4–6P.

———; MacGibbon, R.; Davies, L.; Woodward, P.M. (1973b) 'Problem of the old and the cold.' *Br. Med. J.*, *i*, 21–4.

———; Solman, A.J.; Isaacs, R.; Fry, A.J.; MacDonald, I.E. (1973c) 'A new method for monitoring deep body temperature from the skin surface.' *Clin. Sci.*, *44*, 81–6.

———; Woodward, P.M.; Exton-Smith, A.N.; Green, M.F.; Donnison, D.V.; Wicks, M.H. (1973d) 'Body temperature in the elderly: a national study of physiological, social and environmental conditions.' *Br. Med. J.*, *i*, 200–6.

———; Woodward, P.M.; Fry, A.J.; Collins, J.C.; MacDonald, I.C. (1971) 'Diagnosis of accidental hypothermia of the elderly.' *Lancet*, *i*, 424–7.

Fox, V.F. (1967) 'Human performance in the cold.' *Hum. Factors*, *9*, 203–20.

Francis, T.J.R. (1984) 'Non freezing cold injury: a historical review.' *J. Roy. Nav. Med. Serv.*, *70*, 134–9.

———; Golden, F. St. C. (1985) 'Non-freezing cold injury: the pathogenesis.' *J. Roy. Nav. Med. Serv.*, *71*, 3–8.

Francois, B.; Cahen, R.; Gravejat, M.F.; Estrade, M. (1984) 'Do betablockers prevent pressor responses to mental stress and physical exercise?' *Eur. Heart. J.*, 5, 348–53.

Frankland, J.C. (1975) 'Medical aspects of cave rescue.' *Trans. Br. Cave Res. Ass.*, *2*, 53–63.

——— (1977) 'Caving: problems and pleasures.' *Practitioner*, *219*, 211–18.

——— (1981) 'How I would treat hypothermia and exposure.' *Br. Med. J.*, *i*, 369–70.

——— (1983) 'The Blackpool tragedy.' *J. Brit. Ass. for Immediate Care*, *6*, 34–5.

Franz, D.R.; Berberich, J.J.; Blake, S.; Mills, W.J. (1978) 'Evaluation of fasciotomy and vasodilators for treatment of frostbite in the dog.' *Cryobiology*, *15*, 659–69.

Fraser, I.C.; Loftus, J.A. (1979a) '"Trench foot" caused by the cold.' *Br. Med. J.*, *i*, 414.

———; Loftus, J.A. (1979b) '"Trench foot" caused by the cold.' *Br. Med. J.*, *i*, 1017.

Fraser-Darling, A. (1981) 'Electrocution, drowning and burns.' *Br. Med. J.*, *i*, 530–1.

Frederiksen, P.X. (1977) 'Hypothermia in the newborn.' *Ugeskr. Laeger.*, *139*, 193–6.

Freedman, R.R.; Ianni, P. (1983) 'Role of cold and emotional stress in Raynaud's disease and scleroderma.' *Br. Med. J.*, *ii*, 1499–1502.

Freeman, J.; Pugh, L.G.C.E. (1969) 'Hypothermia in mountain accidents.' *Int. Anaesthesiol. Clin.*, *7*, 997–1007.

Frens, J. (1980) 'Neurotransmitter mapping in central thermoregulation.' In B. Cox, P. Lomax, A.S. Milton, E. Schonbaum (eds.) *Thermoregulatory Mechanisms and Their Therapeutic Implications.* S. Karger, Basel, pp. 1–5.

Friedman, F.; Adams, F.H.; Emmanouilides, G. (1967) 'Regulation of body temperature of premature infants with low-energy radiant heat.' *J. Pediatrics*, *70*, 270–3.

Froese, G.; Burton, A.C. (1957) 'Heat losses from the human head.' *J. Appl. Physiol.*, *10*, 235–41.

Froggatt, P.; Lynas, M.A.; MacKenzie, G. (1971) 'Epidemiology of sudden unexpected death in infants ('cot death') in Northern Ireland.' *Br. J. Prev. Soc. Med.*, *25*, 119–34.

Fuller, J. (1977) 'Rescue on granite mountain.' *Readers' Digest*, *Aug.*, 98–102.

Fuller, R.H. (1963) 'Drowning and the post-immersion syndrome: a clinico-pathological study.' *Mil. Med.*, *128*, 22–36.

Gaillard, J–M. (1983) 'Biochemical pharmacology of paradoxical sleep.' *Br. J. Clin. Pharmac.*, *16*, 205–30S.

Gale, E.A.M.; Tattersal, R.B. (1978) 'Hypotherma: a complication of diabetic ketoacidosis.' *Br. Med. J.*, *ii*, 1387–9.

Gandy, G.M.; Adamson, S.K.; Cunningham, N.; Silverman, W.A.; James, L.S. (1964) 'Thermal environment and acid base homeostasis in human infants during the first few hours of life.' *J. Clin. Invest.*, *43*, 751–8.

Garg, G.P. (1973) 'Humidification of the Rees–Ayre T-piece system for neonates.'

Anesth. Analg. (Cleve.), *52*, 207–9.

Garland, M.H. (1978a) 'Problems in the elderly. 1. Non-specific presentation of disease.' *Hospital Update*, *4*, 111–13.

——— (1978b) 'Problems in the elderly. 2. Falls.' *Hospital Update*, *4*, 241–4.

Garrow, J.S. (1983) 'Luxuskonsumption, brown fat, and human obesity.' *Br. Med. J.*, *i*, 1684–6.

Gavshon, A.; Rice, D. (1984) *The Sinking of the 'Belgrano'.* New English Library, London, p. 106.

Geevarghese, K.P.; Aldrete, J.A.; Patel, J.C. (1976) 'Inspired air temperature with immersion heater humidifiers.' *Anesth. Analg. (Cleve.)*, *55*, 331–4.

Gilston, A. (1978) 'Cerebral function and blood flow during resuscitation.' *Anaesthesia*, *33*, 273–4.

——— (1984) 'Hygroscopic condenser humidifiers: value for money?' *Anaesthesia*, *39*, 1030–1.

Glanvill, P. (1980) 'Medical aspects of caving.' *Medisport*, *2*, 87–9.

Glaser, E.M.; Holmes-Jones, R. (1951) 'The initiation of shivering by cooled blood returning from the lower limbs.' *J. Physiol. (Lond.)*, *114*, 277–82.

Glass, L.; Silverman, W.A.; Sinclair, J.C. (1968) 'Effect of the thermal environment on cold resistance and growth of small infants after the first week of life.' *Paediatrics*, *41*, 1033–46.

Glauser, F.L.; Smith, W.R. (1975) 'Pulmonary interstitial fibrosis following near-drowning and exposure to short-term high oxygen concentrations.' *Chest*, *68*, 373–5.

Glennie, H.R.R. (1969) 'Shipwreck in harbour.' *N.Z. Med. J.*, *70*, 299–301.

Goldberg, M.J.; Roe, C.F. (1966) 'Temperature changes during anaesthesia and surgery.' *Arch. Surg.*, *93*, 365–9.

Goldblatt, A.; Miller, R. (1972) 'Prevention of accidental hypothermia in neurosurgical patients.' *Anesth. Analg. (Cleve.)*, *51*, 536–43.

Golden, F. StC. (1972) 'Immersion hypothermia in hazards of aquatics.' *Br. Med. J.*, *ii*, 344–5.

——— (1973a) 'Recognition and treatment of immersion hypothermia.' *Proc. R. Soc. Med.*, *66*, 1058–1061.

——— (1973b) 'Death after rescue from immersion in cold water.' *J. Roy. Nav. Med. Ser.*, *59*, 5–8.

——— (1974) 'Notes on survival at sea.' *J. Roy. Nav. Med. Serv.*, *60*, 8–19.

——— (1976) 'Hypothermia: a problem for North Sea industries.' *J. Soc. Occupat. Med.*, *26*, 85–8.

——— (1979) 'Why rewarm?' In P. Matter, P. Braun, M. deQuervain, W. Good (eds.) *Skifahren und Sicherheit III.* Buchdruckerei Davos AG, Davos, pp. 163–7.

——— (1980) 'Problems of immersion.' *Br. J. Hosp. Med.*, *24*, 371–4.

——— (1983) 'Rewarming.' In R.S. Pozos and L.E. Wittmers (eds.) *The Nature and Treatment of Hypothermia*, Croom Helm, London/University of Minnesota Press, Minneapolis, pp. 194–208

———; Hervey, G.R. (1972) 'A class experiment on immersion hypothermia.' *J. Physiol. (Lond.)*, *227*, 35–6.

———; Hervey, G.R. (1977) 'The mechanism of the "after-drop" following immersion hypothermia in pigs.' *J. Physiol. (Lond.)*, *272*, 26–7P.

———; Hervey, G.R. (1981) 'The "after-drop" and death after rescue from immersion in cold water.' In J.N. Adams (ed.) *Hypothermia Ashore and Afloat.* Aberdeen University Press, Aberdeen, pp. 37–56.

———; Rivers, J. (1975) 'The immersion incident.' *Anaesthesia*, *30*, 364–73.

———; Hervey, G.R.; Wheeler, J.M. (1977) 'Evidence from computer simulation for a conductive mechanism for the "after-drop" of body temperature after immersion hypothermia.' *J. Physiol. (Lond.)*, *271*, 66P.

Goldman, A.; Exton-Smith, A.N.; Francis, G.; O'Brien, A. (1977) 'A pilot study of low body temperature in old people admitted to hospital.' *J. R. Coll. Phys. Lond.*, *11*, 291–306.

Goldsmith, R.; Minard, D. (1976) 'Cold, cold work.' *Occupational Health & Safety.* International Labour Office, Geneva, Vol. 1, A–K, pp. 319–20.

Goode, R.C.; McDonald, A. (1982) 'Cold water immersion and survival.' In B. Harvald and J.P. Hart Hansen (eds.) *Circumpolar Health 81.* Nordic Council for Arctic Medical Research, Copenhagen, pp. 595–600.

Gooden, B.A. (1982) 'The diving response in clinical medicine.' *Aviat. Space Environ. Med.*, *53*, 273–6.

Gordon, P. (1979) 'Steps to winter survival.' *J. Winter Emerg. Care, 4*, 52–4.

Gorlin, R. (1966) 'Physiology of the coronary circulation.' In J.W. Hurst and R.B. Logan (eds.) *The Heart*. McGraw-Hill, New York, pp. 653–8.

Goudsouzian, N.G.; Morris, R.H.; Ryan, J.F. (1973) 'The effects of a warming blanket on the maintenance of body temperatures in anesthetised children and infants.' *Anesthesiology*, *39*, 351–3.

Gourlay, J. (1979) *The Great Lakes Triangle*. Fontana/Collins, Glasgow, pp. 133–7.

Graham, J.M.; Keatinge, W.R. (1978) 'Deaths in cold water.' *Br. Med. J.*, *ii*, 18–19.

Graham, T.; Baulk, K. (1980) 'Effect of alcohol ingestion on man's thermoregulatory responses during cold water immersion.' *Aviat. Space Environ. Med.*, *51*, 155–9.

———; Dalton, J. (1980) 'Effect of alcohol on man's response to mild physical activity in a cold environment.' *Aviat. Space Environ. Med.*, *51*, 793–6.

Graham, T.E. (1981) 'Thermal and glycemic responses during mild exercise in +5 to −15 °C environments following alcohol ingestion.' *Aviat. Space Environ. Med:*, *52*, 517–22.

Grant, G.C.; Dawson, J.J.W.; Roberts, B.E. (1976) 'A new humidifier.' *Anaesth. Intensive Care*, *4*, 205–10.

Gray, A. (1970) *The Big Grey Man of Ben Macdhui.* Impulse Books, Aberdeen.

Grayson, J.; Kuehn, L.A. (1979) 'Heat transfer and heat loss.' In P. Lomax and E. Schonbaum (eds.) *Body Temperature: Regulation, Drug Effects, and Therapeutic Implications.* Marcel Dekker, New York, pp. 71–87.

Green, A. (1978) 'Working in a cold environment.' *Occupational Health*, *Aug.*, 366–71.

Green, L. (1980) 'Flying doctors of the North Sea.' *BMA News Rev.*, *March*, 30–7.

Green, L.F.; Bagley, R. (1972) 'Ingestion of a glucose syrup drink during long distance canoeing.' *Br. J. Sports Med.*, *6*, 125–8.

Greenfield, A.D.M.; Shepherd, J.T.; Whelan, R.F. (1950) 'The average internal temperatures of fingers immersed in cold water.' *Clin. Sci.*, *9*, 349–54.

Greenhouse, H.B. (1972) *Premonitions: a leap into the future.* Pan Books, London.

Greenleaf, J.E. (1979) 'Hyperthermia and exercise.' In D. Robertshaw (ed.) *Environmental Physiology III.* University Park Press, Baltimore, pp. 157–208.

———; Castle, B.L. (1972) 'External auditory canal temperature as an estimate of core temperature.' *J. Appl. Physiol.*, *32*, 194–8.

———; Shvartz, E.; Keil, L.C. (1981) 'Hemodilution, vasopressin suppression and diuresis during water immersion in man.' *Aviat. Space Environ. Med.*, *52*, 329–36.

Gregory, R.T. (1977) 'Accidental hypothermia: Part 1. an Alaskan problem.' *Alaska Med.*, *13*, 134–6.

———; Doolittle, W.H. (1973) 'Accidental hypothermia, part 11: clinical implications of experimental studies.' *Alaska Med.*, *15*, 48–52.

———; Patton, J.F. (1972) 'Treatment after exposure to cold.' *Lancet*, *i*, 377.

Greig, W.R.; Maxwell, J.D.; Boyle, J.A.; Lindsay, R.M.; Browning, M.C.K. (1971)

'Steroids in mountain rescue.' *Lancet*, *i*, 599.

Grosse-Brockhoff, F. (1950) 'Pathologic physiology and therapy of hypothermia.' *German Aviation Medicine, World War II*. Surgeon General of the US Air Force, Chap. VIII E, *2*, 828–42.

Grossheim, R.L. (1973) 'Hypothermia and frostbite treated with peritoneal dialysis.' *Alaska Med.*, *15*, 53–5.

Gruner, T. (1979) 'Schicksal am Jubilaumsgrat.' *Bergwacht Jahresbericht 1978*, Bavarian Red Cross.

Guest, D. (1977) 'My night in a crevasse.' *Weekend Scotsman*, *March* 5, 1, Col. 1.

Guezennec, C.Y.; Pesquies, P.C. (1985) 'Biochemical basis for physical exercise fatigue.' In J. Rivolier, P. Cerretelli, J. Foray, P. Segantini (eds.) *High Altitude Deterioration*. Karger, Basel, pp. 79–89.

Guild, W.J. (1976) 'Central body rewarming for hypothermia — possibilities, problems and progress.' *J. Roy. Nav. Med. Ser.*, *62*, 173–5.

——— (1978) 'Rewarming via the airway for hypothermia in the field?' *J. Roy. Nav. Med. Ser.*, *64*, 186–93.

Guleria, J.S.; Talwar, J.R.; Malhotra, O.P.; Pande, J.N. (1969) 'Effects of breathing cold air on pulmonary mechanics in normal man.' *J. Appl. Physiol.*, *27*, 320–2.

Gumaa, K.; El-Mahrouky, S.F.; Mahmoud, N.; Mustafa, M.K.Y.; Khogali, M. (1984) 'The metabolic status of heat stroke patients: the Makkah experience.' In M. Khogali and J.R.S. Hales (eds.) *Heat Stroke and Temperature Regulation*. Academic Press, New York, pp. 157–69.

Gundersen, T.; Havag, K. (1975) 'The significance of the climate in upper respiratory tract infections in children.' *Nordic Council Arct. Med. Res.*, *Rep. No. 12*, pp. 31–47.

Guttman, R.; Gross, M.M. (1956) 'Relationship between electrical and mechanical changes in muscle caused by cooling.' *J. Coll. Comp. Physiol.*, *48*, 421–30.

Guy, A.W.; Lehmann, J.F.; Stonebridge, J.B. (1974) 'Therapeutic applications of electromagnetic power.' *Proc. of IEEE*, *62*, 55–75.

Gyntelberg, F. (1977) 'Coronary heart disease and physical activity.' *Nordic Council Arct. Med. Res.*, *Rep. No. 19*, pp. 64–9.

Haberman, S.; Capildeo, R.; Rose, F. (1981) 'The seasonal variation in mortality from cerebrovascular disease.' *J. Neurol. Sci.*, *52*, 25–36.

Hackett, P.; Creagh, C.E.; Grover, R.F.; Honigman, B.; Houston, C.S.; Reeves, J.T.; Sophocles, A.M.; van Hardenbroek, M. (1980) 'High altitude pulmonary oedema in persons without the right pulmonary artery.' *New Engl. J. Med.*, *302*, 1070–3.

Hackett, P.H.; Rennie, D.; Grover, R.F.; Reeves, J.T. (1981) 'Acute mountain sickness and edemas of high altitude: a common pathogenesis?' *Resp. Physiol.*, *46*, 383–90.

Haight, J.S.J.; Keatinge, W.R. (1973) 'Failure of thermoregulation in the cold during hypoglycaemia induced by exercise and ethanol.' *J. Physiol. (Lond.)*, *229*, 87–97.

Hails, F.G. (1973) 'Body temperatures in the elderly.' *Br. Med. J.*, *i*, 421.

Hakansson, C.H.; Toremalm, N.G. (1965) 'Studies on the physiology of the trachea. I. Ciliary activity indirectly recorded by a new "light beam reflex" method.' *Ann. Otol. Rhinol. Laryngol.*, *74*, 954–69.

Hall, G.M. (1978) 'Body temperature and anaesthesia.' *Br. J. Anaesth.*, *50*, 39–44.

Haller, A. (1975) Discussion. *J. Ped. Surg.*, *10*, 591.

Hamilton, R.W. (1981a) 'Design of a combinaion thermal regenerator and carbon dioxide cannister for hyperbaric survival.' In L.A. Kuehn (ed.) *Physiological Criteria for Diving Equipment — Thermal*. UMS. Workshop Report, Undersea Medical Society, Bethesda, MD, pp. 75–82.

——— (1981b) 'Survival in a lost bell: what can be done?' Presentation at *International Diving Symposium*. Association of Diving Contractors, Gretna, LA.

Hamilton, S.J.C. (1980) 'Hypothermia and unawareness of mental impairment.'

Br. Med. J., *i*, 565.

Hamlet, M.P. (1976) 'Thermographic (infra red) evaluation of frostbite.' In R.J. Shephard and S. Itoh (eds.) *Circumpolar Health.* Toronto University Press, Toronto, p. 76.

——— (1983) 'Fluid shifts in hypothermia.' In R.S. Pozos and L.E. Wittmers (eds.) *The Nature and Treatment of Hypothermia.* Croom Helm, London/ University of Minnesota Press, Minneapolis, pp. 94–9.

Hamlin, C.L.; Lydiard, R.B.; Martin, D.; Dackis, C.A.; Pottash, A.C.; Sweeney, D.; Gold, M.S. (1983) 'Urinary excretion of noradrenaline metabolite decreased in panic disorder.' *Lancet*, *ii*, 740–1.

Hammond, E.C.; Garfinkel, L. (1969) 'Coronary heart disease, stroke and aortic aneurysm: factors in the aetiology.' *Arch. Environ. Health*, *19*, 167–82.

Hampton, I.F.G. (1981) 'A laboratory evaluation of the protection against heat loss offered by survival suits for helicopter passengers.' In J.N. Adams (ed.) *Hypothermia Ashore and Afloat.* Aberdeen University Press, Aberdeen, pp. 83–111.

———; Smith, D.; Golden, F. St C. (1979) 'Immersion and thermoregulatory response .' *Br. Med. J.*, *i*, 1566.

Haneda, T.; Nakajima, T.; Shirato, K.; Onedera, S.; Takashima, T. (1983) 'Effects of oxygen breathing on pulmonary vascular input impedance in patients with pulmonary hypertension.' *Chest*, *83*, 520–7.

Hansen, J.P.H. (1977a) 'Medico-legal viewpoints on drowning and floating bodies.' *Nordic Council Arct. Med. Res.*, *Rep. No. 18*, pp. 46–7.

Hansen, P.F. (1977b) 'The Glostrup study.' *Nordic Council Arct. Med. Res.*, *Rep. No. 19*, pp. 58–63.

Hanson, P.G.; Johnson, R.E. (1965) 'Variations in plasma ketones and free fatty acids during cold exposure in man.' *J. Appl. Physiol.*, *20*, 56–60.

Hanson, P.J.V.; Loughridge, L.W.; Mulhall, B.P.; Packham, D.K. (1984) 'Hypothermia in hypoglycaemia.' *Br. Med. J.*, *i*, 1212–13.

Harding, R.M.; Mills, F.J. (1983) 'Problems of altitude. 1: Hypoxia and hyperventilation.' *Br. Med. J.*, *i*, 1408–10.

Harnett, R.M.; O'Brien, E.M.; Sias, F.R.; Pruitt, J.R. (1980) 'Initial treatment of profound accidental hypothermia.' *Aviat. Space Environ. Med.*, *51*, 680–7.

———; Pruitt, J.R., Sias, F.R. (1983a) 'A review of the literature concerning resuscitation from hypothermia: Part 1 — The problem and general approaches.' *Aviat. Space Environ. Med.*, *54*, 425–34.

———; Pruitt, J.R., Sias, F.R. (1983b) 'A review of the literature concerning resuscitation from hypothermia: Part 11 — Selected rewarming protocols.' *Aviat. Space Environ. Med.*, *54*, 487–95.

———; Sias, F.R.; Pruitt, J.R. (1979) 'Resuscitation from hypothermia: a literature review.' *US Department of Transportation, US Coast Guard. Rep. No. CG-D-26-79.* Office of Research and Development, Washington, DC.

Harper, A.E. (1983) 'Coronary heart disease — an epidemic related to diet?' *Am. J. Clin. Nut.*, *37*, 669–81.

Harper, F.W.J. (1981) 'Hypothermia and mountain rescue in Scotland.' In J.N. Adams (ed.) *Hypothermia Ashore and Afloat.* Aberdeen University Press, Aberdeen, pp. 15–21.

Harpin, V.A.; Chellappah, G.; Rutter, N. (1983) 'Responses of the newborn infant to overheating.' *Bil. Neonate*, *44*, 65–75.

Harries, M.G. (1982) 'Survival of prolonged submersion is explained by the protection afforded by hypothermia accelerated by an intact circulation rather than by the diving reflex.' In P. Koch and M. Kohfahl (eds.) *Unterkuhlung im Seenotfall. 2nd Symposium.* Deutsche Gesellschaft zur Rettung Schiffbruchiger, Cuxhaven, pp. 96–100.

——— (1984) 'New developments in external chest compression.' *J. Brit. Ass.*

Immediate Care, *7*, 62–4.
Harriman, D.G.F.; Ellis, F.R. (1983) 'Sudden infant death syndrome — a possible cause.' *Br. Med. J.*, *i*, 391.
Harris, L.; Kirimili, B.; Safar, P. (1967) 'Augmentation of artificial circulation during cardiopulmonary resuscitation.' *Anesthesiology*, *28*, 730.
Hartung, G.H.; Myhre, L.G.; Nunneley, S.A. (1980) 'Physiological effects of cold air inhalation during exercise.' *Aviat. Space Environ. Med.*, *51*, 591–4.
———; Myhre, L.G.; Nunneley, S.A.; Tucker, D.M. (1984) 'Plasma substrate response in men and women during marathon running.' *Aviat. Space Environ. Med.*, *55*, 128–31.
Hasan, S.; Avery, W.G.; Fabian, C.; Sackner, M. (1971) 'Near-drowning in humans. A report of 36 patients.' *Chest*, *59*, 191–7.
Hassi, J. (1982) 'Working in cold conditions.' *Nordic Council for Arctic Medical Research*, *Rep. No. 30*, pp. 20–2.
———; Virokannas, H.; Anttonen, H.; Jarvenpaa, I. (1984) 'Health hazards in snow mobile usage.' *Presentation at Sixth International Symposium on Circumpolar Health. May 13–18, 1984. Anchorage, Alaska.* Abstracts, p. 142.
Hatcher, J.D. (1965) 'Acute anoxic anoxia.' In O.G. Edholm and A.L. Bacharach (eds.) *The Physiology of Human Survival.* Academic Press, London, pp. 81–120
Hattenhauer, M.; Neill, W.A. (1975) 'The effect of cold air inhalation on angina pectoris and myocardial oxygen supply.' *Circulation*, *51*, 1053–8.
Hawthorne, V.M.; Smalls, M. (1980) 'Blood pressure and ambient temperature.' *Br. Med. J.*, *i*, 567–8.
Hayes, B.; Robinson, J.S. (1970) 'An assessment of methods of humidification of inspired gas.' *Br. J. Anaesth.*, *42*, 94–104.
Hayes, P. (1985) 'Thermal protection equipment.' In L. Rey (ed.) *Arctic Underwater Operations.* Graham & Trotman, London, pp. 193–216.
Hayes, P.A. (1977) 'Energy balance and heat loss during saturation diving.' *Royal Naval Physiological Laboratory, Alverstoke.* Report No. 277.
——— (1979) 'Psychophysical studies of thermoperception during prolonged hyperbaric oxyhelium exposures.' *J. Physiol.*, *293*, 80–1P.
———; Padbury, E.H.; Atherton, P.J. (1981) 'Astronaut trial. Section one passive systems validation of emergency procedures, the lost bell situation.' *Admiralty Marine Technology Establishment.* Report AMTE(E) R81 403.
———; Padbury, E.H.; Florio, J.T.; Fyfield, T.P. (1982) 'Respiratory heat transfer in cold water and during rewarming.' *J. Biomechanical Eng.*, *104*, 45–9.
Hayward, J.S. (1979) *The UVIC Heat-Treat. Rescue Treatment for Accidental Hypothermia.* Scitech Products, 570 Linnet Lane, Victoria, BC.
——— (1982) 'Protection against immersion hypothermia.' In P. Koch and M. Kohfahl (eds.) *Unterkuhlung im Seenotfall. 2nd Symposium.* Deutsche Gesellschaft zur Rettung Schiffbruchiger, Cuxhaven, pp. 72–9.
——— (1983) 'The physiology of immersion hypothermia.' In R.S. Pozos and L.E. Wittmers (eds.) *The Nature and Treatment of Hypothermia.* Croom Helm, London/University of Minnesota, Minneapolis, pp. 3–19.
——— (1984) 'Thermal protection performance of survival suits in ice-water.' *Aviat. Space Environ. Med.*, 55, 212–15.
———; Eckerson, J.D. (1984) 'Physiological responses and survival time prediction for humans in ice water.' *Aviat. Space Environ. Med.*, 55, 206–12.
———; Steinman, A.M. (1975) 'Accidental hypothermia: an experimental study of inhalation rewarming.' *Aviat. Space Environ. Med.*, *46*, 1236–40.
———; Collis, M.L.; Eckerson, J.D. (1973) 'Thermographic evaluation of relative heat loss areas of man during cold water immersion.' *Aerospace Med.*, *44*, 708–11.
———; Collis, M.L.; Eckerson, J.D. (1975b) 'Effect of behavioural variables on cooling rate of man in cold water.' *J. Appl. Physiol.*, *38*, 1073–7.

———; Eckerson, J.D.; Collis, M.L. (1975a) 'Thermal balance and survival time prediction of man in cold water.' *Can. J. Physiol. Pharmacol.*, *53*, 21–32.

———; Eckerson, J.D.; Collis, M.L. (1977) 'Thermoregulatory heat production in man; prediction equation based on skin and core temperatures.' *J. Appl. Physiol.*, *42*, 377–84.

———; Eckerson, J.D.; Kemna, D. (1984a) 'Thermal and cardiovascular changes during three methods of resuscitation from mild hypothermia.' *Resuscitation*, *11*, 21–33.

———; Hay, C.; Matthews, B.R.; Overweel, C.H.; Radford, D.P. (1984b) 'Temperature effect on the human dive response in relation to cold water near-drowning.' *J. Appl. Physiol.*, *56*, 202–6.

Hayward, M.G.; Keatinge, W.R. (1979) 'Progressive symptomless hypothermia in water; possible cause of diving accidents.' *Br. Med. J.*, *i*, 1182.

Health and Safety Executive (1978) *One Hundred Fatal Accidents in Construction.* Health and Safety Executive, HMSO, London.

Health Education Council (1977) *Keep Baby Warm*. Health Education Council, London.

Heath, D.; Williams, D.R. (1981) *Man at High Altitude.* Churchill Livingstone, Edinburgh.

———; Brewer, D.; Hicken, P. (1968) *Cor pulmonale in Emphysema*. Charles C. Thomas, Springfield, Ill.

Heaton, R.W.; Guy, R.J.C.; Gray, B.J.; Watkins, P.J.; Costello, J.F. (1984) 'Diminished bronchial reactivity to cold air in diabetic patients with autonomic neuropathy.' *Br. Med. J.*, *ii*, 149–51.

Hedley-White, J.; Burgess, G.E.; Feeley, T.W.; Miller, M.C. (1976) *Applied Physiology, Respiratory Care*. Little, Brown & Co., Boston.

Hegnauer, A.H.; D'Amato, H.D.; Flynn, J. (1951) 'Influence of intraventricular catheters on the course of immersion hypothermia in dogs.' *Am. J. Physiol.*, *167*, 63–8.

———; Shriber, W.J.; Haterius, H.O. (1950) 'Cardiovascular responses of the dog to immersion hypothermia.' *Am. J. Physiol.*, *161*, 455–65.

Heino, M.E. (1980a) 'Ambiguous responses of lung lamellar bodies to sauna-like heat stress in two age groups of adult male rats.' *Aviat. Space Environ. Med.*, *51*, 542–3.

——— (1980b) 'Effects of sauna-like heat stress on the respiratory tract ciliogenesis and cilia in adult male rats.' *Aviat. Space Environ. Med.*, *51*, 885–91.

———; Laitinen, L.A.; Tervo, T. (1981) 'Early polmotoxic effects of oxygen on the rat type II epithelial cell.' *Aviat. Space Environ. Med.*, *52*, 294–8.

Helgason, T. (1977) 'Psychiatric problems in a fishing population.' *Nordic Council Arct. Med. Res., Rep. No. 18*, 7–21.

Hellstrom, B.; Andersen, K.L. (1960) 'Heat output in the cold from hands of arctic fishermen.' *J. Appl. Physiol.*, *15*, 771–5.

———; Berg, K.; Lorentzen, F.V. (1966) 'Human peripheral rewarming during exercise in the cold.' *J. Appl. Physiol.*, *29*, 191–9.

Helweg-Larsen, K. (1984) 'The validity of the mortality statistics in Greenland with special reference to ischaemic heart disease.' *Arct. Med. Res.*, *Report 38*, 43–5.

Hemingway, A. (1941) 'The effect of barbital anaesthesia on temperature regulation.' *Am. J. Physiol.*, *134*, 350–8.

Hendren, H. (1975) Discussion. *J. Ped. Surg.*, *10*, 591–2.

Hercus, W. (1960) 'Temperature changes during thoracotomy in children, infants and the newborn.' *Br. J. Anaesth.*, *32*, 476–80.

Herligkoffer, K.M. (1954) *Nanga Parbat.* Elek Books, London.

Hermansen, M.C.; Perlstein, P.H.; Edwards, N.K. (1984) 'A baffling case of hypothermia.' *Lancet*, *i*, 40–1.

Hernandez, M.J. (1983) 'Cerebral circulation during hypothermia.' In R.S. Pozos and

L.E. Wittmers (eds.) *The Nature and Treatment of Hypothermia*, Croom Helm, London/University of Minnesota, Minneapolis, pp. 61–8.

Hertzman, A.B. (1957) 'Individual differences in regional sweating patterns.' *J. Appl. Physiol.*, *10*, 242–8.

Hervey, G.R. (1973) 'Physiological changes encountered in hypothermia.' *Proc. Roy. Soc. Med.*, *66*, 1053–7.

Hey, E.N. (1972) 'Thermal regulation in the newborn.' *Br. J. Hosp. Med.*, *8*, 51–64.

———; Mount, L.E. (1966) 'Temperature control in incubators.' *Lancet*, *ii*, 202–3.

———; Katz, G.; O'Connell, B. (1970) 'Total thermal insulation of the newborn baby.' *J. Physiol. (Lond.)*, *207*, 683–98.

Hicks, C.E.; McCord, M.C.; Blaunt, S.G. (1956) 'Electrocardiographic changes during hypothermia and circulatory occlusion.' *Circulation*, *13*, 21–8.

Higenbottom, C.; Marcus, P.; Waddell, J. (1977) 'Thermal data from helicopters operating in a sub-arctic environment.' *Aviat. Space Environ. Med.*, *48*, 640–4.

Higgens, R.; Buguet, A.; Kuehn, L. (1978) 'Measurement of skin temperatures of active subjects by wireless telemetry.' *Aviat. Space Environ. Med.*, *49*, 1352–4.

Hill, D.W. (1980) 'Metallized plastic sheeting.' *Br. J. Anaesth.*, *52*, 359.

Hill, R.G.; Hughes, J. (1984) 'Endogenous opioid peptides — biological and clinical significance.' In W.S. Nimmo and G. Smith (eds.) *Opioid Agonist/Antagonist Drugs in Clinical Practice*, Exerpta Medica, Amsterdam, pp. 15–23.

Hillary, Sir E. (1979) 'Three adventurous journeys.' *Br. Med. J.*, *ii*, 1613–16.

Hillman, H. (1971) 'Treatment after exposure to cold.' *Lancet*, *ii*, 1257.

Hilton, S.M. (1965) 'Emotion.' In O.G. Edholm and A.L. Bacharach (eds.) *The Physiology of Human Survival.* Academic Press, London, pp. 479–81.

Hirvonen, J. (1977) 'Fatal accidents in water: a survey.' *Nordic Council Arct. Med. Res., Rep. No. 18*, pp. 38–45.

——— (1979) 'Accidental hypothermia.' In P. Lomax and E. Schonbaum (eds.) *Body Temperature: Regulation, Drug Effects, and Therapeutic Implications.* Marcel Dekker, New York, pp. 561–86.

——— (1982) 'Accidental hypothermia.' *Nordic Council Arct. Med. Res., Rep. No. 30*, pp. 15–19.

Hochachka, P.W.; Murphy, B. (1979) 'Metabolic status during diving and recovery in marine mammals.' In D. Robertshaw (ed.) *Environmental Physiology III*, University Park Press, Baltimore, pp. 253–88.

Hockaday, T.D.R. (1969) 'Accidental hypothermia.' *Br. J. Hosp. Med.*, *2*, 1083–93.

Hodgson, W.C.; Cotton, D.J.; Werner, G.D.; Cockroft, D.W.; Dosman, J.A. (1984) 'Relationship between bronchial response to respiratory heat exchange and nonspecific airways reactivity in asthmatic patients.' *Chest*, *85*, 465–70.

Hoff, H.E.; Stansfield, H. (1949) 'Ventricular fibrillation induced by cold.' *Am. Heart J.*, *38*, 193–201.

Hoke, B.; Jackson, D.L.; Alexander, J.H.; Flynn, E.T. (1976) 'Respiratory heat loss and pulmonary function during cold-gas breathing at high pressure.' In C.J. Lambertsen (ed.) *Underwater Physiology V.* FASEB, Bethesda, pp. 725–40.

Holaday, J.W.; Loh, H.H. (1981) 'Neurobiology of β-Endorphin and related peptides.' In C.H. Li (ed.) *Hormonal Proteins and Peptides. Vol. X, β-Endorphin*, Academic Press, London, pp. 204–92.

Holdcroft, A. (1981) *Body Temperature Control in Anaesthesia, Surgery and Intensive Care.* Baillière Tindall, London.

———; Hall, G.M. (1978) 'Heat loss during anaesthesia.' *Br. J. Anaesth.*, *50*, 157–64.

———; Hall, G.M.; Cooper, G.M. (1979) 'Redistribution of body heat during anaesthesia.' *Anaesthesia*, *34*, 758–64.

Holti, G. (1985) 'Vascular reactivity in patients with Raynaud's phenomenon.' *Scot. Med. J.*, *30*, 120–1.

Holzloehner, E.; Rascher, S.; Finke, E. (1942) 'Report of 10 October 1942 on cooling experiments on human beings.' In *Trials of War Criminals: Vol. 2.* US Govt Print Office, Washington, DC, pp. 226–41.

Hong, S.I.; Nadel, E.R. (1979) 'Thermogenic control during exercise in a cold environment.' *J. Appl. Physiol.*, *47*, 1084–9.

Horak, A.; Raine, R.; Opie, L.H.; Lloyd, E.A. (1983) 'Severe myocardial ischaemia induced by intravenous adrenaline.' *Br. Med. J.*, *i*, 519.

Horita, A.; Snow, A.E. (1980) 'Stress and apomorphine induced hyperthermia in rabbits.' In B. Cox, P. Lomax, A.S. Milton, E. Schonbaum (eds.) *Thermoregulatory Mechanisms and Their Therapeutic Implications.* S. Karger, Basel, pp. 41–2.

Hornback, N.B. (1984) 'Complications of hyperthermia.' In N.B. Hornback (ed.) *Hyperthermia and Cancer. Human Clinical Trial Experience. Vol. II.* CRC Press, Florida, pp. 121–51.

Horton, B.T.; Brown, G.E. (1929) 'Systemic histamine-like reactions in allergy due to cold.' *Am. J. Med. Sci.*, *198*, 191–202.

Horvath, S.M. (1981) 'Exercise in a cold environment.' *Exercise, Sport Sci. Rev.*, *9*, 221–63.

———; Rochelle, R.P. (1977) 'Hypothermia in the aged.' *Environ. Health Perspect.*, *20*, 127–30.

———; Spurr, G.B.; Hutt, B.K.; Hamilton, L.H. (1956) 'Metabolic cost of shivering.' *J. Appl. Physiol.*, *8*, 595–602.

Hossli, G. (1979) 'Pathophysiology of asphyxia during hypothermia.' In P. Matter, P. Braun, M. deQuervain, W. Good (eds.) *Skifahren und Sicherheit III.* Buchdruckerei Davos AG, Davos, pp. 143–50.

Houdas, Y.; Carette, G.; Lecroart, J.L. (1985) 'Cold tolerance.' In J. Rivolier, P. Cerretelli, J. Foray, P. Segantini (eds.) *High Altitude Deterioration.* Karger, Basel, pp. 203–12.

Houk, V.N. (1959) 'Transient pulmonary insufficiency caused by cold.' *US Armed Forces Med. J.*, *10*, 1354–7.

Houlsby, W.T. (1979) 'Accidental hypothermia and low reading thermometers.' *Br. Med. J.*, *i*, 1284.

House, F., Vale, R. (1972) 'Nomograms for calculation of heat loss.' *Br. Med. J.*, *iv*, 20–1.

Howe, G.M. (1972) *Man, Environment and Disease in Britain.* Penguin Books, Harmondsworth.

Howitt, L.F. (1971) 'Death in Scotland from malnutrition and/or hypothermia 1968.' *Health Bull.*, *29*, 43–9.

Hsieh, A.C.L.; Nagasaka, T.; Carlson, L.D. (1965) 'Effect of immersion of the hand in cold water on digital blood flow.' *J. Appl. Physiol.*, *20*, 61–4.

Hsieh, Y.C.; Frayser, R.; Ross, J.C. (1968) 'The effect of cold air inhalation on ventilation in normal subjects and in patients with chronic obstructive pulmonary disease.' *Am. Rev. Resp. Dis.*, *98*, 613–22.

Hudson, M.C.; Robinson, G.J. (1973) 'Treatment of accidental hypothermia.' *Med. J. Austr.*, *1*, 410–11.

Hughes, D.S. (1976) 'An approach to offshore underwater work.' *J. Soc. Underwater Tech.*, *2*, 13–15.

——— (1977) 'Automatic control of ppO_2 in breathing apparatus.' *J. Soc. Underwater Tech.*, *3*, 5.

Humble, B.H. (1969) 'Bothies in the hills.' *Scots Magazine, Nov.*, 170–82.

——— (1972) *Accident Survey for 1971.* Mountain Rescue Committee for Scotland.

Hume, D.M.; Egdahl, R.H.; Nelson, D.H. (1956) 'The effect of hypothermia on pituitary ACTH release and on adrenal cortical and medullary secretion in the dog.' In R.D. Dripps (ed.) *The Physiology of Induced Hypothermia.* National Academy of Sciences — National Research Council, Publication 451, Washington, pp. 170–6.

Hunt, Lord (1977) 'Everest: recollections and reflections.' *Ann. Roy. Coll. Surg. Eng.*, *59*, 160–3.

Hunter, A.R. (1971) 'Reversible death.' *Lancet*, *i*, 140.

Hunter, J.; Kerr, E.H.; Whillans, M.G. (1952) 'The relation between joint stiffness upon exposure to cold and the characteristics of synovial fluid.' *J. Can. Med. Sci.*, *39*, 367–77.

Hutchison, J.H. (1969) 'Hypothermia in infancy.' *Med. Sci. & Law*, *9*, 224–7.

Iampietro, P.F.; Bass, D.E. (1962) 'Heat exchanges of men during caloric restriction in the cold.' *J. Appl. Physiol.*, *17*, 947–9.

———; Bass, D.E.; Buskirk, E.R. (1958) 'Heat exchanges of nude men in the cold: effect of humidity temperature and windspeed.' *J. Appl. Physiol.*, *12*, 351–6.

———; Vaughan, J.A.; Goldman, R.F.; Kreider, M.B.; Masucci, F.; Bass, D.E. (1960) 'Heat production from shivering.' *J. Appl. Physiol.*, *15*, 632–4.

Irravni, J. (1967) 'Flimmerbewelgung in den intrapulmonalen Luftwegen der Ratte.' *Pfleugers Arch.*, *297*, 221–37.

Irvine, R.E. (1974) 'Hypothermia in old age.' *Practitioner*, *213*, 795–800.

Irving, M.H. (1968) 'The sympatho-adrenal factor in haemorrhagic shock.' *Ann. Roy. Coll. Surg. Eng.*, *42*, 367–86.

Isomaki, H.; Virsiheimo, B. (1982) 'Cold and rheumatic diseases.' *Nordic Council Arct. Med. Res.*, *Rep. No. 30*, pp. 29–31.

Item (1976a) 'His shipmate was a ghost.' *Look and Learn Magazine No. 772*, *Oct. 30*, pp. 2–4.

——— (1976b) 'Diagnosis of brain death.' *Br. Med. J.*, *ii*, 1187–8.

Jacob, J.J.; Girault, J-M.T. (1979) '5-hydroxytryptamine.' In P. Lomax and E. Schonbaum (eds.) *Body Temperature: Regulation, Drug Effects, and Therapeutic Implications*. Marcel Dekker, New York, pp. 183–230.

Jacobs, I., Romet, T., Frim, J., Hynes, A. (1984) 'Effects of endurance fitness on responses to cold water immersion.' *Aviat. Space Environ. Med.*, 55, 715–20.

Jacobsen, W.K.; Mason, L.J.; Briggs, B.A.; Schneider, S.; Thompson, J.C. (1983) 'Correlation of spontaneous respiration and neurologic damage in near-drowning.' *Crit. Care Med.*, *11*, 487–9.

Jago, R.H.; Restall, J. (1983) 'Postoperative dreaming.' *Anaesthesia*, *38*, 438–41.

———; Restall, J.; Thompson, M.C. (1984) 'Ketamine and military anaesthesia. The effect of heavy papaveretum premedication and Althesin induction on the incidence of emergence phenomena.' *Anaesthesia*, *39*, 925–7.

James, P.D.; Gothard, J.W.W. (1984) 'Possible hazard from the inserts of condenser humidifiers.' *Anaesthesia*, *39*, 70.

Jansky, L. (1979) 'Heat production.' In P. Lomax and E. Schonbaum (eds.) *Body Temperature: Regulation, Drug Effects, and Therapeutic Implications*. Marcel Dekker, New York, pp. 89–118.

Jasinski, D.R. (1984) 'Opioid receptors and classification.' in W.S. Nimmo and G. Smith. (eds.) *Opioid Agonist/Antagonist Drugs in Clinical Practice*, Exerpta Medica, Amsterdam, pp. 24–30.

Jenkins, J.; Fox, J.; Sharwood-Smith, G. (1983) 'Changes in body heat during transvesical prostatectomy.' *Anaesthesia*, *38*, 748–53.

Jensen, C. (1977) 'Pertinent facts about warm-up.' In E.J. Burke (ed.) *Toward an understanding of Human Performance.* Movement Publications, New York, pp. 58–60.

Jequier, E.; GyGax, P.; Pittet, P.; Vannotti, A. (1974) 'Increased thermal body insulation: relationship to the development of obesity.' *J. Appl. Physiol.*, *36*, 476–78.

Jessen, K.; Hagelsten, J.O. (1972) 'Search and rescue services in Denmark with special reference to accidental hypothermia.' *Aerospace Med.*, *43*, 787–91.

———; Hagelsten, J.O. (1978) 'Peritoneal dialysis in the treatment of profound accidental hypothermia.' *Aviat. Space Environ. Med.*, *49*, 426–9.

——; Hagelsten, J.O.; Graae, J.; Lokkegaard, F.; Lokkegaard, H. (1974) 'Behandling af dyb accidentel hypotermi.' *Ugeskr. Laeger.*, *136*, 2590–5.

Johnson, C.D. (1983) 'Hypothermia in the tropics.' *Bol. Assoc. Med. P. Rico*, *75*, 549–50.

Johnson, D.G.; Hayward, J.S.; Jacobs, T.P.; Collis, M.L.; Eckerson, J.D.; Williams, R.H. (1977) 'Plasma norepinephrine responses of man in cold water.' *J. Appl. Physiol.*, *43*, 216–20.

Johnson, L.A. (1977) 'Accidental hypothermia: peritoneal dialysis.' *J. Am. Coll. Emerg. Phys.*, *6*, 556–61.

Jolly, H.; Molyneux, P.; Newell, D.J. (1962) 'A controlled study of the effect of temperature on premature babies.' *J. Pediat.*, *60*, 889–94.

Jones, J.H. (1971) 'Peritoneal dialysis.' *Br. Med. Bull.*, *27*, 165–9.

Jude, J.R.; Kouwenhoven, W.B.; Knickerbocker, C.G. (1961) 'Cardiac arrest: report of application of external massage in 118 patients.' *J. Am. Med. Ass.*, *178*, 1063.

Juhlin-Dannfelt, A.; Ahlborg, G.; Hagenfeldt, L.; Jorfeldt, L.; Felig, P. (1977) 'The influence of ethanol on splanchnic and skeletal muscle substrate turnover.' *Am. J. Physiol.*, *233*, E195–202.

Jung, R.T.; James, W.P.T. (1980) 'Is obesity metabolic?' *Br. J. Hosp. Med.*, *24*, 503–9.

Juniper, C.P. (1980) 'Exercise-induced asthma.' *Br. Med. J.*, *i*, 565.

Kafer, E.R. (1971) 'Pulmonary oxygen toxicity.' *Br. J. Anaesth.*, *43*, 687–95.

Kanter, G.S. (1962) 'Renal clearance of sodium and potassium in hypothermia.' *Can. J. Biochem. Physiol.*, *40*, 113–22.

Kanwisher, J.W.; Gabrielsen, G.W. (1985) 'The diving response in man.' In L. Rey (ed.) *Arctic Underwater Operations*. Graham & Trotman, London, pp. 81–96.

——; Gabrielsen, G.; Kanwisher, N. (1981) 'Free and forced dives in birds.' *Science*, *211*, 717–19.

Kaplan, A.P. (1984) 'Unusual cold-induced disorders: cold-dependent dermatographism and systemic cold urticaria.' *J. Allergy Clin. Immunol.*, *73*, 453–6.

Kappacoda, C.T.; Macartney, F.J. (1976) 'Effect of environmental temperatures on oxygen consumption in infants with congenital disease of the heart.' *Br. Heart J.*, *38*, 1–4.

Kappes, B.M.; Mills, W.J. (1984) 'Thermal biofeedback training with frostbite patients.' *Presentation at Sixth International Symposium on Circumpolar Health. May 13–18, 1984. Anchorage, Alaska.* Abstracts p. 100.

Karhunen, U.; Cazanitis, D.A. (1983) 'Hypothermia diagonsed as near-drowning in a child.' *J. R. Soc. Med.*, *76*, 967–9.

Karvonen, M.J. (1977) '15-year incidence of coronary heart disease in the east–west population study.' *Nordic Council Arct. Med. Res.*, *Rep. No. 19*, pp. 78–83.

Katz, B.; Miledi, R. (1965) 'The effect of temperature on the synaptic delay at the neuromuscular junction.' *J. Physiol. (Lond.)*, *181*, 656–70.

Kaufman, W.C. (1983) 'The development and rectification of hiker's hypothermia.' In R.S. Pozos and L.E. Wittmers (eds.) *The Nature and Treatment of Hypothermia*, Croom Helm, London, pp. 46–57.

Kaul, S.V.; Beard, A.J.; Millar, R.A. (1973) Preganglionic sympathetic activity and baroreceptor responses during hypothermia.' *Br. J. Anaesth.*, *45*, 433–9.

Kavanagh, T. (1976) *Heart Attack? Counter Attack!* Van Nostrand Reinhold, Toronto.

Kawakami, Y.; Natelson, B.H.; DuBois, A. (1967) 'Cardiovascular effects of face immersion and factors affecting diving reflex in man.' *J. Appl. Physiol.*, *23*, 964–70.

Keatinge, W.R. (1965) 'Death after shipwreck.' *Br. Med. J.*, *ii*, 1537–41.

—— (1969) *Survival in Cold Water*. Blackwell, Edinburgh.

—— (1973) 'Cooling rates of young people swimming in cold water.' *J. Appl.*

Physiol., *45*, 371–5.

——— (1977) 'Accidental immersion hypothermia and drowning.' *Practitioner*, *219*, 183–7.

———; Cannon, P. (1960) 'Freezing point of human skin.' *Lancet*, *i*, 11–14.

———; Evans, M. (1960) 'Effect of food, alcohol and hyoscine on body-temperature and reflex responses of men immersed in cold water.' *Lancet*, *ii*, 176–8.

———; Evans, M. (1961) 'The respiratory and cardiovascular response to immersion in cold water.' *Q. J. Exp. Physiol.*, *46*, 83–9.

———; Hayward, M.G. (1981) 'Sudden death in cold water and ventricular arrhythmia.' *J. Forensic Sci.*, *26*, 459–61.

———; Sloan, R.E.G. (1975) 'Deep body temperature from aural canal with servo-controlled heating to outer ear.' *J. Appl. Physiol.*, *38*, 919–21.

———; Coleshaw, S.R.K.; Cotter, F.; Mattock, M.; Murphy, M.; Chelliah, R. (1984) 'Increases in platelet and red cell counts, blood viscosity, and arterial pressure during mild surface cooling; factors in mortality from coronary and cerebral thrombosis in winter.' *Br. Med. J.*, *ii*, 1405–8.

———; Hayward, M.G.; McIver, N.K. (1980) 'Hypothermia during saturation diving in the North Sea.' *Br. Med. J.*, *i*, 291.

———; Prys-Roberts, C.; Cooper, K.E.; Haight, J.; Honour, A.G. (1969) 'Sudden failure of swimming in cold water.' *Br. Med. J.*, *i*, 480–3.

Kehlet, H.; Binder, C. (1973) 'Adrenocortical function and clinical course during and after surgery in unsupplemented glucocorticoid-treated patients.' *Br. J. Anaesth.*, *45*, 1043–8.

———; Nikki, P.; Jaattela, A.; Takki, S. (1974) 'Plasma catecholamine concentrations during surgery in unsupplemented glucocorticoid-treated patients.' *Br. J. Anaesth.*, *46*, 73–7.

Kempson, G.E.; Coggan, D.; Acheson, E.D. (1983) 'Electrically heated gloves for intermittent digital ischaemia.' *Br. Med. J.*, *i*, 268.

Kennaird, D.L. (1973) 'Hypothermia in infancy.' *Guy's Hosp. Rep.*, *122*, 9–15.

Kenyon, J.R. (1961) 'Experimental deep hypothermia.' *Br. Med. Bull.*, *17*, 43–7.

Kerslake, D.M. (1969) 'Climate and clothing. The value of reflecting layers in clothing.' *Proc. Roy. Soc. Med.*, *62*, 283–4.

Kerslake, D. McK. (1972) *The Stress of Hot Environments*. Cambridge University Press, Cambridge.

Kettle, M.P. (1975) 'Diver's equipment.' *J. Soc. Underwater Tech.*, *1*, 14–17.

Kew, M.C. (1976) 'The effects of temperature change on the human body.' *Br. J. Hosp. Med.*, *16*, 502–15.

Khalil, H.H. (1958) 'Hypothermia by internal cooling in man.' *Lancet*, *i*, 1092–4.

———; MacKeith, R.C. (1954) 'A simple method of raising and lowering body temperature.' *Br. Med. J.*, *ii*, 734–6.

Khogali, M.; Hales, J.R.S. (eds.) (1984) *Heat Stroke and Temperature Regulation*. Academic Press, London.

———; Gumaa, K.; Mustafa, M.K.Y. (1983) 'Fatal heat stroke in a long distance runner.' *Br. Med. J.*, *ii*, 1549.

Killian, H. (1966) *Der Kalte-Unfall. Algemeine Unterkuhlung*. Dustri-Verlag, Munchen.

——— (1981) *Cold and Frost Injuries*. Springer-Verlag, Berlin.

Kinnersley, P. (1974) *The Hazards of Work: How to Fight Them*. Pluto Press, Surrey.

Kirch, T.J.; de Kornfeld, T.J. (1967) 'An unexpected complication (hypothermia) while using the Emerson postoperative ventilator.' *Anesthesiology*, *28*, 1106–7.

Klarskov, P.; Amter, F. (1976) 'Hypotermi efter drukning, korrektion med peritoneal-dialyse.' *Ugeskr. Leger*, *138*, 1937–40.

Klein, E.F.; Graves, S.A. (1974) '"Hot pot" tracheitis.' *Chest*, *65*, 225–6.

Knight, J.G. (1982) 'Dopamine-receptor-stimulating autoantibodies: a possible cause of schizophrenia.' *Lancet*, *ii*, 1073–6.

Koehler, R.C.; Chandra, N.; Guerci, A.D.; Tsitlik, J.; Traystman, R.J.; Rogers, M.C.; Weisfeldt, M.L. (1983) 'Augmentation of cerebral perfusion by simultaneous chest compression and lung inflation with abdominal binding after cardiac arrest in dogs.' *Circulation*, *67*, 266–75.

Kouwenhoven, W.B.; Judge, J.P.; Nickerbocker, S.G. (1960) 'Closed chest cardiac massage.' *J. Am. Med. Ass.*, *173*, 1064–7.

Krarup, N.; Larsen, J.A. (1972) 'The effect of slight hypothermia on liver function as measured by the elimination rate of ethanol, the hepatic uptake and excretion of indocyanine green and bile formation.' *Acta Physiol. Scand.*, *84*, 396–407.

Krebs, H.A.; Freedland, R.A.; Hems, R.; Stubles, M. (1969) 'Inhibition of hepatic gluconeogenesis by ethanol.' *Biochem. J.*, *112*, 117–24.

Krejci, V.; Koch, P. (1980) *Muscle and Tendon Injuries in Athletes*. (Trans. D. leVey.) YB Medical Publishers, London.

Kuehn, L.A. (1985) 'Medical and physiological problems.' In L. Rey (ed.) *Arctic Underwater Operations*. Graham & Trotman, London, pp. 7–18.

——; Ackles, K.N.; Cole, J.D. (1977) 'Survival test of submersible life support systems.' *Aviat. Space Environ. Med.*, *48*, 332–8.

——; Tikuisis, P.; Livingstone, S.; Limmer, R. (1980) 'Body cooling after death.' *Aviat. Space Environ. Med.*, *51*, 965–9.

Kugelberg, J.; Schuller, H.; Berg, B.; Kallum, B. (1967) 'Treatment of accidental hypothermia.' *Scand. J. Thorac. Cardiovasc. Surg.*, *1*, 142–6.

Kugler-Podelleck, I.; Rodewald, G.; Horatz, K.; Kugler, S.; Muller-Brunotte, P. (1965) 'Erfolgreich Wiederbelebung bei Ertrinken im Eiswasser.' *Dtsch. Med. Wschr.*, *90*, 74–80.

Kumar, R.; Hedge, K.S.; Krishna, B.; Sharma, R.S. (1980) 'Combined effect of hypoxia and cold on the phospholipid composition of lung surfactant in rats.' *Aviat. Space Environ. Med.*, *51*, 459–62.

Kurtz, K.J. (1982) 'Hypothermia in the elderly: the cold facts.' *Geriatrics*, *37*, 85–93.

Kvittingen, T.D.; Naess, A. (1963) 'Recovery from drowning in fresh water.' *Br. Med. J.*, *i*, 1315–17.

Lacey, D.J. (1983) 'Sleep EEG abnormalities in children with near-miss sudden infant death syndrome, in siblings, and in infants with recurrent apnea.' *J. Pediatr.*, *102*, 855–9.

Lacoumenta, S.; Hall, G.M. (1984) 'Liquid crystal thermometry during anaesthesia.' *Anaesthesia*, *39*, 54–6.

Laessing, C.J. (1982) 'Report of experiences gathered in the treatment of hypothermic victims.' In P. Koch and M. Kohfahl (eds.) *Unterkuhlung im Seenotfall. 2nd Symposium*. Deutsche Gesellschaft zur Rettung Schiffbruchiger, Cuxhaven, pp. 154–9.

Lagerspetz, K.Y.H. (1982) 'Reactions and adaptations of organisms to cold.' *Nordic Council Arct. Med. Res., Rep. No. 30*, pp. 7–14.

Lahti, A. (1982) 'Cutaneous reactions to cold.' *Nordic Council Arct. Med. Res., Rep. No. 30*, pp. 32–5.

Laitinen, L.A.; Tokola, O.; Gothoni, G.; Vapaatalo, H. (1981) 'Scopolamine alone or combined with ephedrine in seasickness: a double-blind, placebo-controlled study.' *Aviat. Space Environ. Med.*, *52*, 6–10.

Lambertsen, C.J. (ed.) (1976) *Underwater Physiology V*. FASEB, Bethesda.

Lancet (1972a) 'Severe accidental hypothermia.' *Lancet*, *i*, 237.

—— (1972b) 'Treatment after exposure to cold.' *Lancet*, *i*, 378.

—— (1979) 'Sleep apnoea syndrome.' *Lancet*, *i*, 25–6.

—— (1981a) 'Social class and ischaemic heart disease.' *Lancet*, *ii*, 347.

—— (1981b) 'The diving reflex.' *Lancet*, *i*, 1403–4.

—— (1982) 'Stress, hypertension and the heart: the adrenaline trilogy.' *Lancet*, *ii*,

1440–1.

——— (1983) 'Twenty-four hour blood pressure control: does it matter?' *Lancet*, *i*, 222–3.

——— (1985) 'Asthma and the weather.' *Lancet*, *i*, 1079–80.

Lapidus, L.; Bengtsson, C.; Larsson, B.; Pennert, K.; Rybo, E.; Sjostrom, L. (1984) 'Distribution of adipose tissue and risk of cardiovascular disease and death: a 12 year follow up of participants in the population study of women in Gothenburg, Sweden.' *Br. Med. J.*, *ii*, 1257–61.

Larsson, B.; Svardsudd, K.; Welin, L.; Wilhelmsen, L.; Bjorntorp, P.; Tibblin, G. (1984) 'Abdominal adipose tissue distribution, obesity and risk of cardiovascular disease: a 13 year follow up of participants in the study of men born in 1913.' *Br. Med. J.*, *i*, 1401–4.

Lash, R.F.; Burdette, J.A.; Ozdil, T. (1967) 'Accidental profound hypothermia and barbiturate intoxication. A report of rapid 'core' rewarming by peritoneal dialysis.' *J. Am. Med. Ass.*, *201*, 269–70.

Latcham, R.W., Kreitman, N., Plant, M.A., Crawford, A. (1984) 'Regional variations in British alcohol morbidity rates: a myth uncovered? 1: Clinical surveys.' *Br. Med. J.*, *ii*, 1341–3.

Lathrop, T.G. (1972) *Hypothermia: Killer of the Unprepared*. Mazamas, Portland, Oregon.

Laufman, H. (1951) 'Profound accidental hypothermia.' *J. Am. Med. Ass.*, *147*, 1201–12.

Lawless, J.; Lawless, M.M. (1972) 'Malnutrition and body temperature.' *Br. Med. J.*, *i*, 566–7.

Lawrence, F.H. (1984) Letter. *Aviat. Space Environ. Med.*, 55, 500.

Lawson, A.A.H. (1976) 'Intensive therapy of acute poisoning.' *Br. J. Hosp. Med.*, *16*, 333–48.

Leathart, G.L. (1971) 'Treatment after exposure to cold.' *Lancet*, *ii*, 1257.

Le Blanc, J. (1966) 'Adaptive mechanisms in humans.' *Ann. N.Y. Acad. Sci.*, *134*, 721–31.

——— (1976) 'Physiological responses to cooling of the face.' In R.J. Shephard and S. Itoh (eds.) *Circumpolar Health*. University Press, Toronto, pp. 72–73.

———; Dulac, S.; Cote, J.; Girard, B. (1975) 'Autonomic nervous system and adaptation to cold in man.' *J. Appl. Physiol.*, *39*, 181–6.

Ledingham, I. McA. (1979) 'Internal or external rewarming.' In P. Matter, P. Braun, M. deQuervain, W. Good (eds.) *Skifahren und Sicherheit III*. Buchdruckerei Davos AG, Davos, pp. 168–71.

——— (1981) 'Management of urban hypothermia.' In J.N. Adams (ed.) *Hypothermia Ashore and Afloat*. Aberdeen University Press, Aberdeen, pp. 151–7.

——— (1983a) 'Clinical management of elderly hypothermic patients.' In R.S. Pozos and L.E. Wittmers (eds.) *The Nature and Treatment of Hypothermia*. Croom Helm, London/University of Minnesota Press, Minneapolis, pp. 165–81.

——— (1983b) Discussion. In R.S. Pozos and L.E. Wittmers (eds.) *The Nature and Treatment of Hypothermia*. Croom Helm, London/University of Minnesota Press, Minneapolis, p. 258.

———; Mone, J.G. (1972) 'Treatment after exposure to cold.' *Lancet*, *i*, 534–5.

———; Mone, J.G. (1978) 'Accidental hypothermia.' *Lancet*, *i*, 391.

———; Mone, J.G. (1980) 'Treatment of accidental hypothermia: a prospective clinical study.' *Br. Med. J.*, *i*, 1102–5.

———; Mone, J.G. (1982) 'Hypothermia in the elderly.' *Br. J. Hosp. Med.*, *27*, 317.

———; Norman, J.N. (1964) 'Immersion hypothermia re-explored.' *Br. J. Surg.*, *51*, 69.

———; Douglas, I.H.; Routh, G.S.; MacDonald, A.M. (1980) 'Central rewarming system for treatment of hypothermia.' *Lancet*, *i*, 1168–9.

——; MacVicar, S.; Watt, I.; Weston, G.A. (1982) 'Early resuscitation after marathon collapse.' *Lancet*, *ii*, 1096–7.

Lee, H.A.; Ames, A.C. (1965) 'Haemodialysis in severe barbiturate poisoning.' *Br. Med. J.*, *i*, 1217–19.

Lee, E.C.B.; Lee, K. (1971) *Survival and Safety at Sea*. Cassell, London.

Lee, T.H.; Assoufi, B.K.; Kay, A.B. (1983) 'The link between exercise, respiratory heat exchange, and the mast cell in bronchial asthma.' *Lancet*, *i*, 520–2.

Leese, D.E.; Schuette, W. (1980) 'Microwave rewarming.' *Anesth. Analg. (Cleve.)*, *59*, 161.

——; Schuette, W.; Bull, J.M.; Whang-Peng, J.; Atkinson, E.B.; Macnamara, T.E. (1978) 'An evaluation of liquid-crystal thermometry as a screening device for intraoperative hyperthermia.' *Anesth. Analg. (Cleve.)*, *57*, 669–74.

Leese, W.L.B. (1981) 'Considerations of disaster caused by helicopter ditching.' In J.N. Adams (ed.) *Hypothermia Ashore and Afloat*, Aberdeen University Press, Abderdeen, pp. 75–82.

——; Norman, J.N. (1979) 'Helicopter passenger survival suits standards in the U.K. offshore oil industry.' *Aviat. Space Environ. Med.*, *50*, 110–14.

Legrand, V. (1984) 'Les rechauffeurs d'air.' *These pour le Doctorat en Medecine*, Lille.

Lehmann, J.F. (1971) 'Diathermia.' In *Handbook of Physical Medicine and Rehabilitation. 2nd Ed.* W.B. Saunders, Philadelphia, pp. 1397–1442.

Lehrmann, H. (1982) '12 hours in distress in tide-waters.' In P. Koch and M. Kohfahl (eds.) *Unterkuhlung im Seenotfall. 2nd Symposium*. Deutsche Gesellschaft zur Rettung Schiffbruchiger, Cuxhaven, pp. 22–5.

Leigh, D.A. (1974) 'The treatment of infection in peritoneal dialysis.' *Br. J. Hosp. Med.*, *12*, 389–403.

Leitch, D.R. (1981) 'A study of unusual incidents in a well-documented series of dives.' *Aviat. Space Environ. Med.*, *52*, 618–24.

——; Pearson, R.R. (1978) 'Decompression sickness or cold injury?' *Undersea Biomed. Res.*, 5, 363–7.

Leithead, C.S. (1965) 'Hot climates.' In O.G. Edholm and A.L. Bacharach (eds.) *Exploration Medicine*. John Wright, Bristol, pp. 197–244.

Leon, D.F.; Amidi, M.; Leonard, J.J. (1970) 'Left heart work and temperature responses to cold exposure in man.' *Am. J. Cardiol.*, *26*, 38–45.

Lepesckin, E. (1951) 'Role of temperature gradients within ventricular muscle in genesis of normal T wave of electrocardiogram and ventricular gradient responsible for it.' *Fed. Proc.*, *10*, 81.

Leppaluoto, J. (1984) 'Cold as a disabling factor in northern countries.' *Nordic Council Arct. Med. Res.*, *Rep. No. 37*,·pp. 10–12.

——; Hassi, J.; Paakkonen, R. (1984) 'Seasonal variation of blood pressure, basal metabolism rate and skin temperature in outdoor workers in northern Finland.' *Presentation at Sixth International Symposium on Circumpolar Health. May 13–18, 1984. Anchorage, Alaska.* Abstracts p. 74.

Levack, I.D. (1983) 'Oxygen hazards in divers' breathing helium and oxygen mixtures.' *Br. Med. J.*, *ii*, 1594–5.

Levison, H.; Linsao, L.; Swyer, P.R. (1966) 'A comparison of infra-red and convective heating for newborn infants.' *Lancet*, *ii*, 1346–8.

Lewis, D.G.; Mackenzie, A. (1972) 'Cooling during major vascular surgery.' *Br. J. Anaesth.*, *44*, 859–64.

Lewis, R.A.; Lewis, M.N.; Tattersfield, A.E. (1984) 'Asthma induced by suggestion. Is it due to airway cooling?' *Am. Rev. Respir. Dis.*, *129*, 691–5.

Lewis, T.; Landis, E.M. (1929) 'Some physiological effects of sympathetic ganglionectomy in the human being and its effect in a case of Raynaud's malady.' *Heart*, *15*, 151–76.

Light, I.M.; Norman, J.N. (1980) 'The thermal properties of a survival bag incorporating metallised plastic sheeting.' *Aviat. Space Environ. Med.*, *51*, 367–70.

———; Dingwall, R.H.M.; Norman, J.N. (1980) 'The thermal protection offered by lightweight survival systems.' *Aviat. Space Environ. Med.*, *51*, 1100–3.

———; Norman, J.N.; Stoddart, M. (1983) 'Rewarming from immersion hypothermia: reduction of afterdrop.' *Scot. Med. J.*, *28*, 80–1.

Lightman, S.L. (1978) 'Dialysis in renal failure.' *Br. J. Clin. Equip.*, *3*, 236–7.

Lilja, G.P. (1983) 'Emergency treatment of hypothermia.' In R.S. Pozos and L.E. Wittmers (eds.) *The Nature and Treatment of Hypothermia*. Croom Helm, London/University of Minnesota Press, Minneapolis, pp. 143–51.

Lim, T.P.K. (1960) 'Central and peripheral control mechanisms of shivering and its effect on respiration.' *J. Appl. Physiol.*, *15*, 567–74.

Linderholm, H. (1977) 'The cold environment and coronary insufficiency.' *Nordic Council Arct. Med. Res., Rep. No. 18*, pp. 48–56.

——— (1982) 'Coronary insufficiency and cold.' *Nordic Council Arct. Med. Res., Rep. No. 30*, pp. 23–8.

———; Lagerkvist, B. (1984) 'Increased tendency to cold induced vasospasm in the fingers (Raynaud's phenomenon) in copper smelter workers exposed to arsenic (As).' *Presentation at Sixth International Symposium on Circumpolar Health. May 13–18, 1984. Anchorage, Alaska.* Abstracts p. 72.

Lindner, K.H.; Dick, W.; Lotz, P. (1983) 'The delayed use of positive end-expiratory pressure (PEEP) during respiratory resuscitation following near-drowning with fresh or salt water.' *Resuscitation*, *10*, 197–211.

Linklater, M. (1982) *Massacre: The Story of Glencoe*. Collins, London.

Linton, A.L.; Ledingham, I. McA. (1966) 'Severe hypothermia with barbiturate intoxication.' *Lancet*, *i*, 24–6.

Lippitt, M.W.; Nuckols, M.L. (1983) 'Active diver thermal protection requirements for cold water diving.' *Aviat. Space Environ. Med.*, *54*, 644–8.

Livingstone, S.D.; Kuehn, L.A.; Limmer, R.E.; Weatherson, B. (1980) 'The effect of alcohol on body heat loss.' *Aviat. Space Environ. Med.*, *51*, 961–4.

Lloyd, E.L. (1971) 'Treatment after exposure to cold.' *Lancet*, *ii*, 1376.

——— (1972) 'Diagnostic problems and hypothermia.' *Br. Med. J.*, *iii*, 417.

——— (1973) 'Accidental hypothermia treated by central rewarming via the airway.' *Br. J. Anaesth.*, *45*, 41–8.

——— (1977) 'Accidental hypothermia.' *Outdoors*, *8*, 9–10.

——— (1979a) 'Treatment of accidental hypothermia.' *Br. Med. J.*, *i*, 413–14.

——— (1979b) 'Practical prospects for central rewarming from hypothermia.' In P. Matter, P. Braun, M. deQuervain, W. Good (eds.) *Skifahren und Sicherheit III*. Buchdruckerei Davos AG, Davos, pp. 172–81.

——— (1979c) 'Oral temperature and hypothermia.' *Br. Med. J.*, *i*, 1221.

——— (1979d) 'Diving and hypothermia.' *Br. Med. J.*, *ii*, 668.

——— (1979e) 'Temperature sensations in veins.' *Anaesthesia*, *34* 919.

——— (1981a) 'Hypothermia in the elderly. 1. Risk factors and prevention.' *Edinburgh Medicine, Jan,*, 5–6.

——— (1981b) 'Hypothermia in the elderly. 2. Identification and treatment.' *Edinburgh Medicine, Mar.*, 5.

——— (1981c) 'A rational regimen for peri-operative steroid supplements and a clinical assessment of the requirement.' *Ann. R. Coll. Surg. Eng.*, *63*, 54–7.

——— (1982) 'Hallucinations and misinterpretations in hypothermia and cold stress.' In B. Harvald and J.P. Hart Hansen (eds.) *Circumpolar Health 81*. Nordic Council for Arctic Medical Research, Copenhagen, pp. 612–16.

——— (1983a) 'Hallucinations in hypothermia and cold stress and their neurochemical basis.' In P. Lomax and E. Schonbaum (eds.) *Environment, Drugs and Thermoregulation*. Karger, Basel, pp. 40–2.

——— (1983b) 'Marathon medicine.' *Lancet*, *i*, 69–70.

——— (1986) 'Treatment of accidental hypothermia.' MD Thesis, submitted University of Edinburgh.

———; Croxton, D. (1981) 'Equipment for the provision of airway warming (insulation) in the treatment of accidental hypothermia.' *Resuscitation*, *9*, 61–5.

———; Frankland, J.C. (1974) 'Accidental hypothermia treated by central rewarming in the field.' *Br. Med. J.*, *iv*, 717.

———; MacRae, W.R. (1971) 'Respiratory tract damage in burns, case reports and a review of the literature.' *Br. J. Anaesth.*, *43*, 365–79.

———; Mitchell, B. (1974) 'Factors affecting the onset of ventricular fibrillation in hypothermia: a hypothesis. *Lancet*, *ii*, 1294–6.

———; Conliffe, N; Orgel, H.; Walker, P. (1972) 'Accidental hypothermia: an apparatus for central rewarming as a first-aid measure.' *Scot. Med. J.*, *17*, 83–91.

———; Mitchell, B.; Williams, J.T. (1976a) 'Rewarming from immersion hypothermia. A comparison of three methods.' *Resuscitation*, 5, 5–18.

———; Mitchell, B.; Williams, J.T. (1976b) 'The cardiovascular effects of three methods of rewarming from immersion hypothermia.' *Resuscitation*, 5, 229–33.

Lloyd, O.C. (1964) 'Cavers dying of cold.' *Bristol Med. Chir. J.*, *79*, 1–5.

Lockhart, J.M. (1960) 'Extreme body cooling and psychomotor performance.' *Ergonomics*, *11*, 249–60.

———; Keiss, O.K. (1971) 'Auxilliary heating of hands during cold exposure and manual performance.' *Hum. Factors*, *13*, 457–65.

Logan, R.L.; Riemersma, R.A.; Thomson, M.; Oliver, M.F.; Olsson, A.G.; Walldius, G.; Rossner, S.; Kaijser, L.; Callmer, E.; Carlson, L.A.; Lockerbie, L.; Lutz, W. (1978) 'Risk factors for ischaemic heart-disease in normal men aged 40. Edinburgh-Stockholm study.' *Lancet*, *i*, 949–55.

Lomax, P. (1983) 'Neuropharmocological aspects of thermoregulation.' In R.S. Pozos and L.E. Wittmers (eds.) *The Nature and Treatment of Hypothermia*, Croom Helm, London University of Minnesota Press, Minneapolis, pp. 81–93.

——— (1985) 'Environmental stress.' In L. Rey (ed.) *Arctic Underwater Operations*, Graham & Trotman, London, pp. 29–40.

———; Green, M.D. (1979) 'Histamine.' In P. Lomax and E. Schonbaum (eds.) *Body Temperature: Regulation, Drug Effects, and Therapeutic Implications*. Marcel Dekker, New York, pp. 289–304.

———; Schonbaum, E. (eds.) (1979) *Body Temperature: Regulation, Drug Effects and Therapeutic Implications*. Marcel Dekker, New York.

———; Schonbaum, E. (eds.) (1983) *Environment, Drugs and Thermoregulation*. Karger, Basel.

Lougheed, W.M. (1961) 'The central nervous system in hypothermia.' *Br. Med. Bull.*, *17*, 61–5.

Lovel, T.W.I. (1962) 'Myxoedema coma.' *Lancet*, *i*, 823–7.

Low, A. (1982) 'The "ELMA TRES" tragedy: real life drama in a hurricane.' In P. Koch and M. Kohfahl (eds.) *Unterkuhlung im Seenotfall. 2nd Symposium*. Deutsche Gesellschaft zur Rettung Schiffbruchiger, Cuxhaven, pp. 26–33.

Lunn, H.F. (1967) 'Effect of humidity of inspired air on aural temperature.' *J. Physiol. (Lond.)*, *189*, 51–2.

——— (1969) 'Observations on heat gain and loss in surgery.' *Guy's Hosp. Rep.*, *118*, 117–27.

McAllister, T.W. (1975) 'A single-use clinical thermometer.' *Scot. Med. J.*, *20*, 300–4.

McAniff, J.J. (1980) 'The incidence of hypothermia in scuba diving fatalities.' Presented at *International Hypothermia Conference and Workshop*, Univ. of Rhode Is., USA. Jan., 1980.

McCaffrey, T.V.; Geis, G.S.; Chung, J.M.; Wurster, R.D. (1975a) 'Effect of isolated head heating and cooling on sweating in man.' *Aviat. Space Environ. Med.*, *46*, 1353–7.

———; McCook, R.D.; Wurster, R.D. (1975b) 'Effect of head skin temperature on

tympanic and oral temperature in man.' *J. Appl. Physiol.*, *39*, 114–18.
McCook, R.D.; Peiss, C.N.; Randall, W.C. (1961) 'Hypothalamic temperature responses to blood flow and anesthesia. *Fed. Proc.*, *20*, 213–17.
McCrone, R.O.O. (1978) 'Swimming dangers.' *Scotsman*, *June 19*, 8, Col. 6.
McDonald, I.H.; Stocks, J.G. (1965) 'Prolonged nasotracheal intubation: a review of its development in a paediatric hospital.' *Br. J. Anaesth.*, *37*, 161–73.
McDonald, P. (1979) 'Immersion injury and frostbite.' *Br. Med. J.*, *i*, 958.
McFadden, E.R. (1981) 'An analysis of exercise as a stimulus for the production of airway obstruction.' *Lung*, *159*, 3–11.
——— (1983) 'Respiratory heat and water exchange: physiological and clinical implications.' *J. Appl. Physiol.*, *54*, 331–6.
McHardy, V.U.; Inglis, J.M.; Calder, M.A.; Crofton, J.W.; Gregg, I.; Ryland, D.A.; Taylor, P.; Chadwick, M.; Coombs, D.; Riddell, R.W. (1980) 'A study of infective and other factors in exacerbations of chronic bronchitis.' *Br. J. Dis. Chest*, *74*, 228–38.
McHarg, J.F. (1980) 'A vision of Nechtansmere.' *The Scots Magazine*, *Jan.*, 379–87.
MacInnes, C. (1971) 'Steroids in mountain rescue.' *Lancet*, *i*, 599.
——— (1979) 'Treatment of accidental hypothermia.' *Br. Med. J.*, *i*, 130–1.
———; Rothwell, R.I.; Jacobs, R.S.; Nabarro, J.D.N. (1971) 'Plasma 11-hydroxy-corticosteroid and growth-hormone levels in climbers.' *Lancet*, *i*, 49–51.
McKean, W.I.; Dixon, S.R.; Gwynne, J.F.; Irvine, R.O.H. (1970) 'Renal failure after accidental hypothermia.' *Br. Med. J.*, *ii*, 463–4.
McKee, A. (1966) *Black Saturday*. New English Library, London.
McKee, J.I.; Finlay, W.E.I. (1983) 'Cortisol replacement in severely stressed patients.' *Lancet*, *i*, 484.
Mackenzie, A. (1973) 'Hazards in the operating theatre; environmental control.' *Ann. R. Coll. Surg.*, *52*, 361–5.
Mackuanying, N.; Chalon, J. (1974) 'Humidification of anaesthetic gases for children.' *Anesth. Analg. (Cleve.)*, *53*, 387–91.
Maclean, D.; Emslie-Smith, D. (1977) *Accidental Hypothermia*, Blackwell, Edinburgh.
———; Griffiths, P.D.; Emslie-Smith, D. (1968) 'Serum enzymes in relation to electrocardiographic changes in accidental hypothermia.' *Lancet*, *ii*, 1266–70.
McMichael, J. (1974) 'Diet and exercise in coronary heart disease.' *Lancet*, *i*, 1340–1.
McNicholas, W.T.; Fitzgerald, M.X. (1984) 'Nocturnal deaths among patients with chronic bronchitis and emphysema.' *Br. Med. J.*, *ii*, 878.
McNicol, M.W.; Smith, R. (1964) 'Accidental hypothermia.' *Br. Med. J.*, *i*, 19–21.
McOwan, R. (1979) 'The hills are alive.' *The Scots Magazine*, *Dec.*, 258–67.
——— (1985) 'Beneath the shelter stone.' *The Scots Magazine*, *122*, 420–8.
Masden, J.V. (1983) 'Svaer accidentel hypotermi behandlet med varmeloft.' *Ugeskr. Laeger.*, *145*, 3409–11.
Mager, M.; Francesconi, R. (1983) 'The relationship of glucose metabolism to hypothermia.' In R.S. Pozos and L.E. Wittmers (eds.) *The Nature and Treatment of Hypothermia*, Croom Helm, London/University of Minnesota Press, Minneapolis, pp. 100–20.
Maier, G.W.; Tyson, G.S.; Olsen, C.O.; Kernstine, K.H.; Davies, J.W.; Conn, E.H.; Sabiston, D.C.; Rankin, S.J. (1984) 'The physiology of external cardiac massage; high impulse cardiopulmonary resuscitation.' *Circulation*, *70*, 86–101.
———; Tyson, G.S.; Olsen, C.O.; Kernstine, K.H.; Murrah, R.; Rankin, S.J.; Sabiston, D.C. (1982) 'Optimal techniques of external cardiac massage.' *Am. Coll. Surgeons Surg. Forum*, *33*, 282–4.
Malamos, B.; Moulopoulos, S.; Konstandinidis, K.; Panayotopoulos, E. (1962) 'Blood pH changes and ventricular fibrillation in deep hypothermia.' *J. Thor.*

Cardiovasc. Surg., *43*, 453–8.
Malhotra, M.S.; Mathew, L. (1978) 'Effect of rewarming at various water bath temperatures in experimental frostbite.' *Aviat. Space Environ. Med.*, *49*, 874–6.
Malmros, I. (1977) 'Some aspects about frostbites among patients in the northern part of Sweden.' *Nordic Council Arct. Med. Res.*, *Rep. No. 18*, pp. 72–5.
Maningas, P.A. (1985) 'Cardiac output using ECM in hypothermic dogs.' Presentation at 4th World Congress on Emergency and Disaster Medicine. Brighton 4–7 June 1985.
Mann, J.S.; Howarth, P.H.; Holgate, S.T. (1984) 'Bronchoconstriction induced by iprotropium bromide in asthma: relation to hypotonicity.' *Br. Med. J.*, *ii*, 469.
Mann, T.P. (1955) 'Hypothermia in the newborn: a new syndrome?' *Lancet*, *i*, 613–14.
——— (1967) 'Hypothermia in the newborn.' In K. Simpson (ed.) *Modern Trends in Forensic Medicine. Vol. 2*. Butterworth, London, pp. 197–223.
Marcus, P. (1973a) 'Some effects of cooling and heating areas of the head and neck on body temperature measurement at the ear.' *Aerospace Med.*, *44*, 397–402.
——— (1973b) 'Some effects of radiant heating of the head on body temperature measurement at the ear.' *Aerospace Med.*, *44*, 403–6.
——— (1978) 'Laboratory comparison of techniques for rewarming hypothermic casualties.' *Aviat. Space Environ. Med.*, *49*, 692–7.
——— (1979a) 'The treatment of acute accidental hypothermia; proceedings of a symposium held at the RAF Institute of Aviation Medicine.' *Aviat. Space Environ. Med.*, *50*, 834–43.
——— (1979b) '"Trench foot" caused by the cold.' *Br. Med. J.*, *i*, 622.
———; Richards, S. (1978) 'Effect of clothing insulation beneath an immersion coverall on the rate of body cooling in cold water.' *Aviat. Space Environ. Med.*, *49*, 480–3.
———; Robertson, D.; Langford, R. (1977) 'Metallised plastic sheeting for use in survival.' *Aviat. Space Environ. Med.*, *48*, 50–2.
Marfatia, S.; Donahoe, P.K.; Hendren, W.H. (1975) 'Effect of dry and humidified gases on the respiratory epithelium in rabbits.' *J. Ped. Surg.*, *10*, 583–90.
Marmot, M.G.; Adelstein, A.M.; Robinson, N.; Rose, G.A. (1978) 'Changing social-class distribution of heart disease'. *Br. Med. J.*, *ii*, 1109–12.
Marshall, H.C.; Goldman, R.F.; (1976) 'Electrical response of nerve to freezing injury.' In R.J. Shephard and S. Itoh (eds.) *Circumpolar Health*, University Press, Toronto, p. 77.
Martin, S.; Diewold, R.J.; Cooper, K.E. (1977) 'Alcohol respiration skin and body temperature during cold water immersion.' *J. Appl. Physiol.*, *43*, 211–15.
———; Diewold, R.J.; Cooper, K.E. (1978) 'The effect of clothing on the initial ventilatory responses during cold water immersion.' *Can. J. Physiol. Pharmacol.*, *56*, 886–8.
Matter, P. (1979) 'Injuries in the avalanche.' In P. Matter, P. Braun, M. deQuervain, W. Good (eds.) *Skifahren und Sicherheit III*. Buchdruckerei Davos AG, Davos, pp. 133–6.
Matthew, H. (1975) 'Barbiturates.' *Clin. Tox.*, *8*, 495–513.
Matthews, H.R.; Meade, J.B.; Evans, C.C. (1974a) 'Peripheral vasoconstriction after open-heart surgery.' *Thorax*, *29*, 338–42.
———; Meade, J.B.; Evans, C.C. (1974b) 'Significance of prolonged peripheral vasoconstriction after open-heart surgery.' *Thorax*, *29*, 343–8.
Mattocks, A.M.; El-Bassiouni, E.A. (1971) 'Peritoneal dialysis; a review.' *J. Pharmacol. Sci.*, *60*, 1767–82.
Maughan, R.J. (1984) 'Temperature regulation during marathon competition.' *Br. J. Sports Med.*, *18*, 257–60.
———; Light, I.M.; Whiting, P.H.; Miller, J.D.B. (1982) 'Hypothermia, hyperkalaemia, and marathon running.' *Lancet*, *ii*, 1336.
MDC (1982) *Report over the Swedish Navy diving center and test with personal*

survival equipment for deep divers in distressed diving bells (lost Bell). Marinens Dykeri Centrum, Sweden.

Medical Tribune, (1978) '"Sneaky" hypothermia will kill old with cool, not cold.' *Medical Tribune and Medical News, Jan. 11*, pp. 1, 8, 9.

Meikeir, K. de; Arantz, T.; Hollman, W.; Vanhaelst, L. (1985) 'The role of endogenous opiates in thermal regulation of the body during exercise.' *Br. Med. J.*, *i*, 739–40.

Meldrum, K.I. (1972) 'Margins of safety in mountaineering.' *Health Bull.*, *30*, 204–5.

Mellett, P. (1980) 'Current views on the psychophysiology of hypnosis.' *Br. J. Hosp. Med.*, *25*, 441–6.

Mersey, Lord (Wreck commissioner) (1912) *Report of a Formal Investigation into the Circumstances Attending the Foundering on 15th April 1912 of the British Steamship 'Titanic' of Liverpool after Striking Ice in or near Latitude 41° 46' N, Longitude 50° 14' North Atlantic Ocean, whereby Loss of Life Ensued*. HMSO, London.

Michael, J.R.; Guerci, A.D.; Koehler, R.C.; Shi, A.-Y.; Tsitlik, J.; Chandra, N.; Niedermeyer, E.; Rogers, M.C.; Traystman, R.J.; Weisfeldt, M.L. (1984) 'Mechanisms whereby epinephrine augments cerebral and myocardial perfusion during cardiopulmonary resuscitation in dogs.' *Circulation*, *69*, 822–35.

Mikat, M.; Peters, J.; Zindler, M.; Arndt, J.O. (1984) 'Whole body oxygen consumption in awake, sleeping, and anesthetized dogs.' *Anesthesiology*, *60*, 220–7.

Miles, S. (1974) 'Water.' *Scot. Med. J.*, *19*, 245.

——— (1975) 'Drowning and hypothermia.' *Br. J. Sports Med.*, *9*, 142–3.

Millar, J.S.; Nairn, J.R.; Unkles, R.D.; McNeill, R.S. (1965) 'Cold air and ventilatory function.' *Br. J. Dis. Chest*, *59*, 23–7.

Miller, A.T. (1974) 'Altitude.' In N.B. Slomin (ed.) *Environmental Physiology*. C.V. Mosby & Co., St. Louis, Mo., pp. 350–75.

Miller, J.D.; Speciale, S.G.; McMillen, B.A.; German, D.C. (1984) 'Naloxone antagonism of stress-induced augmentation of frontal cortex dopamine metabolism.' *Europ. J. Pharmac.*,, *98*, 437–9.

Miller, J.W.; Danzl, D.F.; Thomas, D.M. (1980) 'Urban accidental hypothermia: 135 cases.' *Ann. Emerg. Med.*, *9*, 456–61.

Miller, M.G. (1984) 'Visual hallucinations in children receiving decongestants.' *Br. Med. J.*, *i*, 1688.

Mills, G.L. (1973d) 'Accidental hypothermia in the elderly.' *Br. J. Hosp. Med.*, *10*, 691–9.

Mills, G.L. (1979) 'Accidental hypothermia and low-reading thermometers.' *Br. Med. J.*, *i*, 1082–3.

Mills, W.J. (1966) 'Frostbite.' *Northwest Med.*, *65*, 119–25.

——— (1968) 'Disturbances due to cold.' In H.F. Conn (ed.) *Current Therapy*. Saunders, New York, pp. 817–20.

——— (1973a) 'Frostbite and hypothermia – current concepts.' *Alaska Med.*, *15*, 26.

——— (1973b) 'Frostbite.' *Alaska Med.*, *15*, 27–47.

——— (1973c) 'Summary of treatment of the cold injured patient.' *Alaska Med.*, *15*, 56–9.

——— (1977) 'When your patient suffers frostbite.' *Patient Care*, *Feb. 1*, 132–8.

——— (1980) 'Accidental hypothermia: management approach.' *Alaska Med.*, *22*, 9–11.

——— (1983a) 'General hypothermia.' *Alaska Med.*, *25*, 29–32.

——— (1983b) 'Frostbite.' *Alaska Med.*, *25*, 33–8.

——— (1983c) 'Accidental hypothermia.' In R.S. Pozos and L.E. Wittmers (eds.) *The Nature and Treatment of Hypothermia*. Croom Helm, London/University of Minnesota Press, Minneapolis, pp. 182–93.

———; Rau, D. (1983) 'University of Alaska, Anchorage-section of high latitude study, and the Mt. McKinley project.' *Alaska Med.*, *25*, 21–8.

Milton, A.S. (ed.) (1982) *Pyretics and Antipyretics*. Springer-Verlag, Berlin.

Mitchell, J.R.A. (1984) 'Hearts and minds.' *Br. Med. J.*, *ii*, 1557–8.

Modell, J.H. (1971) *Pathophysiology and Treatment of Drowning and Near-drowning*. Charles C. Thomas, Springfield, Ill.

——— (1976) 'A case of drowning.' *Anaesthesia*, *31*, 1296–7.

———; Davis, J.H. (1969) 'Electrolyte changes in human drowning victims.' *Anesthesiology*, *30*, 414–20.

———; Giammona, M.; Davis, J.H. (1967) 'Effect of chronic exposure to ultrasonic aerosols on the lung.' *Anesthesiology*, *28*, 680–8.

———; Graves, S.A.; Ketover, A. (1976) 'Clinical course of 91 consecutive near-drowning victims.' *Chest*, *70*, 231–8.

Mognoni, P.; Lafortuna, C.L. (1985) 'Respiratory mechanics at altitude.' In J. Rivolier, P. Cerretelli, J. Foray, P. Segantini (eds.) *High Altitutde Deterioration*. Karger, Basel, pp. 64–72.

Molnar, G.W. (1946) 'Survival of hypothermia by men immersed in the ocean.' *J. Am. Med. Ass.*, *131*, 1046–50.

Moore, T.O.; Morlock, J.F.; Lally, D.A.; Hong, S.K. (1976) 'Thermal cost of saturation diving: respiratory and whole body heat loss at 16.1 ATA.' In C.J. Lambertsen (ed.) *Underwater Physiology V*. FASEB, Bethesda, pp. 741–54.

Moore-Ede, M.C. (1983) 'Hypothermia: a timing disorder of circadian thermoregulatory rhythms?' In R.S. Pozos and L.E. Wittmers (eds.) *The Nature and Treatment of Hypothermia*. Croom Helm, London/University of Minnesota Press, Minneapolis, pp. 69–80.

Morgan, A.P. (1968) 'The pulmonary toxicity of oxygen.' *Anesthesiology*, *29*, 570–9.

Morgan, J.; York, D.A. (1983) 'The elderly, hypothermia, and thermogenesis.' *Lancet*, *i*, 592.

Moritz, A.R.; Weisiger, J.R. (1945) 'Effects of cold air on the air passages and lungs: an experimental investigation.' *Arch. Int. Med.*, *75*, 233–40.

———; Henriques, F.C.; McLean, R. (1945) 'The effects of inhaled heat on the air passages and lungs: an experimental investigation.' *Am. J. Path.*, *21*, 311–25.

Moriya, K. (1984) 'Cross adaptation mechanisms between exercise training and cold adaptation; assessment of free fatty acids metabolism in norepinephrine-induced heat production and finger temperature responses to local cooling.' *Presentation at Sixth International Symposium on Circumpolar Health. May 13–18, 1984. Anchorage, Alaska.* Abstracts p. 75.

Morris, J.N. (1983) 'Exercise, health, and medicine.' *Br. Med. J.*, *i*, 1597–8.

Morris, R.H. (1971a) 'Operating room temperature and the anaesthetised, paralysed patient.' *Arch. Surg.*, *102*, 95–7.

——— (1971b) 'Influence of ambient temperature on patient temperature during intra-abdominal surgery.' *Ann. Surg.*, *173*, 230–3.

———; Kumar, A. (1972) 'The effect of warming blankets on maintenance of body temperature of the anesthetized paralyzed adult patient.' *Anesthesiology*, *36*, 408–11.

———; Wilkie, B.R. (1970) 'The effects of ambient temperature on patient temperature during surgery not involving body cavities.' *Anesthesiology*, *32*, 102–7.

Morrison, J.B.; Conn, M.L.; Hayward, J.S. (1979) 'Thermal increment provided by inhalation rewarming from hypothermia.' *J. Appl. Physiol.*, *46*, 1061–5.

Moss, G. (1966) 'Systemic hypothermia via gastric cooling.' *Arch. Surg.*, *92*, 80–2.

Mountain Rescue (1968) *Training Handbook for the Royal Air Force Mountain Rescue Teams*. PAM (Air) HMSO, London, p. 299.

Mountain Rescue and Cave Rescue (1972) *Issued by the Mountain Rescue Committee*. A. Taylor & Sons, Barnsley.

Mouritzen, C.V.; Andersen, M.N. (1965) 'Myocardial temperature gradients and ventricular fibrillation during hypothermia.' *J. Thorac. Cardiovasc. Surg.*, *49*, 937–44.

Moyer, J.H.; Morris, G.C.; DeBakey, M.E. (1956) 'Renal functional response to hypothermia and ischaemia in man and dog.' In R.D. Dripps (ed.) *Physiology of Induced Hypothermia*. National Academy of Science – National Research Council, Publication 451, Washington, pp. 199–213.

MRC (1981) 'Medical Research Council Working Party. Long-term domiciliary oxygen therapy in chronic hypoxic cor pulmonale complicating chronic bronchitis and emphysema.' *Lancet*, *i*, 641–85.

Mudge, G.H.; Grossman, W.; Mills, R.M.; Lesch, M.; Braunwald, E. (1976) 'Reflex increase in coronary vascular resistance in patients with ischaemic heart disease.' *New Engl. J. Med.*, *295*, 1333–7.

Muhlemann, W. (1979) 'Drei Mal tiefe akzidentielle Hypothermie Voraussetzungen und Besonderheiten einer adaquaten Therapie.' In P. Matter, P. Braun, M. deQuervain, W. Good (eds.) *Skifahren und Sicherheit III*. Buchdruckerei Davos AG. Davos, pp. 202–8.

Murazian, R.I.; Smirnov, S.V.; Panchenkov, N.R. (1978) 'Diagnosis and treatment of frostbite of the extremities.' *Vestn. Khir.*, *121*, 74–8.

Murray, J.C.; Campbell, D.; Reid, J.M.; Telfer, A.B.M. (1974) 'Severe self-poisoning — a ten year experience in the Glasgow area.' *Scot. Med.J.*, *19*, 279–85.

Murray, M.J. (1962) 'Effect of inspiration of cold air on electrocardiograms of normal dogs and normal humans with angina pectoris.' *Circulation*, *26*, 765–6.

Myers, R.A.M.; Britten, J.S.; Cowley, R.A. (1979) 'Hypothermia: quantitative aspects of therapy.' *J. Am. Coll. Emerg. Phys.*, *8*, 523–7.

Nadel, E.R.; Horvath, S.M. (1970) 'Comparison of tympanic membrane and deep body temperature in man.' *Life Sci.*, *9*, 868–75.

Nair, C.S.; Singh, I.; Malhotra, M.S.; Mathew, L.; Dasgupta, A.; Purakayastha, S.S.; Shankar, J. (1977) 'Studies on heat output from the hands of frostbite subjects.' *Aviat. Space Environ. Med.*, *48*, 192–4.

Nash, G.; Blennerhasset, J.B.; Potopiddan, H. (1967) 'Pulmonary lesions associated with oxygen therapy and artificial ventilation.' *New Engl. J. Med.*, *276*, 368–74.

Nayha, S. (1984a) 'The cold season and deaths in Finland.' *Nordic Council Arct. Med. Res.*, *Rep. No. 37*, pp. 20–4.

——— (1984b) 'Seasonal variation in suicide and mental depression in Finland.' *Presentation at Sixth International Symposium on Circumpolar Health. May 13–18, 1984. Anchorage, Alaska.* Abstracts p. 138.

Negovskii, V.A. (1962) *Resuscitation and Artificial Hypothermia*. Consultants Bureau, New York.

Nemiroff, M.J.; Saltz, G.R.; Weg, J.G. (1977) 'Survival after cold-water near-drowning; the protective effect of the diving reflex.' *Am. Rev. Resp. Dis.*, *115*, 45.

Neureuther, G. (1979) 'Die Warmepackung.' In P. Matter, P. Braun, M. deQuervain, W. Good (eds.) *Skifahren und Sicherheit III*. Buchdruckerei Davos AG, Davos, p. 182.

Newburgh, L.H. (1949) *Physiology of Heat Regulation and the Science of Clothing*. W.B. Saunders, Philadelphia.

Newman, B.J. (1971) 'Control of accidental hypothermia. Occurrence and prevention of accidental hypothermia during vascular surgery.' *Anaesthesia*, *26*, 177–87.

Newton, D.E.F. (1975) 'The effect of anaesthetic gas humidificationon body temperature.' *Br. J. Anaesth.*, *47*, 1026.

——— (1976) 'Temperature control in the operating theatre.' *Anaesthesia*, *31*,

834.

——— (1980) 'Routine humidification of anaesthetic gases for major surgery.' *Anaesthesia*, *35*, 120–1.

NHS (1974) 'Accidental hypothermia.' *NHS Memorandum No. 1974 (GEN) 7.* Scottish Home and Health Department.

Niazi, S.A.; Lewis, F.J. (1957) 'Profound hypothermia in monkey with recovery after long periods of cardiac standstill.' *J. Appl. Physiol.*, *10*, 137–8.

———; Lewis, F.J. (1958) 'Profound hypothermia in man; report of a case.' *Ann. Surg.*, *147*, 254–66.

Nickerson, M.; Collier, B. (1975) 'Propranolol and related drugs.' In L.S. Goodman and A. Gilman (eds.) *The Pharmacological Basis of Therapeutics, 5th Ed.* Macmillan, London, pp. 547–52.

Nicolas, F.; Desjars, Ph. (1979) 'Haemodynamic and cardiac disturbances in accidental hypothermia.' In P. Matter, P. Braun, M. deQuervain, W. Good (eds.) *Skifahren und Sicherheit III.* Buchdruckerei Davos AG, Davos, pp. 151–4.

Nigro, G.; Pastoris, M.C.; Fantasia, M.M.; Midulla, M. (1983) 'Legionellosis and cot deaths.' *Lancet*, *ii*, 1034–5.

Nilsson, J.L.G.; Carlsson, A. (1982) 'Dopamine-receptor agonist with apparent selectivity for autoreceptors: a new principle for antipsychotic action?' In J.W. Lamble (ed.) *More About Receptors*. Elsevier Biomedical, Amsterdam, pp. 98–104.

Nilsson, S. (1984) 'Heat stroke during running in a cold climate.' *Tidsskr. Nor. Laegeforen.*, *104*, 1286–9.

Ninneman, J.; Ozkan, N.; Stewart, G.L.; Mills, W. (1984) 'Immunologic changes in frostbite.' *Presentation at Sixth International Symposium on Circumpolar Health. May 13–18, 1984. Anchorage, Alaska.* Abstracts p. 98.

Norberg, J.; Foster, J.; Bryant, E.; Lewbel, N. (1979) 'Blizzard '78, Indiana, Michigan, Ohio, New York.' *J. Winter Emerg. Care*, *4*, 47–51.

Northcote, R.J.; Ballantyne, D. (1983) 'Sudden death in a marathon runner.' *Lancet*, *i*, 417.

Nunn, J.F.; Payne, J.P. (1962) 'Hypoxaemia after general anaesthesia.' *Lancet*, *ii*, 631–2.

Nystrom, S.H.M.; Heikkinen, E.R. (1984) 'Thermocoagulation of ganglion gasseri in trigeminal neuralgia: experiences in northern Finland.' *Nordic Council Arct. Med. Res.*, *Rep. No. 37*, pp. 43–7.

Oakley, E.H.N. (1984) 'The design and function of military footwear: a review following experiences in the South Atlantic.' *Ergonomics*, *6*, 631–7.

O'Cain, C.F.; Dowling, N.B.; Slutsky, A.S.; Strohl, K.P.; McFadden, E.R.; Ingram, R.H. (1980) 'Airway effects of respiratory heat loss in normal subjects.' *J. Appl. Physiol.*, *49*, 875–80.

O'Donnell, B. (1980) 'The Fastnet race 1979.' *Br. Med. J.*, *ii*, 1665–7.

Offermeier, J.; van Rooyen, J.M. (1982) 'Is it possible to integrate dopamine receptor terminology?' In J.W. Lamble (ed.) *More About Receptors*. Elsevier Biomedical, Amsterdam, pp. 93–7.

Ogilvie, J. (1977) 'Exhaustion and exposure.' *Climber and Rambler*, *Sept.*, pp. 34–9, and *Oct.*, pp. 52–5.

Ogston, S.A.; Florey, C. duV.; Walker, C.H.M. (1985) 'The Tayside infant morbidity and mortality study: effect on health of using gas for cooking.' *Br. Med. J.*, *i*, 957–60.

O'Keefe, K.M. (1977) 'Outdoor health care: how not to be a babe in the woods or mountains.' *Am. J. Nurs.*, *77*, 974–9.

Oliver, M.F. (1983) 'Should we not forget about mass control of coronary risk factors?' *Lancet*, *ii*, 37–8.

———; Nimmo, I.A.; Cooke, M.; Carlson, L.A.; Olsson, A.G. (1975) 'Ischaemic heart disease and associated risk factors in 40 year old men in Edinburgh and

Stockholm.' *Europ. J. Clin. Invest.*, 5, 507–14.

Olsen, R.G.; David, T.D. (1984) 'Hypothermia and electromagnetic rewarming in the rhesus monkey.' *Aviat. Space Environ. Med.*, *55*, 1111–17.

Olson, N.C.; Robinson, N.E.; Scott, J.B. (1983) 'Effects of brain hypoxia on pulmonary haemodynamics.' *J. Surg. Res.*, *35*, 21–7.

Olsson, A.G.; Walldius, G.; Carlson, L.A.; Logan, R.L.; Riemersmaa, R.A.; Oliver, M.F. (1977) 'Differences in lipid metabolism in relation to ischaemic heart disease in Edinburgh and Stockholm.' *Nordic Council Arct. Med. Res.*, *Rep. No. 19*, pp. 135–42.

Osborn, J. (1953) 'Experimental hypothermia: respiratory and blood pH changes in relation to cardiac function.' *Am. J. Physiol.*, *175*, 389–98.

———; Gerbode, F.; Johnston, J.B.; Ross, J.K.; Ogata, T.; Kerth, W.J. (1961) 'Blood chemical changes in perfusion hypothermia for cardiac surgery.' *J. Thorac. Cardiovasc. Surg.*, *42*, 462–76.

Osborne, L.; Kamal El-Din, A.S.; Smith, J.E. (1984) 'Survival after prolonged cardiac arrest and accidental hypothermia.' *Br. Med. J.*, *ii*, 881–2.

Oswald, I. (1975) 'Sleep research and mental illness.' *Psychol. Med.*, 5, 1–3.

Overstall, P.W.; Exton-Smith, A.N.; Imms, F.T.; Johnson, A.L. (1977) 'Falls in the elderly related to postural imbalance.' *Br. Med. J.*, *i*, 261–4.

Oyama, T. (1969) 'Hazards of steroids in association with anaesthesia.' *Can. Anaesth. Soc. J.*, *16*, 361–71.

Park, W.M.; Reece, B.L. (1976) *Fundamental Aspects of Medical Thermography*. British Institute of Radiology, London.

Patel, K.R. (1984) 'Terfenadine in exercise in exercise induced asthma.' *Br. Med. J.*, *i*, 1496–7.

Paton, B.C. (1983a) 'Cardiac function during accidental hypothermia.' In R.S. Pozos and L.E. Wittmers (eds.) *The Nature and Treatment of Hypothermia*. Croom Helm, London/University of Minnesota Press, Minneapolis, pp. 133–42.

——— (1983b) 'Accidental hypothermia.' *Pharmac. Ther.*, *22*, 331–77.

Patton, J.F. (1974) 'Accidental hypothermia: a matter of turning the scoreboard around.' *The Medical Post (Canada)*, *10*, No. 23, 4–5.

——— (1976) 'Renal function after core and surface rewarming of hypothermic dogs.' In R.J. Shephard and S. Itoh (eds.) *Circumpolar Health*. Toronto University Press, Toronto, pp. 55–61.

———; Doolittle, W.H. (1972) 'Core rewarming by peritoneal dialysis following induced hypothermia in the dog.' *J. Appl. Physiol.*, *33*, 800–4.

Pausescu, E.; Lugojan, R.; Chirvasie, R.; Diocescu, R. (1969) 'Cerebral metabolic aspects in post-hypothermic brain edema.' *Rev. Roum. Physiol.*, *6*, 299–306.

Pavlin, E.; Hornbein, T.F.; Chaney, R. (1976) 'Rewarming of hypothermic dogs with the use of heated nebulized ventilation.' *Proceedings of the American Association of Anesthesiologists*, Annual meeting, San Francisco, pp. 105–6.

Payne, K.; Ireland, P. (1984) 'Plasma glucose levels in the peri-operative period in children.' *Anaesthesia*, *39*, 868–72.

Payne, R. (1984) 'Lessons of the Falklands.' *World Med.*, *19*, 26–7.

Payne, R.B. (1959) 'Tracking proficiency as a function of thermal balance.' *J. Appl. Physiol.*, *14*, 387–9.

Pearn, J.H. (1980) 'Secondary drowning in children.' *Br. Med. J.*, *ii*, 1103–5.

Pelizzo, C.; Franchi, G.L. (1978) 'Frostbite. Clinical note.' *Minerva Anestesiol.*, *44*, 41–4.

Pelto, J.M. (1984) 'Birthweight and maternal age specific infant mortality rates in Alaska.' *Presentation at Sixth International Symposium on Circumpolar Health. May 13–18, 1984. Anchorage, Alaska.* Abstracts, p. 250.

Pemberton, J. (1984) 'Factors in mortality from coronary and cerebral thrombosis in winter.' *Br. Med. J.*, *ii*, 1693.

Penrod, K.E. (1951) 'Cardiac oxygenation during severe hypothermia in dogs.' *Am. J.*

Physiol., *164*, 79–85.

Penttinen, K. (1982) 'Cold and viral infections. A review.' *Nordic Council Arct. Med. Res.*, *Rep. No. 30*, 36–8.

Perlstein, P.H.; Edwards, N.K.; Sutherland, J.M. (1970) 'Apnea in premature infants and incubator-air-temperature changes.' *New Engl. J. Med.*, *282*, 461–6.

Petrofsky, J.S.; Lind, A.R. (1975) 'Insulative power of body fat on deep muscle temperatures and isometric endurance.' *J. Appl. Physiol.*, *39*, 639–42.

Pfenninger, J.; Sutter, M. (1982) 'Intensive care after fresh water immersion accidents in children.' *Anaesthesia*, *37*, 1157–62.

Phillips, M. (1982) 'Fuel policy: a national disaster.' *World Med.*, *Jan. 23*, 19.

Phillipson, E.A. (1978) 'Control of breathing during sleep.' *Am. Rev. Respir. Dis.*, *118*, 909–39.

———; Herbert, F.A. (1967) 'Accidental exposure to freezing; clinical and laboratory observations during convalescence from near-fatal hypothermia.' *Can. Med. Ass. J.*, *97*, 786–92.

Pickering, B.G.; Bristow, G.K.; Craig, D.B. (1977) 'Core rewarming by peritoneal irrigation in accidental hypothermia.' *Anesth. Analg. (Cleve.)*, *56*, 574–7.

Piersol, G.M.; Schwan, H.P.; Pennell, R.B.; Carstenson, E.L. (1952) 'Mechanism of absorption of ultrasonic energy in blood.' *Arch. Phys. Med.*, *33*, 327–32.

Piironen, P. (1970) 'Sinusoidal signals in the analysis of heat transfer in the body.' In J.G. Hardy, A.P. Gagge, J.A.J. Stolwijk (eds.) *Physiological and Behavioural Temperature Regulation*. Charles C. Thomas, Springfield, Ill., pp. 358–66.

Platner, W.S.; Hosko, M.J. (1953) 'Mobility of serum magnesium in hypothermia.' *Am. J. Physiol.*, *174*, 273–6.

Platt, S.; Kreitman, N. (1984) 'Trends in parasuicide and unemployment among men in Edinburgh, 1968–82.' *Br. Med. J.*, *ii*, 1029–32.

Pleuvry, B.J. (1983) 'An update on opioid receptors.' *Br. J. Anaesth.*, 55, 143–6S.

Popovic, V.; Popovic, P. (1974) *Hypothermia in Biology and Medicine*. Academic Press, London.

Porter, A.M.W. (1984) 'Marathon running and adverse weather conditions.' *Br. J. Sports Med.*, *18*, 261–4.

Poulton, E.C.; Hutchings, N.B.; Brooke, R.B. (1965) 'Effect of cold and rain upon the vigilance of lookouts.' *Ergonomics*, *8*, 163–8.

Powell, J.; Machin, D.; Kershaw, C.R. (1983) 'Unexpected sudden infant deaths in Gosport — some comparisons between service and civilian families.' *J. Roy. Nav. Med. Serv.*, *69*, 141–50.

Pozner, H. (1965) 'Mental fitness.' In O.G. Edholm and A.L. Bacharach (eds.) *Exploration Medicine*. John Wright & Sons, Bristol, pp. 77–97.

Pozos, R.S.; Wittmers, L.E. (1983) 'The relationship between shiver and respiratory parameters in humans.' In R.S. Pozos and L.E. Wittmers (eds.), *The Nature and Treatment of Hypothermia*. Croom Helm, London/University of Minnesota Press, Minneapolis, pp. 121–30.

Prescott, L.F.; Peard, M.C.; Wallace, I.R. (1962) 'Accidental hypothermia: a common condition.' *Br. Med. J.*, *ii*, 1367–70.

Primrose, W.R.; Smith, L.R.N. (1981) 'Urban hypothermia.' *Br. Med. J.*, *i*, 474.

Provins, K.A.; Clarke, R.S.J. (1960) 'The effect of cold on manual performance.' *J. Occup. Med.*, *2*, 169–76.

Pugh, L.G.C.E. (1964) 'Deaths from exposure on Four Inns walking competition.' *Lancet*, *i*, 1210–12.

——— (1966) 'Accidental hypothermia in walkers, climbers and campers: report to the medical commission on accident prevention.' *Br. Med. J.*, *i*, 123–9.

——— (1967) 'Cold stress and muscular exercise with special reference to accidental hypothermia.' *Br. Med. J.*, *ii*, 333–7.

——— (1968) 'Isafjordur trawler disaster. Medical aspects.' *Br. Med. J.*, *i*, 826–9.

Pyorala, K.; Punsar, S.; Siltanen, P.; Savolainen, E.; Sarna, S. (1977) 'The coronary heart disease morbidity of Helsinki policemen born in western and eastern Finland.' *Nordic Council Arct. Med. Res., Rep. No. 19*, pp. 70–7.

Questions in the Commons (1973) 'Hypothermia in the elderly.' *Br. Med. J.*, *i*, 367.

Racini, J.; Jarjoui, E. (1982) 'Severe hypothermia in infants.' *Helv. Paediatr. Acta*, *37*, 317–22.

Radford, P.; Thurlow, A.C. (1979) 'Metallized plastic sheeting in prevention of hypothermia during surgery.' *Br. J. Anaesth.*, *51*, 237–9.

Raffe, M.R.; Martin, F.B. (1983) 'Effect of inspired air heat and humidification on anaesthetic-induced hypothermia in dogs.' *Am. J. Vet. Res.*, *44*, 456–8.

Ramanathan, N.L. (1964) 'A new weighting system for mean surface temperature of the human body.' *J. Appl. Physiol.*, *19*, 531–3.

Ramanathan, S.; Chalon, J.; Turndorf, H. (1975) 'Humidity output of the Bloomquist infant circle.' *Anesthesiology*, *43*, 679–82.

———; Chalon, J.; Turndorf, H. (1976) 'A compact well-humidified breathing circuit for the circle system.' *Anesthesiology*, *44*, 238–42.

Ramirez-Lassepas, M.; Hans, E.; Lakarua, D. (1980) 'Seasonal (circannual) periodicity of spontaneous intracerebral hemorrhage in Minnesota.' *Ann. Neurol.*, *8*, 539–41.

Randall, W.C.; Rawson, R.O.; McCook, R.D.; Peiss, C.N. (1963) 'Central and peripheral factors in dynamic thermoregulation.' *J. Appl. Physiol.*, *18*, 61–4.

Rankin, A.C.; Rae, A.P. (1984) 'Cardiac arrhythmias during rewarming of patients with accidental hypothermia.' *Br. Med. J.*, *ii*, 874–7.

Rashad, K.F.; Benson, D.W. (1967) 'Role of humidity in prevention of hypothermia in infants and children.' *Anesth. Analg. (Cleve.)*, *46*, 127–33.

Ravenas, B.; Lindholm, C.E. (1979) 'The foam nose — a new disposable heat and moisture exchanger. A comparison with other similar devices.' *Acta Anaesth. Scand.*, *23*, 34–9.

Rawlins, J. (1981) 'Thermal protection for divers.' In J.N. Adams (ed.) *Hypothermia Ashore and Afloat*. Aberdeen University Press, Aberdeen, pp. 112–18.

Rawlinson, G. (1910) *The History of Herodotus Translated. Vol. 2*. J.M. Dent & Sons, London.

Raymond, L.W. (1975) 'Temperature regulation in helium-oxygen atmospheres.' *Lancet*, *i*, 807.

RCP (1966) *Report of Committee on Accidental Hypothermia*. Royal College of Physicians, London.

Read, A.E.; Emslie-Smith, D.; Gough, K.R.; Holmes, R. (1961) 'Pancreatitis and accidental hypothermia.' *Lancet*, *ii*, 1219–21.

Reaves, T.A.; Hayward, J.N. (1979) 'Hypothalamic and extrahypothalamic thermoregulatory centers.' In P. Lomax and E. Schonbaum (eds.) *Body Temperature: Regulation, Drug Effects, and Therapeutic Implications*. Marcel Dekker, New York, pp. 39–70.

Reed, L.D.; Livingstone, S.D.; Limmer, R.E. (1984) 'Patterns of skin temperature and surface heat flow in man during and after cold water immersion.' *Aviat. Space Environ. Med.*, 55, 19–23.

Rees, J. (1984) 'ABC of asthma: precipitating factors.' *Br. Med. J.*, *i*, 1512–14.

Rees, J.R. (1958) 'Accidental hypothermia.' *Lancet*, *i*, 556–9.

Reeves, J.T.; Grover, R.F. (1975) 'High altitude pulmonary hypertension and pulmonary oedema.' *Progress in Cardiology*, *4*, 99–118.

———; Wagner, W.W.; McMurty, I.F.; Grover, R.F. (1979) 'Physiological effects of high altitude on the pulmonary circulation.' In D. Robertshaw (ed.) *Environmental Physiology III*. University Park Press, Baltimore, pp. 289–310.

Reinke, J.J. (1985) 'Beobachtung uber die Korpertemperatur Betrunkener.' *Deut. Arch. Klin. Med.*, *16*, 12.

Renstrom, B.S-E. (1982) 'Why did eight young people die from hypothermia?' In B. Harvald and J.P. Hart Hansen (eds.) *Circumpolar Health 81*. Nordic Council for Arctic Medical Research, Copenhagen, pp. 610–11.

Reuler, J.B.; Parker, R.A. (1978) 'Peritoneal dialysis in the management of hypothermia.' *J. Am. Med. Ass.*, *240*, 2289–90.

Rey, L. (ed.) (1985) *Arctic Underwater Operations*. Graham & Trotman, London.

Rhind, G.B.; Catterall, J.R.; Douglas, N.J. (1985) 'Nocturnal asthma is not reduced by blocking vagal tone.' *Scot. Med. J.*, *30*, 125.

Ricci, D.R.; Orlick, A.E.; Cipriano, P.R.; Guthauer, D.F.; Harrison, D.C. (1979) 'Altered adrenergic activity in coronary arterial spasm: insight into mechanism based on study of coronary haemodynamics and the electrocardiogram.' *Am. J. Cardiol.*, *43*, 1073–9.

Richardson, W.T. (1981) 'Losses at sea of deep sea fishermen from Hull 1970–1977.' In J.N. Adams (ed.) *Hypothermia Ashore and Afloat*. Aberdeen University Press, Aberdeen, pp. 119–24.

Rickham, P.P. (1957) *Metabolic response to neonatal surgery*. Harvard University Press, Massachusetts.

Riggs, C.E.; Johnson, D.J.; Kilgour, R.D.; Konopka, B.J. (1983) 'Metabolic effects of facial cooling in exercise.' *Aviat. Space Environ. Med.*, *54*, 22–6.

Rimpela, A.H.; Rimpela, M.K. (1985) 'Increased risk of respiratory symptoms in young smokers of low tar cigarettes.' *Br. Med. J.*, *i*, 1461–3.

Rivers, J.F. (1972) 'Near-drowning.' *Br. J. Hosp. Med.*, *8*, 299–300.

———; Orr, G.; Lee, H.A. (1970) 'Drowning: its clinical sequelae and management.' *Br. Med. J.*, *ii*, 157–61.

Rivolier, J.; Bachelard, C.; Regnard, J. (1984) 'Cooling power and heat exchange.' *International Biomedical Expedition to the Antarctic*. Poster abstracts presented at 6th International Symposium on Circumpolar Health, Anchorage May 1984, pp. 67–8.

Robert-Lamblin, J. (1984) 'Causes of death, age at death, changes in mortality in the 20th century in Ammassalik (East Greenland).' *Presentation at Sixth International Symposium on Circumpolar Health. May 13–18, 1984. Anchorage, Alaska*. Abstracts p. 14.

Roberts, A.; Robinson, J.L. (1970) 'Disposable heat exchanger.' *Br. Med. J.*, *iv*, 742.

Roberts, D.E.; Patton, J.F.; Kerr, D.W. (1983) 'The effect of airway warming on severe hypothermia.' In R.S. Pozos and L.E. Wittmers (eds.) *The Nature and Treatment of Hypothermia*. Croom Helm, London/University of Minnesota, Minneapolis, pp. 209–20.

———; Barr, J.C.; Kerr, D.; Murray, C.; Harris, R. (1985) 'Fluid replacement during hypothermia.' *Aviat. Space Environ. Med.*, *56*, 333–7.

Roberts, J.; Golding, J.; Keeling, J.; Sutton, B.; Lynch, M.A. (1984) 'Is there a link between cot death and child abuse?' *Br. Med. J.*, *ii*, 789–91.

Robinson, E. (1984) 'Mortality among the James Bay Cree, Quebec.' *Presentation at Sixth International Symposium on Circumpolar Health. May 13–18, 1984. Anchorage, Alaska.* Abstracts p. 15.

Robson, R.H.; Fluck, D.C. (1977) 'Effect of isometric exercise on catecholamines in the coronary circulation.' *Europ. J. Appl. Physiol.*, *37*, 289–95.

Rode, A.; Shephard, R. (1984) 'Lung function in a cold environment — a current perspective.' *Presentation at Sixth International Symposium on Circumpolar Health. May 13–18, 1984. Anchorage, Alaska.* Abstracts p. 99.

Rodriguez, J.L.; Weissman, C.; Damask, M.C.; Askanazi, J.; Hyman, A.I.; Kinney, J.M. (1983) 'Physiologic requirements during rewarming: suppression of the shivering response.' *Crit. Care Med.*, *11*, 490–7.

Roe, C.F.; Goldberg, M.J.; Blair, C.S.; Kinney, J.M. (1966a) 'The influence of body temperature on early postoperative oxygen consumption.' *Surgery*, *60*, 85–92.

———; Santulli, T.V.; Blair, C.S. (1966b) 'Heat loss in infants during general anaesthesia and operations.' *J. Paediat. Surg.*, *1*, 266–74.

Roe, P.F. (1963) 'Accidental hypothermia.' *Irish Med. J.*, *454*, 459–63.

Rogers, M.C.; Greenberg, M.; Alpert, J.J. (1971) 'Cold injury of the newborn.' *New Engl. J. Med.*, *285*, 332–4.

Rogers, T.A. (1971) 'The clinical course of survival in the arctic.' *Hawaii Med. J.*, *30*, 31–4.

Romanova, N.P. (1956) 'Dynamics of histopathological changes in the brain in experimental hypoxia.' *Zhur. Neuropat. i Psikhiat*, *56*, 49–55.

Rosch, P.J. (1983) 'Stress, cholesterol, and coronary heart disease.' *Lancet*, *ii*, 851–2.

Rose, G. (1966) 'Cold weather and ischaemic heart disease.' *Br. J. Prev. Soc. Med.*, *20*, 97–100.

Rose, J.C.; McDermott, T.F.; Lilienfiled, L.S.; Porfido, F.A.; Kelly, R.T. (1957) 'Cardiovascular response in hypothermic anaesthetised man.' *Circulation*, *15*, 512–17.

Rothwell, N.J.; Stock, M.J. (1979) 'A role for brown adipose tissue in diet-induced thermogenesis.' *Nature (Lond.)*, *281*, 31–8.

Roythorne, C. (1981) 'Cold in North Sea oil operations.' In J.N. Adams (ed.) *Hypothermia Ashore and Afloat*. Aberdeen University Press, Aberdeen, pp. 66–74.

Rudikoff, M.T.; Maugham, L.W.; Effron, M.; Freund, P.; Weisfeldt, M.L. (1980) 'Mechanisms of blood flow during cardiopulmonary resuscitation.' *Circulation*, *61*, 345–52.

Russel, W.J. (1974) 'A review of blood warmers for massive transfusion.' *Anaesth. Intens. Care*, *2*, 109–30.

Sabiston, D.C.; Theilen, E.O.; Gregg, D.E. (1955) 'The relationship of coronary blood flow and cardiac output and other parameters in hypothermia.' *Surgery*, *38*, 498–505.

Sadikali, F.; Owor, R. (1974) 'Hypothermia in the tropics. A review of 24 cases.' *Trop. Geog. Med.*, *26*, 265–70.

Salvosa, C.B.; Payne, R.R.; Wheeler, E.F. (1971) 'Environmental conditions and body temperature of women living alone or in Local Authority home.' *Br. Med. J.*, *iv*, 656–9.

Samuelson, T., Doolittle, W., Hayward, J., Mills, W., Nemiroff, M. (1982) 'Hypothermia and cold water near drowning: treatment guidelines.' *Alaska Med.*, *24*, 106–11.

Satinoff, E. (1979) 'Drugs and thermoregulatory behavior.' In P. Lomax and E. Schonbaum (eds.) *Body Temperature: Regulation, Drug Effects, and Therapeutic Implications*. Marcel Dekker, New York, pp. 151–82.

Sato, M. (1978) 'Studies on hypertension: changes of blood pressure and catecholamine under various environments.' *Nichidai Igaku Zasshi*, *37*, 1199–1210.

Savard, G.K.; Cooper, K.E.; Veale, W.L. (1984) 'Possible mechanisms for the after-drop of core temperature upon rewarming from mild hypothermia.' *Presentation at Sixth International Symposium on Circumpolar Health. May 13–18, 1984. Anchorage, Alaska.* Abstracts p. 77.

Schaefer, O.; Eaton, R.D.P.; Timmermans, F.J.W.; Hildes, J.A. (1980) 'Respiratory function impairment and cardiopulmonary consequences in long-term residents of the Canadian Arctic.' *Can. Med. Ass. J.*, *123*, 997–1004.

Schalekamp, M.A.D.H., Vincent, H.H., Man in't Veld, A.J. (1983) 'Adrenaline, stress and hypertension.' *Lancet*, *i*, 362.

Schell, F. (1978) 'Prisoners of the ice.' *Readers Digest*, *Feb.*, 97–103.

Scherf, D.; Blumenfeld, S.; Terranova, R. (1953) 'Ventricular fibrillation elicited by focal cooling.' *Am. Heart J.*, *46*, 741–53.

Schissler, P.; Parker, M.A.; Scott, S.J. (1981) 'Profound hypothermia: value of prolonged cardiopulmonary resuscitation.' *South. Med. J.*, *74*, 474–7.

Schmid-Schonbein, H.' Neumann, F.J. (1985) 'Pathophysiology of cutaneous frost injury: disturbed microcirculation as a consequence of abnormal flow behavior of the blood. Application of new concepts of blood rheology.' In J. Rivolier, P. Cerretelli, J. Foray, P. Segantini (eds.) *High Altitude Deterioration*, Karger, Basel, pp. 20–38.

Schneider, M.F.; Brooke, J.D. (1979) 'Bimodal relationship of human tremor and shivering on introduction to cold exposure.' *Aviat. Space Environ. Med.*, *50*, 1016–19.

Schonle, Ch. (1982) 'Studies on body temperature in wind-surfing.' In P. Koch and M. Kohfahl (eds.) *Unterkuhlung im Seenotfall. 2nd Symposium*. Deutsche Gesellschaft zur Rettung Schiffbruchiger, Cuxhaven, pp. 192–203.

Schwartz, E.; Glick, Z.; Magazanik, A. (1977) 'Responses to temperate, cold and hot environments and the effect of physical training.' *Aviat. Space Environ. Med.*, *48*, 254–60.

Scotsman (1977) 'Prevention of shoplifting.' *Scotsman*, *Dec. 28*, 5, Col. 5.

——— (1978) 'Woman died of exposure.' *Scotsman*, *Jan.* 5, 5, Col. 3.

——— (1981) 'Cairngorm climber freezes to death.' *Scotsman*, *Jan. 3*, 1, Col. 1.

Scott-Daniell, D. (1965) *World War I. An Ilustrated History.* Ernest Benn, London.

Searle, J.F. (1971) 'Incidental hypothermia during surgery for peripheral vascular disease.' *Br. J. Anaesth.*, *43*, 1095–8.

Sefrin, P. (1982) 'Hypothermia and injury.' In P. Koch and M. Kohfahl (eds.) *Unterkuhlung im Seenotfall. 2nd Symposium*. Deutsche Gesellschaft zur Rettung Schiffbruchiger, Cuxhaven, pp. 112–23.

Segantini, P. (1979) 'Kasuistik der Lawinenunfalle in der Schweiz 1976–77 und 1977–78.' In P. Matter, P. Braun, M. deQuervain, W. Good (eds.) *Skifahren und Sicherheit III*. Buchdruckerei Davos AG, Davos, pp. 111–15.

Sekar, T.S.; MacDonnell, K.F.; Namsirikul, P.; Herman, R.S. (1980) 'Survival after prolonged submersion in cold water without neurological sequelae. Report of two cases.' *Arch. Intern. Med.*, *140*, 775–9.

Sellers, E.M.; Martin, P.R.; Roy, M.L.; Sellers, E.A. (1979) 'Amphetamines.' In P. Lomax and E. Schonbaum (eds.) *Body Temperature: Regulation, Drug Effects, and Therapeutic Implications*. Marcel Dekker, New York, pp. 461–98.

Sellick, B.A. (1963) 'Hypothermia.' In C.L. Hewer (eds.) *Recent advances in anaesthesia and analgesia*. Churchill, London, pp. 111–24.

Shakoor, M.A.; Sabean, J.; Wilson, K.M.; Hurt, H.H.; Graff, T.D. (1968) 'High density water environment by ultrasonic humidification: pulmonary and systemic effects.' *Anesth. Analg. (Cleve.)*, *46*, 638–46.

Shanks, C.A. (1973) 'The effects of inspiration of gases saturated with water vapour on heat and moisture exchange during endotracheal intubation.' *Br. J. Anaesth.*, *45*, 887–90.

——— (1974a) 'Clinical anaesthesia and the multiple-gauze condenser humidifier.' *Br. J. Anaesth.*, *46*, 773–7.

——— (1974b) 'Humidification and loss of body heat during anaesthesia. 1. Quantification and correlation in the dog.' *Br. J. Anaesth.*, *46*, 859–62.

——— (1974c) 'Humidification and loss of body heat during anaesthesia. 2. Effects on surgical patients.' *Br. J. Anaesth.*, *46*, 863–6.

——— (1975a) 'Heat balance during surgery involving body cavities.' *Anaesth. Intensive Care*, *3*, 114–17.

——— (1975b) 'Control of heat balance during arterial surgery.' *Anaesth. Intensive Care*, *3*, 118–21.

——— (1975c) 'Mean skin temperature during anaesthesia: an assessment of formulae in the supine surgical patient.' *Br. J. Anaesth.*, *47*, 871–5.

——— (1975d) 'Heat gain in the treatment of accidental hypothermia.' *Med. J. Aust.*,

2, 346–9.

——— (1977) 'Humidifiers and humidification.' *Br. J. Clin. Equip.*, *2*, 21–5.

———; Gibbs, J.M. (1975) 'A comparison of two heated water-bath humidifiers.' *Anaesth. Intensive Care*, *3*, 41–7.

———; Marsh, H.M. (1973) 'Simple core rewarming in accidental hypothermia.' *Br. J. Anaesth.*, *45*, 522–5.

———; Sara, C. (1973a) 'Airway heat and humidity during endotracheal intubation. I Inspiration of arid gases via a non-rebreathing circuit.' *Anaesth. Intensive Care*, *1*, 211–14.

———; Sara, C. (1973b) 'Airway heat and humidity during endotracheal intubation. II Partial rebreathing via a circle absorber system.' *Anaesth. Intensive Care*, *1*, 215–17.

———; Sara, C. (1973c) 'Airway heat and humidity during endotracheal intubation. III Rebreathing from the circle absorber system at low fresh gas flow.' *Anaesth. Intensive Care*, *1*, 415–17.

———; Sara, C. (1974) 'Airway heat and humidity during endotracheal intubation. IV Connotation of delivered water vapour content.' *Anaesth. Intensive Care*, *2*, 212–20.

Shannon, D.C.; Kelly, D.H. (1982) 'SIDS and near-SIDS.' *New Engl. J. Med.*, *306*, 1022–8.

Shapiro, C.M.; Parry, M.R. (1984) 'Is unemployment a cause of parasuicide?' *Br. Med. J.*, *ii*, 1622.

———; Goll, C.C.; Cohen, G.R.; Oswald, I. (1984) 'Heat production during sleep.' *J. Appl. Physiol.*, *56*, 671–7.

Shaw, A.; Franzel, I.; Borduik, J. (1971) 'Prevention of neonatal hypothermia by a fiber-optic "hot pipe" system. A new concept.' *J. Paed. Surg.*, *6*, 354–8.

Shibolet, S.; Lancaster, M.C.; Danon, Y. (1976) 'Heat stroke: a review.' *Aviat. Space Environ. Med.*, *47*, 280–301.

Shimizu, H.J.; Alton, J.D.M. (1982) 'Burn/frostbite syndrome.' In B. Harvald and J.P. Hart Hansen (eds.) *Circumpolar Health 81*. Nordic Council for Arctic Medical Research, Copenhagen, pp. 608–9.

Shukla, R.B.; Kelly, D.G.; Daly, L.; Guiney, E.J. (1982) 'Association of cold weather with testicular torsion.' *Br. Med. J.*, *ii*, 1459–1560.

Shulzhenko, E.B.; Panfilov, V.E.; Gogolev, K.I.; Aleksandrova, E.A. (1979) 'Comparison of physiological effects of head-down tilting and immersion in the human body.' *Aviat. Space Environ. Med.*, *50*, 1020–2.

Siebke, H.; Breivik, H.; Rod, T.; Lind, B. (1975) 'Survival after 40 minutes' submersion without cerebral sequelae.' *Lancet*, *i*, 1275–9.

Sillanpaa, M.L. (1982) 'Treatment of alcohol withdrawal symptoms.' *Br. J. Hosp. Med.*, *30*, 343–50.

Silverman, W.A.; Sinclair, J.C. (1966) 'Temperature regulation in the newborn infant.' *New Engl. J. Med.*, *274*, 92–4.

———; Fertig, J.W.; Berger, A.P. (1958) 'The influence of the thermal environment upon the survival of newly born premature infants.' *Paediatrics*, *22*, 876–86.

Simpson, H. (1983) 'Sudden unexpected infant death. II home monitoring.' *Arch. Dis. Child.*, *58*, 469–71.

Simpson, H.W. (1972) 'The exploring scientist.' *Br. J. Sports Med.*, *6*, 100–7.

——— (1981) 'Variations in body rhythms.' Presentation in *Hypothermia and Hyperthermia in Anaesthesia and Intensive Care*. Faculty of Anaesthetists Scientific Meeting, Nov. 5 and 6.

Simpson, R.G. (1974) 'Disease patterns in the elderly.' *Br. J. Hosp. Med.*, *12*, 660–77.

Singh, S.P.; Patel, D.G. (1978) 'Effect of ethanol on carbohydrate metabolism. II Influence on glucose tolerance in diabetic rats.' *J. Stud. Alcoholism*, *39*, 1206–12.

———; Patel, D.G.; Snyder, H.K. (1980) 'Ethanol inhibition of insulin secretion by perfused rat islets.' *Acta Endocrinol.*, *93*, 61–6.

Siple, P.A.; Passel, C.F. (1945) 'General principles governing selection of clothing for cold climates.' *Proc. Am. Phil. Soc.*, *89*, 177–99.

Sloan, R.E.G.; Keatinge, W.G. (1975) 'Depression of sublingual temperature by cold saliva.' *Br. Med. J.*, *i*, 718–20.

Smith, A.P.; Loh, H.H. (1981) 'The opiate receptor.' In C.H.Li (ed.) *Hormonal Proteins and Peptides. Vol. X, β-Endorphin.* Academic Press, London, pp. 89–170.

Smith, A.U. (1959) 'Viability of supercooled and frozen mammals.' *Ann. N.Y. Acad. Sci.*, *80*, 291–300.

Smith, D.J. (1952) 'Constriction of isolated arteries and their vasa vasorum produced by low temperatures.' *Am. J. Physiol.*, *171*, 528–37.

Smith, D.K.; Ovesen, L.; Chu, R.; Sackel, S.; Howard, L. (1983) 'Hypothermia in a patient with anorexia nervosa. *Metabolism*, *32*, 1151–4.

Smith, H.S. (1983) 'Dangers of heated water blankets and small children.' *Anaesthesia*, *38*, 1006–7.

SMJ (1972) 'Accidental hypothermia.' *Scot. Med. J.*, *17*, 81–2.

Smythe, F.S. (1956) *Camp IV.* Camelot Press, London, pp. 186–9.

Snider, G.L. (1981) 'Pathogenesis of emphysema and chronic bronchitis.' *Med. Clin. N. Am.*, *65*, 647–65.

Sniderman, A.; Burdon, T.; Homa, J.; Salerno, T.A. (1984) 'Pulmonary blood flow – a potential factor in the pathogenesis of pulmonary edema.' *J. Thor. Cardiovasc. Surg.*, *87*, 130–5.

Snyder, S.H. (1983) 'Schizophrenia.' In *Neurotransmitters and CNS Disease. Lancet, London*, pp. 6–10.

Social Work (1977) *Old and cold? How to keep warm this winter.* Social Work Dept, Edinburgh.

Soininen, L.; Lunden, J. (1982) 'A mask saving warmth of breathing air. An appliance for cold climate.' In B. Harvald and J.P. Hart Hansen (eds.) *Circumpolar Health 81.* Nordic Council Arctic Medical Research, Copenhagen, pp. 576–7.

Soulski, R.; Polin, R.A.; Baumgart, S. (1983) 'Respiratory water loss and heat balance in intubated infants receiving humidified air.' *J. Pediat.*, *103*, 307–10.

Soung, I.S.; Swank, I.; Ing, T.S.; Said, R.A.; Goldman, J.W.; Perez, J.; Geis, W.P. (1977) 'Treatment of accidental hypothermia with peritoneal dialysis.' *Can. Med. Ass. J.*, *117*, 1415–16.

Southall, D.P.; Levitt, G.A.; Richards, J.M.; Jones, R.A.; King, C.; Farndon, P.A.; Alexander, J.R.; Wilson, A.J. (1983) 'Undetected episodes of prolonged apnoea and severe bradycardia in preterm infants.' *Pediatrics*, *72*, 541–51.

Sprunt, J.G.; Maclean, D.; Browning, M.C.K. (1970) 'Plasma corticosteroid levels in accidental hypothermia.' *Lancet*, *i*, 324–6. .

Stanley, M.; Mann, J.J. (1983) 'Increased serotonin-2 binding sites in frontal cortex of suicide victims.' *Lancet*, *i*, 214–16.

Stanton, A.N. (1982) ' "Near-miss" cot deaths and home monitoring.' *Br. Med. J.*, *ii*, 1441–2.

Steegman, A.T. (1979) 'Human facial temperatures in natural and laboratory cold.' *Aviat. Space Environ. Med.*, *50*, 227–32.

Steele, P. (1972) *Doctor on Everest.* Hodder & Stoughton, London, pp. 191–2.

Steinman, A. (1982) 'Triage problems in disasters at sea.' In P.Koch and M. Kohfahl (eds.) *Unterkuhlung im Seenotfall. 2nd Symposium.* Deutsche Gesellschaft zur Rettung Schiffbruchiger, Cuxhaven, pp. 66–71.

Stephens, D.H. (1982) 'Sleeping snugly in cold damp bedrooms.' *J. Roy. Soc. Health*, *6*, 272–5.

Stephenson, J.M.; Du, J.N.; Oliver, T.K. (1970) 'The effect of cooling on blood gas tensions in newborn infants.' *J. Paediat.*, *76*, 848–52.

Steward, D.J. (1976) 'A disposable condenser humidifier for use during anaesthesia.'

Can. Anaesth. Soc. J., *23*, 191–5.

Stewart, M.; Graham, E. (1984) 'Darkness-related secondary amenorrhea.' *Presentation at Sixth International Symposium on Circumpolar Health. May 13–18, 1984. Anchorage, Alaska.* Abstracts p. 162.

Stewart, T. (1972) 'Treatment after exposure to cold.' *Lancet*, *i*, 140.

——— (1977) 'Clinical signs of exposure to cold.' *General Practitioner, Feb. 23*, 23–5.

——— (1981) 'Mountain rescue and the exposure syndrome: some case reports and observations.' In J.N. Adams (ed.) *Hypothermia Ashore and Afloat.* Aberdeen University Press, Aberdeen, pp. 22–7.

Stine, R.J. (1977) 'Accidental hypothermia.' *J. Am. Coll Emerg. Phys.*, *6*, 413–16.

Stoddart, J.C. (1976) 'Drowning, exposure and hypothermia. *Anaesthesia*, *31*, 833.

Stone, D.R.; Downs, J.B.; Paul, W.L.; Perkins, H.M. (1981) 'Adult body temperature and heated humidification of anesthetic gases during general anesthesia.' *Anesth. Analg.*, *60*, 736–41.

Stradling, J.R.; Lane, D.J. (1983) 'Nocturnal hypoxaemia in chronic obstructive pulmonary disease.' *Clin. Sci.*, *64*, 213–22.

Strauss, R.H.; McFadden, E.R.; Ingram, R.H.; Deal, E.C.; Jaeger, J.J. (1978) 'Influence of heat and humidity on the airway obstruction induced by exercise in asthma.' *J. Clin. Invest.*, *61*, 433–40.

Stromme, S.B.; Ingjer, F. (1978) 'Comparison of diving bradycardia and maximal aerobic power.' *Aviat. Space Environ. Med.*, *49*, 1267–70.

Stupfol, M.; Severinghaus, J.W. (1956) 'Internal body temperature gradients during anaesthesia and hypothermia and effect of vagotomy.' *J. Appl. Physiol.*, *9*, 380–6.

Sumner, D.S.; Strandness, D.E. (1972) 'An abnormal finger pulse associated with cold sensitivity.' *Ann. Surg.*, *175*, 294–8.

Sun (1977) 'Mum saves man trapped in the deep freeze.' *Sun*, *Aug.* 5, 5, Col. 3.

Sunday Post (1978) 'Frozen to death in Glasgow.' *Sunday Post*, *Dec. 3*, 18, Col. 1.

Surwit, R.S.; Allen, L.M.; Gilgor, R.S.; Schanberg, S.; Kuhn, C.; Duvic, M. (1983) 'Neuroendocrine response to cold in Raynaud's syndrome.' *Life Sci.*, *32*, 995–1000.

SUT (1975a) *Submersibles.* Society for Underwater Technology, London.

——— (1975b) *The Principles of Safe Diving Practice.* Society for Underwater Technology, London.

——— (1976) *The Principles of Safe Diving Practice: Helium Diving.* Society for Underwater Technology, London.

Sutton, J.R. (1983) 'The chilliness of a long-distance runner.' *Lancet*, *i*, 600.

———; Lassen, N. (1979) 'Pathophysiology of acute mountain sickness and high altitude pulmonary oedema: an hypothesis.' *Bull. Eur. Physiopathol. Respir.*, *15*, 1045–52.

Swan, H.; Virtue, R.W.; Blount, S.G.; Kircher, L.T. (1955) 'Hypothermia in surgery. Analysis of 100 clinical cases.' *Ann. Surg.*, *142*, 383–400.

———; Zearin, I.; Holmes, J.H.; Montgomery, V. (1953) 'Cessation of circulation in general hypothermia. I Physiologic changes and their control.' *Ann. Surg.*, 138, 360–76.

Swann, H. (1950) 'Studies in resuscitation.' *AF Tech. Rep.*, p. 6006.

——— (1951) 'Studies in resuscitation.' *AF Tech. Rep.*, p. 6696

Swann, H.G.; Spafford, N.R. (1951) 'Body salt and water changes during fresh water and sea water drowning.' *Tex. Rep. Biol. Med.*, *9*, 356–82.

Tabeling, B.B. (1983) 'Near-drowning and its treatment.' In R.S. Pozos and L.E. Wittmers (eds.) *The Nature and Treatment of Hypothermia*. Croom Helm, London/University of Minnesota Press, pp. 221–31.

Tabeling, B.B.; Modell, J.H. (1983) 'Fluid administration increases oxygen delivery during continuous positive pressure ventilation after freshwater near-drowning.' *Crit. Care Med.*, *11*, 693–6.

Taggart, P.; Parkinson, P; Carruthers, M. (1972) 'Cardiac responses to thermal, physical and emotional stress.' *Br. Med. J.*, *iii*, 71–6.

Talbot, J.H.; Consolazio, W.V.; Percora, L.J. (1941) 'Hypothermia — report of a case in which the patient died during therapeutic reduction of body temperature, with metabolic and pathological studies.' *Arch. Int. Med.*, *68*, 1120–32.

Talsma, P.; Optroodt, N.; Havill, J.H. (1978) 'Device for humidification and controlled oxygenation during spontaneous breathing.' *Anaesth. Intens. Care*, *6*, 160–1.

Tansey, W.A. (1973) 'Medical aspects of cold water immersion: a review.' *US Nav. Submar. Med. Res. Lab.*, Rep. NSMRL 763. NTIS document AD–775–687.

Tappan, D.V.; Jacey, M.J.; Heyder, E.; Gray, P.H. (1984) 'Blood volume responses in partially dehydrated subjects working in the cold.' *Aviat. Space Environ. Med.*, 55, 296–301.

Tausk, H.C.; Miller, R.; Roberts, R.B. (1976) 'Maintenance of body temperature by heated humidification.' *Anesth. Analg. (Cleve.)*, 55, 719–23.

Taylor, D.E.M. (1972) 'Cold survival.' *Br. J. Sports Med.*, *6*, 111–16.

Taylor, G. (1975) 'Men at risk from cold.' *Viewpoint*, *Nov.*, 2.

——— (1978) 'Death in winter.' Unpublished.

——— (1981) 'Covering up hypothermia.' *World Med.*, *16*, 21.

Taylor, G.J.; Tucker, M.; Greene, H.L.; Rudikoff, M; Weisfeldt, M.L. (1977) 'Importance of prolonged compression duration during cardiopulmonary resuscitation in man.' *N. Engl. J. Med.*, *296*, 1515–17.

Taylor, I.M. (1956) 'The effect of low temperatures upon intracellular potassium in isolated tissues.' In C. Dripps (ed.) *The Physiology of Induced Hypothermia*. Nat. Acad. Sci., New York, pp. 26–9.

Tayyab, M.A.; Ambiavagar, M.; Chalon, J. (1973) 'Water nebulization in an ordinary breathing system during anaesthesia.' *Can. Anaesth. Soc. J.*, *20*, 728–35.

Teichner, W.H. (1954) 'Assessment of mean body surface temperature.' *J. Appl. Physiol.*, *12*, 169–76.

——— (1958) 'Reaction time in the cold.' *J. Appl. Physiol.*, *42*, 54–9.

———; Kobrich, J.L. (1955) 'Effects of prolonged exposure to low temperatures on visual motor performance.' *J. Exp. Psychol.*, *49*, 122–6.

Theilade, D. (1977) 'The danger of fatal misjudgement in hypothermia after immersion. Successful resuscitation following immersion for 25 minutes.' *Anaesthesia*, *32*, 889–92.

Thomas, D.J.; Green, I.D. (1973) 'Periodic hypothermia.' *Br. Med. J.*, *ii*, 696–7.

Thomas, J.E.P.; Gerber, S. (1965) 'Accidental hypothermia.' *Cent. Afr. J. Med.*, *11*, 151–2.

Thompson, J.W. (1984) 'Opioid peptides.' *Br. Med. J.*, *i*, 259–61.

Thompson, M.K. (1977a) 'Helping pensioners to keep warm.' *Br. Med. J.*, *i*, 716.

Thompson, R.L. (1977b) 'Cause of death in aircraft accidents: drowning —v— traumatic injuries.' *Aviat. Space Environ. Med.*, *48*, 924–8.

Thomson, D. (1981) 'Doctor in a cave.' *Br. Med. J.*, *i*, 277–9.

Thornton, R.J.; Blakeney, C.; Feldman, S.A. (1976) 'The effect of hypothermia on neuromuscular conduction.' *Br. J. Anaesth.*, *48*, 264.

Tindall, J.P.; Becker, S.F.; Rosse, W.F. (1969) 'Familial cold urticaria. A generalised reaction involving leukocytosis.' *Arch. Int. Med.*, *124*, 129–34.

Ting, S. (1984) 'Cold-induced urticaria in infancy.' *Pediatrics*, *73*, 105–6.

Tirlapur, V.G. (1984) 'Nocturnal deaths among patients with chronic bronchitis and emphysema.' *Br. Med. J.*, *ii*, 1540.

Tolman, K.G.; Cohen, A. (1970) 'Accidental hypothermia.' *Can. Med. Ass. J.*, *103*, 1357–61.

Tonjum, S.; Hamilton, R.W.; Brubakk, A.O.; Petersen, R.E.; Youngblood, D.A. (1980) *Project Polar Bear. Testing of Diver Thermal Protection in a Simulated 'Lost Bell'*. Norwegian Underwater Institute, Bergen. Report 2–80.

———; Pasche, A.; Onarheim, J.; Hayes, P.; Padbury, H. (1985) 'The case of the lost bell.' In L. Rey (ed.) *Arctic Underwater Operations*. Graham & Trotman, London, pp. 263–7.

Toremalm, N.G. (1901) 'Air-flow patterns and ciliary activity in the trachea after tracheostomy.' *Acta Otolaryngol.*, *53*, 442.

Toung, J.K.; Alvaran, S.B.; Shakoor, M.A.; Graff, T.D.; Benson, D.W. (1970) 'Alveolar surface activity following mechanical endotracheal ventilation with high-density water mist.' *Anesth. Analg. (Cleve.)*, *49*, 851–8.

Towne, W.D.; Geiss, W.P.; Yanes, H.O.; Rahimtoola, S.H. (1972) 'Intractible ventricular fibrillation associated with profound accidental hypothermia — successful treatment with partial cardiopulmonary bypass.' *New Engl. J. Med.*, *287*, 1135–6.

Treasure, T. (1984) 'The safe duration of total circulatory arrest with profound hypothermia.' *Ann. Roy. Coll. Surg. Eng.*, *66*, 235–40.

Trimble, M.R. (1981) 'Visual and auditory hallucinations.' *Trends in Neurosciences*, *42*, 2–4.

Truscott, D.G.; Firor, W.G.; Clein, L.J. (1973) 'Accidental profound hypothermia: successful resuscitation by core rewarming and assisted circulation.' *Arch. Surg.*, *106*, 216–18.

Tufik, S.; Lindsey, C.J.; Carlini, E.A. (1978) 'Does REM sleep deprivation induce a supersensitivity of dopaminergic receptors in the rat brain?' *Pharmacology*, *16*, 98–105.

Tunley, R. (1978) 'The challenge of the Eiger.' *Reader's Digest*, *June*, 144–50.

Turina, M.; Hossli, G. (1979) 'Successful rewarming with the heart-lung-machine after accidental hypothermia.' In P. Matter, P. Braun, M. de Quervain, W. Good (eds.) *Skifahren und Sicherheit III*. Buchdruckerei Davos AG, Davos, pp. 209–14.

Turner, T.H.; Cookson, J.C.; Wass, J.A.H.; Drury, P.L.; Price, P.A.; Besser, G.M. (1984) 'Psychotic reactions during treatment of pituitary tumours with dopamine agonists.' *Br. Med. J.*, *ii*, 1101–3.

Tyrer, P.J. (1984) 'Benzodiazepines on trial.' *Br. Med. J.*, *i*, 1101–2.

Umach, P.; Unterdorfer, H. (1979a) 'Morphology of death due to super-cooling a: before reanimation and warm-up measurements, b: after warm-up measurements and shock treatment.' In P. Matter, P. Braun, M. de Quervain, W. Good (eds.) *Skifahren und Sicherheit III*. Buchdruckerei Davos AG, Davos, pp. 116–26.

———; Unterdorfer, H. (1979b) 'Morphology of death in an avalanche (before reanimation measurements).' In P. Matter, P. Braun, M. de Quervain, W. Good (eds.) *Skifahren und Sicherheit III*. Buchdruckerei Davos AG, Davos, pp. 127–32.

Ungley, C.C.; Channell, G.D.; Richards, R.L. (1945) 'The immersion foot syndrome.' *Br. J. Surg.*, *33*, 17–31.

US Coastguard (1980) *Hypothermia and Cold Water Survival*. Dept of Transportation, US Coastguard.

Vaagenes, P.; Holme, J.A. (1982) 'Accidental deep hypothermia due to exposure. *Anaesthesia*, *37*, 819–24.

Vale, R.J. (1971) 'Control of accidental hypothermia.' *Anaesthesia*, *26*, 526.

——— (1973) 'Normothermia: its place in operative and post-operative care.' *Anaesthesia*, *28*, 241–5.

———; Lunn, H.F. (1969) 'Heat balance in anaesthetised surgical patients.' *Proc. R. Soc. Med.*, *62*, 1017–18.

Valkonen, T.; Notkola, V. (1977) 'Social environment and natural environment in relation to ischaemic heart disease mortality in Finland.' *Nordic Council Arct. Med. Res.*, *Rep. No. 19*, pp. 95–100.

van Praag, H.M. (1983a) 'CSF 5-HIAA and suicide in non-depressed schizophrenics.' *Lancet*, *ii*, 977–8.

——— (1983b) 'Depression.' In *Neurotransmitters and CNS Disease. Lancet*, London, pp. 33–8.

Vanggaard, L. (1975) 'Physiological reactions to wet-cold.' *Aviat. Space Environ. Med.*, *46*, 33–6.

——— (1977) 'Occupational hazards in the Danish North-Sea fishing.' *Nordic Council Arct. Med. Res.*, *Rep. No. 18*, pp. 31–7.

——— (1978) 'Alcohol (ethanol) and cold.' *Nordic Council Arct. Med. Res.*, *Rep. No. 21*, pp. 82–92.

——— (1985) 'Cold-induced changes.' In L. Rey (ed.) *Arctic Underwater Operations*. Graham & Trotman, London. pp. 41–8.

Varene, P.; Timbal, J.; Viellifond, H.; Guenard, H; L'Huillier, J. (1976) 'Energy balance of man in simulated dive from 1.5 to 31 ATA.' In C.J. Lambertsen (ed.) *Underwater Physiology V*. FASEB, Bethesda, pp. 755–64.

Vaughan, M.S.; Vaughan, R.W.; Cork, R.C. (1981) 'Postoperative hypothermia in adults: relationship of age, anaesthesia and shivering to rewarming.' *Anesth. Analg. (Cleve.)*, *60*, 746–51.

Vaughan, W.S. (1977) 'Distraction effect of cold water on performance of high-order tasks.' *Undersea Biomed. Res.*, *4*, 103–16.

Veghte, J.H. (1972) 'Cold sea survival.' *Aerosp. Med.*, *43*, 506–11.

———; Adams, W.C.; Bernauer, E.M. (1979) 'Temperature changes during exercise measured by thermography.' *Aviat. Space Environ. Med.*, *50*, 708–13.

Verlander, J.M.; Beerwinkle, K.; Fife, W.P. (1978) 'Radiotelemetry system for obtaining body temperature during simulated diving to 1000 FSW.' *Aviat. Space Environ. Med.*, *49*, 641–3.

Vernon, H.M. (1939) *Health in Relation to Occupation*. Oxford University Press, London.

Victor, M.; Adams, R. (1958) 'Alcohol.' In J. Harrison (ed.) *Principles of Internal Medicine*. McGraw-Hill, London, pp. 747–55.

Vidal, C.; Suaudeau, C.; Jacob, J. (1983) 'Hyper- and hypothermia induced by non-noxious stress: effects of naloxone, diazepam and Y-acetylenic GABA.' *Life Sci.*, *33 Suppl. 1*, 587–90.

Virr, L.E. (1985) 'Mechanical design and operation of thermal protection equipment.' In L. Rey (ed.) *Arctic Underwater Operations*. Graham & Trotman, London, pp. 217–36.

Vivori, E.; Bush, G.H. (1977) 'Modern aspects in the management of the newborn undergoing operation.' *Br. J. Anaesth.*, *49*, 51–7.

Vogel, G.W. (1975) 'A review of sleep deprivation.' *Arch. Gen. Psychiatry*, *32*, 749–61.

von Kappeler, O. (1880) 'Anaesthetica (monograph).' *Deutsche Chirurgie*, *168*, 33–6.

Wade, C.E.; Veghte, J.H. (1977) 'Thermographic evaluation of the relative heat loss by area in man after swimming.' *Aviat. Space Environ. Med.*, *48*, 16–18.

———; Dacanay, S.; Smith, R.M. (1979) 'Regional heat loss in resting man during immersion in 25.2 °C water.' *Aviat. Space Environ. Med.*, *50*, 590–3.

Wagner, J.A.; Robinson, S.; Marino, R.P. (1974) 'Age and temperature regulation of humans in neutral and cold environments.' *J. Appl. Physiol.*, *37*, 562–5.

Waldron, H.A. (1976) *Lecture Notes on Occupational Medicine*. Blackwell, London.

Walker, E.C.; Wells, R.E.; Merrill, E.W. (1961) 'Heat and water exchange in the respiratory tract.' *Am. J. Med.*, *30*, 259–67.

Wallace, C.T.; Baker, J.D.; Brown, C.S. (1978) 'Heated humidification for infants during anesthesia.' *Anesthesiology*, *48*, 80.

Walther, A. (1862) 'Beitrage zur Lehre von der Thierischen Warme.' *Virchows Arch.*, *25*, 414.

Wanderer, A.A. (1979) 'An "allergy" to cold.' *Hosp. Pract.*, *14*, 136–7.

Wang, L.C.H. (1978) 'Factors limiting maximum cold-induced heat production.' *Life Sci.*, *23*, 2089–98.

Ward, M. (1973) 'Mountains hold no fear — only fascination.' *Pulse*, *Feb. 17*, 35.
——— (1974) 'Frostbite.' *Br. Med. J.*, *i*, 67–70.
——— (1975a) *Mountain Medicine*. Crosby Lockwood Staples, London.
——— (1975b) 'Frostbite.' In C. Clarke; M. Ward; E. Williams (eds.) *Mountain Medicine and Physiology*, Alpine Club, London, pp. 19–27.
Wasserman, S.I.; Soter, N.A.; Center, D.M.; Austen, K.F. (1977) 'Cold urticaria. Recognition and characterization of a neutrophil chemotactic factor which appears in serum during experimental cold challenge.' *J. Clin. Invest.*, *60*, 189–96.
Waterman, A. (1975) 'Accidental hypothermia during anaesthesia in dogs and cats.' *Vet. Rec.*, *96*, 308–13.
Watters, D.D.; Szlachcic, J.; Bonan, R.; Miller, D.D.; Dawe, F.; Theroux, P. (1983) 'Comparative sensitivity of exercise, cold pressor and ergonovine in provoking attacks of variant angina in patients with active disease.' *Circulation*, *67*, 310–15.
Watts, J.M. (1963) 'Tracheotomy in modern practice.' *Br. J. Surg.*, *50*, 954–7.
Wauer, R.R. (1978) 'Heat-protection foil for the prevention of heat loss in newborn infants.' *Kinderaerztl. Prax.*, *46*, 189–90.
Wayne, M.A. (1976) 'Conversion of paroxysmal atrial tachycardia by facial immersion in ice water.' *J. Am. Coll. Emerg. Phys.*, 5, 434–5.
Webb, G.E. (1973a) 'Comparison of esophageal and tympanic temperature monitoring during cardiopulmonary bypass.' *Anesth. Analg. (Cleve.)*, *52*, 729–33.
Webb, P. (1951) 'Air temperature in respiratory tracts of resting subjects in cold.' *J. Appl. Physiol.*, *4*, 378–82.
——— (1955) 'Respiratory heat loss in cold.' *Fed. Proc.*, *14*, 486–7.
——— (1973b) 'Rewarming after diving in cold water.' *Aerospace Med.*, *44*, 1152–7.
——— (1976) 'Thermal stress in undersea activity.' In C.J. Lambertsen (ed.) *Underwater Physiology V*. FASEB, Bethesda, pp. 705–24.
Webster, A.P. (1952) 'Caloric requirement of man in cold climates: theoretical considerations.' *J. Appl. Physiol.*, 5, 134–42.
Webster, D.R.; Woolhouse, F.M.; Johnson, J.L. (1942) 'Immersion foot.' *J. Bone and Joint Surg.*, *24*, 785–94.
Wedin, B. (1976) 'Cases of paradoxical undressing by people exposed to severe hypothermia.' In R.J. Shephard and S. Itoh (eds.) *Circumpolar Health*. Toronto University Press, Toronto, pp. 61–71.
———; Vanggaard, L.; Hirvonen, J. (1979) '"Paradoxical undressing" in fatal hypothermia.' *J. Forensic Sci.*, *24*, 543–53.
Wedley, J. (1978) 'Post-operative temperature control.' *On Call*, *Apr. 27*, 8 and 9.
Wedley, J.R. (1974) 'Incidental hypothermia during surgery for peripheral vascular disease.' *Br. J. Anaesth.*, *46*, 713.
——— (1979) 'Body temperature.' *Br. J. Clin. Equip.*, *4*, 244.
Weeks, D.B. (1975a) 'Higher humidity, an additional benefit of a disposable anesthesia circle.' *Anesthesiology*, *43*, 375–7.
——— (1975b) 'Humidification during anesthesia.' *NY State J. Med.*, *75*, 1216.
Weihe, W.H. (1973) 'The effect of temperature on the action of drugs.' *Am. Rev. Pharmacol.*, *13*, 409–25.
Weihl, A.C.; Langworthy, H.C.; Manalasay, A.R.; Layton, R.P. (1981) 'Metabolic responses of resting man immersed in 25.5 °C and 33 °C water.' *Aviat. Space Environ. Med.*, *52*, 88–91.
Weinberger, S.E.; Weiss, S.T.; Johnson, T.S.; von Gal, E.; Balsavich, L. (1982) 'Naloxone does not affect bronchoconstriction induced by isocapnic hyperpnoea of subfreezing air.' *Am. Rev. Respir. Dis.*, *126*, 468–71.

Weiner, J.S.; Khogali, M. (1980) 'A physiological body cooling unit for treatment of heatstroke.' *Lancet*, *i*, 507–9.

Welch, G.S. (1974) 'Frostbite.' *Practitioner*, *213*, 801–4.

Welford, A.T. (1965) 'Fatigue and monotony.' In O.G. Edholm and A.L. Bacharach (eds.) *The Physiology of Human Survival*. Academic Press, London, pp. 431–64.

Wells, C. (1977) 'Snow shovelling and coronary deaths.' *Br. Med. J.*, *i*, 908.

Wells, R.E.; Walker, J.E.C.; Hickler, R.B. (1960) 'Effects of cold air on respiratory airflow resistance in patients with respiratory tract disease.' *New Engl. J. Med.*, *363*, 268–73.

Wells, R.N. (1973) 'Profound hypothermia with cardiac arrest after immersion.' *Br. Med. J.*, *iv*, 678.

Welton, D.E.; Mattox, K.L.; Miller, R.R.; Petmecky, F.F. (1978) 'Treatment of profound hypothermia.' *J. Am. Med. Ass.*, *240*, 2291–2.

Weltz, G.A.; Wendt, H.J.; Ruppin, H. (1942) 'Warming after severe hypothermia.' *Munch. Med. Wochen.*, *89*, 1092–8.

Werner, H. (1885) *Jean Dominique Larrey*. Ferdinand Enke Verlag, Stugggart.

Werner, J.A.; Greene, L.H.; Janko, C.L.; Cobb, L.A. (1981) 'Visualization of cardiac valve motion in man during external chest compression using two-dimensional echocardiography. Implications regarding the mechanism of blood flow.' *Circulation*, *63*, 1417–21.

Wessel, H.U.; James, G.W.; Paul, M.H. (1966) 'Effects of respiration and circulation on central blood temperature of the dog.' *Am. J. Physiol.*, *211*, 1403–12.

West, J. (1980) 'The chill wind of approaching old age.' *Commun. Nurs.*, *3*, 4 and 5.

West, J.B. (1984) 'Hypoxic man: lessons from extreme altitude.' *Aviat. Space Environ. Med.*, 55, 1058–62.

West, R.R.; Lloyd, S.; Roberts, C. (1973a) 'The old and the cold.' *Br. Med. J.*, *ii*, 50.

———; Lloyd, S.; Roberts, C. (1973b) 'Mortality from ischaemic heart disease — association with weather.' *Br. J. Prev. Soc. Med.*, *27*, 36–40.

———; Lowe, C.R. (1976) 'Mortality from ischaemic heart disease — inter-town variation and its association with climate in England and Wales.' *Int. J. Epidemiol.*, 5, 195–202.

Westenskow, D.R.; Wong, K.C. (1980) 'Microwave rewarming.' *Anesth. Analg. (Cleve.)*, *59*, 161–2.

———; Wong, K.C.; Johnson, C.C.; Wilde, C.S. (1979) 'Physiologic effects of deep hypothermia and microwave rewarming; possible applications for neonatal cardiac surgery.' *Anesth. Analg. (Cleve.)*, *58*, 297–301.

Westmorland, H.; Gate, G.E. (1972) *Report 1971*. Keswick Mountain Rescue Team.

Weyman, A.E.; Greenbaum, D.M.; Grace, W.J. (1974) 'Accidental hypothermia in the alcoholic population.' *Am. J. Med.*, *56*, 13–21.

Whitby, J.D.; Dunkin, L.J. (1969) 'Temperature differences in the oesophagus. The effects of intubation and ventilation.' *Br. J. Anaesth.*, *41*, 615–18.

———; Dunkin, L.J. (1970) 'Oesophageal temperature differences in children.' *Br. J. Anaesth.*, *42*, 1013–15.

———; Dunkin, L.J. (1971) 'Cerebral, oesophageal and nasopharyngeal temperatures.' *Br. J. Anaesth.*, *43*, 673–6.

White, D.; Butterfield, A.B.; Greer, K.A.; Schoem, S.; Johnson, C.; Holloway, R.R. (1984) 'Comparison of rewarming by radio wave regional hyperthermia and warm humidified inhalation.' *Aviat. Space Environ. Med.*, 55, 1103–6.

White, D.G. (1980) 'Anaesthesia in old age.' *Br. J. Hosp. Med.*, *24*, 145–50.

White, E.R.; Roth, N.J. (1979) 'Cold water survival suits for aircrew.' *Aviat. Space Environ. Med.*, *50*, 1040–5.

White-Thomson, S. (1981) 'The endeavour- training groups. 1978 expedition.'

Medisport, *3*, 3 and 4.
Whittington, R.M. (1977) 'Snow shovelling and coronary deaths.' *Br. Med. J.*, *i*, 577.
Whittle, J.L.; Eates, J.H. (1979) 'Thermoregulatory failure secondary to acute illness: complications and treatment.' *Arch. Intern. Med.*, *139*, 418–21.
Whitworth, J.A.G.; Wolfman, M.J. (1983) 'Fatal heat stroke in a long distance runner.' *Br. Med. J.*, *ii*, 948.
Wicks, M. (1978) *Old and Cold. Hypothermia and Social Policy*. Heinemann, London.
Wickstrom, P.; Ruiz, E.; Lilja, G.P.; Hinkerkopf, J.P.; Haglin, J.J. (1976) 'Accidental hypothermia: core rewarming with partial bypass.' *Am. J. Surg.*, *131*, 622–5.
Wigglesworth, R. (1973) 'Hypothermia.' *Br. Med. J.*, *i*, 482.
Wildenthal, K.; Leshin, S.L.; Atkins, J.M.; Skelton, C.L. (1975) 'The diving reflex used to treat paroxysmal atrial tachycardia.' *Lancet*, *i*, 12–14.
Wilkerson, J.; Raven, P.; Boldvan, N.; Horvath, S. (1974) 'Adaptions in man's adrenal function in response to acute cold stress.' *J. Appl. Physiol.*, *36*, 183–9.
Wilkinson, R. (1975) 'North Sea storms a power to be reckoned with.' *Offshore Engineer, Dec.*, 19–22.
Wilkinson, R.T. (1965) 'Sleep deprivation.' In O.G. Edholm and A.L. Bacharach (eds.) *The Physiology of Human Survival*. Academic Press, London, pp. 399–430.
Will, D.H.; McMurty, I.F.; Reeves, J.T.; Grover, R.F. (1978) 'Cold induced pulmonary hypertension in cattle.' *J. Appl. Physiol.*, *45*, 469–73.
Williams, A.L.; Uren, E.C.; Bretherton, L. (1984) 'Respiratory viruses and sudden infant death.' *Br. Med. J.*, *i*, 1491–3.
Williamson, R. (1983) 'Cold weather and testicular torsion.' *Br. Med. J.*, *i*, 1436.
Wilmore, D.W.; Mason, A.D.; Johnson, D.W.; Pruitt, B.A. (1975) 'Effect of ambient temperature on heat production and heat loss in burn patients.' *J. Appl. Physiol.*, *38*, 593–7.
Wilson, A.J.; Stevens, V.; Franks, C.I.; Alexander, J.; Southall, D.P. (1985) 'Respiratory and heart rate patterns in infants destined to be victims of sudden infant death syndrome: average rates and their variability measured over 24 hours.' *Br. Med. J.*, *i*, 497–501.
Wilson, O.; Hedner, P.; Laurell, S.; Nosslin, B.; Rerup, C.; Rosengren, E. (1970) 'Thyroid and adrenal response to acute cold exposure in man.' *J. Appl. Physiol.*, *28*, 543–9.
Wind, J. (1975) 'Survival after drowning.' *Lancet*, *ii*, 656–7.
Witherspoon, J.M.; Goldman, R.F.; Breckenridge, J.R. (1971) 'Heat transfer coefficients of humans in cold water.' *J. Physiol. (Paris)*, *63*, 459–62.
Wolff, H.S. (1961) 'A method of measuring core temperature by a "radio-pill".' *New Scientist*, *12*, 419–23.
Wood, D.L.; Sheps, S.G.; Elveback, L.R.; Shirger, A. (1984) 'Cold pressor test as a predictor of hypertension.' *Hypertension*, *6*, 301–6.
Wood, J.E.; Bass, D.E.; Iampietro, P.F. (1958) 'Responses of peripheral veins of man to prolonged and continuous cold exposure.' *J. Appl. Physiol.*, *12*, 357–60.
Woodruff, L.M. (1941) 'Survival of hypothermia by the dog.' *Anesthesiology*, *2*, 410–20.
Wright, G.R.; Shephard, R.J. (1979) 'Physiological effects of carbon monoxide.' In D. Robertshaw (ed.) *Environmental Physiology III*. University Park Press, Baltimore, pp. 311–68.
Wustmann, Ch.; Fischer, H.-D.; Schmidt, J. (1982) 'Inhibitory effects of hypoxia on dopamine release.' *Acta Biol. Med. Germ.*, *41*, 571–4.
Wylie, W.D.; Churchill-Davidson, H.C. (eds.) (1966) *A Practice of Anaesthesia*. Lloyd-Luke, London.
Wyndham, C.H.; Morrison, J.F.; Ward, J.S.; Bredell, G.A.G.; von Rahden, M.J.E.;

Holdsworth, L.D.; Wenzel, H.G.; Munro, A. (1964) 'Physiological reactions to cold of Bushmen, Bantu and Caucasian males.' *J. Appl. Physiol.*, *19*, 868–76.

Wyon, D.P.; Lidwell, D.M.; Williams, R.E.O. (1968) 'Thermal comfort during surgical operations.' *J. Hygiene (Camb.)*, *66*, 229–48.

Yoder, R.D.; Lees, D.E. (1979) 'Liquid crystal thermometry.' *Anesth. Analg. (Cleve.)*, *58*, 351.

York, D.H. (1979) 'The neurophysiology of dopamine receptors.' In A.S. Horn, J. Korf, B.H.C. Westerlink (eds.) *Neurobiology of Dopamine*. Academic Press, London, pp. 395–413.

Young, M.A.; Rowlands, D.B.; Stallard, T.J.; Watson, R.D.S.; Littler, W.A. (1983) 'Effect of environment on blood pressure: home versus hospital.' *Br. Med. J.*, *i*, 1235–6.

Young, R.S.K.; Marks, K.H. (1983) 'Hypothermia and the pediatric patient.' In R.S. Pozos and L.E. Wittmers (eds.) *The Nature and Treatment of Hypothermia*. Croom Helm, London/University of Minnesota, Minneapolis, pp. 20–34.

Zachau-Christiansen, B. (1975) 'Respiratory tract infections in Greenland children.' *Nordic Council Arct. Med. Res.*, *Rep. No. 12*, pp. 6–8.

Zideman, D. (1984) 'Cardiopulmonary resuscitation — can we do it better?' *Care of the Critically Ill*, *I*, 4–8.

Zingg, W. (1966) 'The management of accidental hypothermia.' *Med. Serv. J. Can.*, *22*, 399–410.

——— (1967) 'The management of accidental hypothermia.' *Can. Med. Ass. J.*, *96*, 214–18.

INDEX